Angiotensin-Converting Enzyme Inhibitors: The Advance Continues

Third Edition

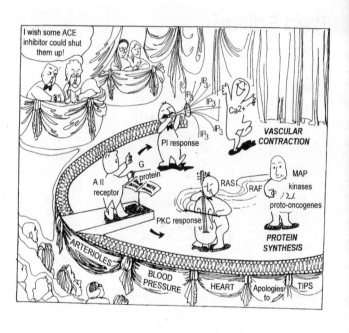

Angiotensin-Converting Enzyme Inhibitors: The Advance Continues

Third Edition

by

Lionel H. Opie, MD, DPhil, FRCP, DSc
Co-Director, Cape Heart Centre and
Medical Research Council
Inter-University Cape Heart Group
University of Cape Town.
Consultant Physician
Groote Schuur Hospital
Cape Town
South Africa.
Visiting Professor (1984-1998)
Stanford University Medical Centre
Stanford, California

Introduction by:
Victor Dzau, MD
Harvard Medical School
Boston, Mass
USA

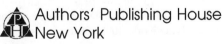 Authors' Publishing House
New York

 University of Cape Town Press

1999

Disclaimer

Although every effort has been made to ensure that the indications and doses for the various drugs are correct, the ultimate legal responsibility for the correct use of drugs lies with prescribing physician. Likewise, the institutions with which the author is or has been associated have no direct nor indirect responsibility for the contents of this book, nor for the mode in which any drugs in this book are used.

The author's aim has been to achieve a totally unbiased text. Readers are requested to communicate any inadvertent bias directly to the author.

ISBN: 1-919713-48-4

First Published 1999
Second Impression 1999

Copyright © 1999 LH Opie

Medical illustrator: Jeanne Walker

Co-published in South Africa by University of Cape Town Press, University of Cape Town, Private Bag, Rondebosch, 7701 Cape Town, South Africa

Printed in South Africa by The Rustica Press, Ndabeni, Western Cape

D7453

CONTENTS

"I hope the author is not tempted to put his pen down because a new edition will soon be required to keep pace with the new developments in this rapidly evolving topic."

Review of the First Edition, British Medical journal, 1992

"Voici mon secret. Il est tres simple: on ne voit bien qu'avec le coeur. L'essentiel est invisible pour les yeux."

Le petit prince, Antoine de Saint-Exupery

"This is my secret. It is very simple: one only sees clearly through the heart. The essentials are invisible to the eyes."

Professor Opie's third edition reflects the astounding and accelerating rate of progress in our knowledge of the renin-angiotensin system and the dominant role of its inhibitors in current cardiovascular therapy. The story started with one of the major discoveries of this century in pharmacology, namely the isolation of the nonapeptide angiotensin-converting enzyme (ACE) inhibitor from the snake venom of *Bothrops jararaca*. This discovery translated into the development of synthetic, orally active drugs that inhibit the renin-angiotensin system in humans. In the early 1980s, the first ACE inhibitor, captopril, was introduced. This was followed by enalapril, lisinopril and by now there are many more with different pharmacological properties as reviewed in this book. Angiotensin-converting enzyme (ACE) inhibitors have now emerged as one of the most important drug class in modern cardiovascular medicine. Their efficacy in the treatment of hypertension, congestive heart failure, early ventricular dysfunction, left ventricular hypertrophy, early stage acute myocardial infarction, postinfarct follow-up, and diabetic nephropathy has been well established. In addition, ACE inhibitors have demonstrated potential in the treatment of myocardial ischemia, reinfarction, as well as in renal and vascular protection (Dzau, 1998).[1]

Modern biology has revolutionized our understanding of physiology and pathophysiology. The powerful tools of molecular and cell biology, applied in concert with traditional physiology and pharmacology, have led to new insights into cardiovascular diseases. One important outcome of this research is an improved understanding of the biology and pharmacology of the renin-angiotensin system (Dzau and Pratt, 1991).[2] Molecular and cell biological studies show that angiotensin is not only a contractile agonist, but also a growth promoter of heart and blood vessels. Angiotensin II growth action is mediated by the expression of proto-oncogenes and autocrine growth factors such as platelet-derived growth factor, basic fibroblast growth factor and transforming growth factor β_1. Angiotensin II also modulates extracellular matrix composition. These trophic effects regulate long-term cardiovascular function and structure and may account for the slow pressor effect of Angiotensin II. Angiotensin II is also produced at local tissue sites and acts on both type 1 and type 2 receptors. For example Angiotensin II may promote vascular injury by a sequence proposed to involve oxidative stress, vascular inflammation, and thrombogenesis (Dzau, 1998).[1] Specifically, it is now appreciated that a major determinant of ACE inhibitor effect is the inhibition of tissue ACE. Accordingly, blockade of local Angiotensin II production may influence cardiac and vascular function and remodeling. Furthermore, tissue ACE inhibition not only suppresses angiotensin II synthesis but may also activate the protective bradykinin-nitric oxide system (Vanhoutte, 1998).[3]

The lethal cardiac chain. Previously, Dr. Eugene Braunwald and I (1991)[4] proposed that organic heart disease is the consequence of a continuous chain of pathophysiological events that is usually initiated by risk factors leading to atherosclerosis, coronary artery disease, myocardial ischemia, and infarction. The ventricular dysfunction and remodeling that develop as a consequence of myocardial infarction may result in ventricular dilatation and, eventually, symptomatic heart failure (see Fig 12-2). Indeed, angiotensin plays an important role in many of these cardiovascular responses and contributes to the pathophysiology of disease expression and progression. Accordingly, it is logical to expect that inhibitors of the renin-angiotensin system may interrupt this chain of pathophysiological events and prevent the progression to significant ischemic heart disease, congestive heart failure, and end-stage cardiac disease (Fig 12-5). The contents of this book specifically address the effects of ACE inhibition on each step of this serious pathophysiological progression with increased fatality at each of the sequential steps.

New aspects of this edition. Given the rapid development of this area of research and the related clinical disciplines, there is a continuing need for a comprehensive and up-to-date book that reviews the scientific basis for clinical use of ACE inhibitors, and extends into the practical clinical realm. Professor Opie has again masterfully accomplished these difficult tasks in this the third Edition of his book. The contents of this book provide proof of the important links from bench to bedside between fundamental research and clinical application in this area. The many excellent explanatory diagrams are an Opie trademark, according to Eugene Braunwald. For example, modern molecular concepts such as the new growth signals including NF-kappa-B (Fig 2-5) and the angiotensin II type II receptor (Fig 12-3) are beautifully illustrated. There is a new chapter on vascular disease and remodelling (Fig 2-2), an area that I feel will become more and more important (Dzau, 1998).[1]

What can we expect in the future? Professor Opie speculates on the impact of the angiotensin II receptor type 1 blockers, the increasing use of combination therapy in hypertension, and the new combinations in heart failure including ACE inhibitors plus beta-adrenergic blockers, spironolactone and AT-blockers. We can also expect much from a rapidly increasing understanding of the function of the angiotensin II type 2 receptor (Horiuchi et al,1999),[5] and from increased genetic profiling of our patients. We can anticipate that as we get the results of preventative trials such as PROGRESS, PEACE, HOPE and EUROPA, the case for cardiovascular protection by ACE inhibitors will become firmly established. In my opinion, this class of drugs has already earned the labelling of the *"cardioprotective drug of the 1990s."* Indeed, with such rapid and impressive progress in this field, as witnessed by the extensive updates between the first three editions of this book, it is certain that we can anticipate the publication of the next edition with excitement and enthusiasm.

1. Dzau VJ. Mechanism of protective effects of ACE inhibition on coronary artery disease. Eur Heart J 1998; 19 (suppl J): J2–J6

2. Dzau VJ, Pratt RE. Renin angiotensin. In: Fozzard HA, Haber E, Jennings B, Katz AM (eds.), *The Heart and Cardiovascular System.* New York: Raven Press, 1991; 1817-1850.

3. Vanhoutte, PM. Endothelial dysfunction and inhibition of converting enzyme. Eur Heart J 1998; 19 (suppl J): J7–J15

4. Dzau VJ, Braunwald E. Resolved and unresolved issues in the prevention and treatment of coronary heart disease: a workshop consensus statement. *Am Heart J* 1991; 121:1244–1263.

5. Horiuchi M, Akishita M, Dzau VJ. Recent progress in angiotensin II type 2 receptor research in the cardiovascular system. Hypertension 1999;33: 613–621.

Victor J. Dzau
*Hersey Professor of the Theory and Practice of Medicine,
Harvard Medical School, Boston, Mass.*

AUTHOR'S PREFACE TO THE THIRD EDITION

First and foremost, there is a change of subtitle of the book, which becomes:

The Advance Continues.

This comes from a series of lectures that I gave in Australia a year or two ago. Yes, the advance continues, and the limits have not been reached. The more I learn, the more confident I feel that we are still far from having reached the limits of what we know about the renin-angiotensin-aldosterone system (RAAS). This pervasive system now seems as fundamental as the adrenergic-autonomic system with which it closely interacts. ACE inhibitors are increasing seen as protectors against endothelial dysfunction, acting by bradykinin and nitric oxide. In growth, the angiotensin receptors play a fundamental role, and the complex signal pathways involved are being clarified by the day.

In particular, our understanding of the pathogenic role of angiotensin II in vascular disease is increasing so rapidly that even since the completion of the text of this book in April, 1999, two new and important articles have appeared in the same issue of Circulation. First, upregulation of the angiotensin type I (AT-I) receptor follows hypercholesterolemia, together with increased vascular superoxide production[4]. This concept, fitting perfectly with Dzau's picture of the pathogenic role of oxidative stress in vascular injury (Fig 2-2 of this book), leads us to consider the following possible sequence:

> Hypercholesterolemia → endothelial damage → initiation of vascular vicious circle → upregulation of AT-1 → receptor pathogenic role for angiotensin II → increased oxidative stress → increased vascular damage (Fig 2-2).

Secondly, ACE inhibitors may interact directly with the bradykinin (B_2) receptor. Ramiprilat interferes with the sequestration of this receptor within the endothelial plasma membrane[1]. Normally, with continued ACE inhibitor therapy, local bradykinin production may be chronically increased so that the bradykinin receptor is down-regulated. By increasing the availability of the bradykinin receptor, the protective effects of bradykinin are sustained. Similar effects have been reported with enalaprilat, while perindoprilat increases bradykinin-mediated vasodilation[3]. Thus, ACE inhibitors probably interact directly with the bradykinin receptor, quite apart from lessening the breakdown of bradykinin:

> ACE inhibitors → direct interaction with bradykinin receptor → promotes sensitivity to bradykinin → vascular effects even in the absence of ACE activity → enhanced nitric oxide protects against vascular vicious circle (Fig 2-2).

For the clinician too, these are exciting times. The advance
continues, and ACE inhibitors are used more and more:

1. *In early phase acute myocardial infarction,* ACE inhibitors
    can improve the outcome and reduce long-term mor-
    tality. These benefits are particularly noted in patients
    at high risk, as in those with diabetes or large anterior
    infarcts or clinical heart failure.

2. *In post-infarct patients,* progressive post-infarct heart
    failure is prevented. Sudden cardiac death is
    decreased[2].

3. *Protection against re-infarction,* found in retrospective
    analyses of large trials, is now being tested in prospec-
    tive mega-trials. Evidence is coming in for a preventa-
    tive fibrinolytic effect, possibly mediated by an
    angiotensin IV receptor.

4. *In heart failure,* the reduction in mortality has now
    been confirmed in thousands of patients, so ACE inhi-
    bitors remain the cornerstone of treatment to which
    other therapies must be added or compared.

5. *In hypertension,* JNC VI (the sixth report of the Ameri-
    can Joint National Committee) recognizes certain
    "compelling indications" for ACE inhibitors such as
    hypertensives with heart failure or diabetes type 1
    with proteinuria or postinfarct hypertension with sys-
    tolic dysfunction. The first outcome study with an
    ACE inhibitor, captopril, was however defective
    because this drug as given too infrequently and blood
    pressure control was less tight than in the comparator
    group.

6. *In diabetes mellitus,* protection against complications
    including nephropathy, retinopathy, and possibly neu-
    ropathy, is now being recognized.

7. *Nephroprotection* in chronic non-diabetic renal changes
    in the intraglomerular pressure, and by enhanced
    blood pressure control. failure may be mediated by
    beneficial

8. *Recurrent cerebrovascular events*: protection is being
    tested in a large trial.

No wonder that I feel excited at the new knowledge and
challenges presented in this the third edition of my book.
Samuel Johnson once said: "He who is tired of London, is
tired of life". My paraphrase is: "Whoever is tired of renin-
angiotensin, is tired of new cardiovascular concepts."

Lionel H. Opie
Cape Heart Center,
University of Cape Town,
South Africa

References:

1. Benzing T, Fleming I, Blaukat A, et al. Angiotensin-converting enzyme inhibitor ramiprilat interferes with the sequestration of the B_2 kinin receptor within the plasma membrane of native endothelial cells. Circulation 1999;99:2034-2040.
2. Domanski MJ, Exner DV, Bordowf CB, et al. Effect of angiotensin converting enzyme inhibition on sudden cardiac death in patients following acute myocardial infarction. A meta-analysis of randomized clinical trials. J Am Coll Cardiol 1999;33:598-604.
3. Vanhoutte PM. Endothelial dysfunction and inhibition of converting enzyme. Eur Heart J 1998;19 (Suppl J):J7-J15.
4. Warnholtz A, Nickenig G, Schulz E, et al. Increased NADH-oxidase-mediated superoxide production in the early stages of atherosclerosis. Evidence for involvement of the renin-angiotensin system. Circulation 1999;99:2027-2033.

FOREWORD TO THE FIRST EDITION

The beginning of the era of hypertension research dates back to 1934, to the classic Goldblatt's experiment on the dog made hypertensive by renal artery stenosis. It may seem surprising, therefore, that antihypertensive therapy had so long ignored the possibility of antagonizing the renin-angiotensin system. The fact is that Goldblatt's experiment was correctly interpreted as a model of renovascular hypertension, rather than of the most common form of hypertension, essential hypertension. As a consequence, any attempt to interfere pharmacologically with the renin-angiotensin system was considered to be aimed at the limited field of renovascular hypertension. Even in 1976, discussing the first experiences with antagonists and inhibitors of the renin-angiotensin system, an authority like Franz Gross wrote: "Undoubtedly, the antagonists and inhibitors of the renin-angiotensin system are most useful tools, but their application will be limited to the share of the renin-dependent forms of high blood pressure in the total field of hypertension."

The advent of the angiotensin-converting enzyme (ACE) inhibitors has reversed this widespread viewpoint and has initiated an entirely new approach to the treatment of hypertension. Not only have ACE inhibitors been shown to be active outside the limited field of renovascular and renal hypertension, but they are widely recognized among the first choice agents for treatment of hypertension. Nor have these compounds remained restricted to the specific area of hypertension: ACE inhibitors are now successfully used in congestive heart failure and are actively being investigated in cardioprotection after myocardial infarction and in renal protection in diabetic nephropathy and other types of nephropathies.

Complexity of research requires simplicity of presentation, especially when the outcome of research has to be quickly translated into useful therapeutic applications, as was, and is still, the case with ACE inhibitors. No one could have accomplished the difficult task of clarifying the scientific basis for the practical use of ACE inhibitors better than Lionel Opie, whose gifts as a scientist and a teacher are testified by the success of his two recent volumes, *Drugs for the Heart and The Clinical Use of Calcium Channel Antagonists.* I am sure that this new volume, where a large body of data has been screened by the critical judgment of the investigator and the experience of the clinician, will meet the same indisputable success. From these pages, the readers will be able to perceive how the new therapeutic advances initiated by ACE inhibition have promoted a deeper understanding of the pathophysiology of hypertension, heart failure, cardiac remodeling, vascular and renal disease. Such advances in knowledge are, in turn, leading to a broadening of the therapeutic applications of these compounds. This story is a further example of the fascinating interaction between science and clinical practice in medicine.

Alberto Zanchetti
Professor of Medicine and Director
Institute of Clinical Medicine and
Center of Clinical Physiology and Hypertension
University of Milan
Italy

APPENDIX 1: SUMMARY OF PHARMACOLOGIC PROPERTIES, CLINICAL INDICATIONS AND DOSES OF ACE INHIBITORS

Drug	Zinc ligand	Active drug	Elim T1/2 (hours)	T/P ratio % (FDA)	Hypertension (usual daily dose)	CHF initial dose	CHF maintenance dose
Class I: captopril-like							
Captopril	SH	Captopril	4-6 (total captopril)	–	25-50 mg 2x or 3X	6.25 mg	Up to 50 mg 3x
Class II: prodrugs							
Alacepril	carboxyl	captopril	8 (total captopril)	–	12.5-25 mg 2×	–	–
Benazepril	carboxyl	benazeprilat	11	-	10-80 mg in 1-2 doses	2 mg	5-20 mg 1×
Cilazepril	carboxyl	cilazeprilat	9	-	2.5-5 mg 1×	-	-
Delapril	carboxyl	delaprilat / 5-OH-delaprilat	1.2-1.4	-	7.5-30 mg in 1-2 doses	-	-
Enalapril	carboxyl	enalaprilat	6; 11 (accum)	-	5-20 mg in 1-2 doses	2.5 mg	Up to 20 mg 2×
Fosinopril	phosphoryl	fosinoprilat	12	50-80	10-40 mg 1× (or 2×)	10 mg	20 40 mg
Perindopril	carboxyl	perindoprilat	3-10	75-100	4-8 mg 1×	2 mg	4 mg 1×
Quinapril	carboxyl	quinaprilat	1.8	50	10-40 mg in 1-2 doses	5 mg	10-40 mg 2×
Ramipril	carboxyl	ramiprilat	13-17	50-60	2.5-10 mg in 1-2 doses	2.5 mg	2.5-5 mg 2×
Spirapril	carboxyl	spiraprilat	<2	-	3-6 mg 1 dose*	-	-
Trandolapril	carboxyl	trandoprilat	10	50-90	0.5-4 mg 1×, then 4 mg 2×	-	1-4 mg 1×
Class III: water-soluble							
Lisinopril	carboxyl	lisinopril	7; 12 (accum)	–	10-40 mg 1× (may need high dose if given 1X)	5 mg	2.5-20 mg 1×

Data based on FDA-approved information where available. Elim T1/2, elimination half-life; accum = accumulation half-life; CHF, congestive heart failure; T/P ratio, trough/peak ratios, FDA-approved values.

*Thurmann, Hypertension, 1996; 28:450. Also see Chapter 8 and Salvetti (ref 126).

APPENDIX 2: ACE INHIBITORS: SIDE-EFFECTS AND
CONTRAINDICATIONS

1. **Side-effects, Class**

   Cough common

   Hypotension variable (renal artery stenosis; severe
   heart failure, especially if excess diuretics)

   Deterioration of renal function (related to hypotension)

   Angioedma (rare)

   Acute renal failure (rare, may be unexpected)

   Hyperkalemia (in renal failure, or with excess
   K-retaining diuretics)

   Skin reactions

2. **Side-effects first described for high dose captopril**

   Neutropenia (cannot exclude Class effect)

   Proteinuria

   Loss of taste

   Oral lesions

   Scalded mouth syndrome (rare)

3. **Contraindications**

   Renal bilateral renal artery stenosis or equivalent
   lesions

   Pre-existing hypotension

   Severe aortic stenosis or obstructive cardiomyopathy

   Pregnancy (NB: prominent FDA warning)

APPENDIX 3: Generic and Trade Names of ACE Inhibitors

Generic name	Trade names
Alacepril	Cetapril
Altiopril	Lowpres
Benazepril	Cibace, Cibacen, Cibacene, Lotensin*
Captopril	Capoten*, Lopril, Lopirin, Captopril
Cilazepril	Inhibace, Inibace, Vascace
Delapril	Adecut
Enalapril	Innovace, Pres, Renitec, Renivace, Vasotec*, Xanef
Fosinopril	Monopril*, Staril
Lisinopril	Longes, Prinivil*, Zestril*
Perindopril	Aceon*, Acertil, Coverene, Coverex, Coversum, Coversyl, Prestarium, Prexanil, Prexum, Procaptan
Quinapril	Accupril*, Accuprin, Accupro, Acuitel
Ramipril	Altace*, Delix, Ramace, Triatec, Tritace
Spirapril	Renpress, Sandopril
Trandolapril	Mavik*, Odrik, Gopten

* in USA

The renin-angiotensin-aldosterone system and its role in cardiovascular regulation

"Angiotensin II activates an array of signaling molecules" – Sadoshima (1998)[66]

HOW IT ALL STARTED

Just over 100 years ago, Tigertstedt and Bergman[75] linked the kidneys to hypertension by their discovery of *renin*, a renal-derived injectable substance that elevated the blood pressure. Next came Goldblatt[24] whose unilateral renal artery clamp produced hypertension. In 1940, the actual pressor agent was identified in North and South America almost simultaneously.[8,64] Its name? After some years of conflict, the two groups decided[9] to call it angiotensin. In the meantime two forms had been identified, and were now renamed angiotensin I and angiotensin II. The enzyme converting the first form to the pressor second form was called the angiotensin converting enzyme. The stage was set for the discovery of teprotide, the first angiotensin converting enzyme (ACE) inhibitor, and then captopril.[17]

HYPERTENSION TO HEART FAILURE TO VASCULAR PROTECTION

Persistent stimulation of the renin-angiotensin-aldosterone system is likely to promote hypertension because of the strong vasoconstrictive qualities of angiotensin II and the sodium retention induced by aldosterone. Thus, when angiotensin-converting enzyme inhibitors first became available, it was logical to test the antihypertensive effect in patients with high renin states such as renovascular hypertension in which arteriolar constriction was playing a prominent role. Not surprisingly, the ACE inhibitors worked very well in these conditions. In addition, we now know that antihypertensive effects are also found when plasma renin is normal, or even sometimes when it is low, suggesting alternate or additional modes of action for these agents. Recognition of the reactive arteriolar vasoconstriction in states of severe heart failure next led to the successful testing of ACE inhibitors in patients refractory to conventional anti-failure therapy. The remarkable therapeutic success of ACE inhibitors in hypertension and in heart failure is based on solid scientific evidence for the role of the renin-angiotensin-aldosterone system in these two common cardiological conditions.

THE RENIN-ANGIOTENSIN-ALDOSTERONE SYSTEM

Angiotensin II, a potent vasoconstrictor, is an octapeptide. It is formed from its precursor, *angiotensin I*, a decapeptide, by the activity of the *angiotensin-converting enzyme* (ACE). Such ACE activity, although chiefly found in the vascular endothelium of the lungs, also occurs in the endothelium of other vascular beds and in many other tissues including the myocardium and the coronary arteries.

Angiotensin I originates from *angiotensinogen* (Fig 1-1) under the influence of the enzyme *renin*, a protease. The activity of this enzyme is rate-limiting for the formation of angiotensin I. This conversion of the angiotensin I occurs in the liver. Renin in turn is formed in the kidney from the juxtaglomerular cells. Classic stimuli to the release of renin include (1) impaired renal blood flow as in ischemia or hypotension; (2) salt depletion or sodium diuresis; and (3) beta-adrenergic stimulation. When renin formation is enhanced for more than 4 hours, then the rate of synthesis of the precursor, *prorenin*, is also increased in the kidney.[18]

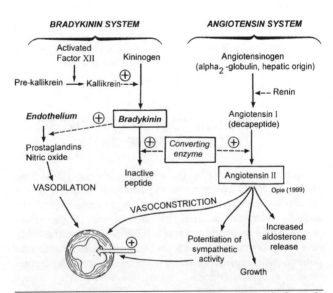

Figure 1-1. ACE inhibitors have dual vasodilatory actions, chiefly on the circulating and tissue renin-angiotensin systems with ancillary effects on the enzymes that inactivate bradykinin. The result of the former action is the inhibition of the vasoconstrictory systems and the result of the latter is the formation of vasodilatory nitric oxide and prostacyclin. Figure © LH Opie, 1999

The angiotensin-converting enzyme. Also called kininase-II and, technically EC 3.4.15.1, ACE is a protease with two zinc groups, hence being a metalloprotease. There is, however, only one zinc atom at the high affinity binding site that interacts with angiotensin II or all the ACE inhibitors.[70] The converting enzyme is nonspecific because it not only converts angiotensin I to angiotensin II but inactivates bradykinin, hence the alternate name of *kininase.* The positively charged ions of the zinc atom and of another lower affinity active site interact with terminal negatively charged carboxyl groups of the ACE inhibitor.[63] Inclusion of the SH group in the structure to replace a -COOH group greatly increases the ACE inhibitory power and thus captopril was born.[63] It is now known, however, that SH groups are not at all essential to achieve ACE inhibition (Fig 1-2).

Angiotensin II receptors and intracellular messenger system. Just as there are many intermediate steps between occupation of the beta-adrenoceptor and increased contractile activity of the myocardium, so there are many complex steps between occupation of the angiotensin II receptor and

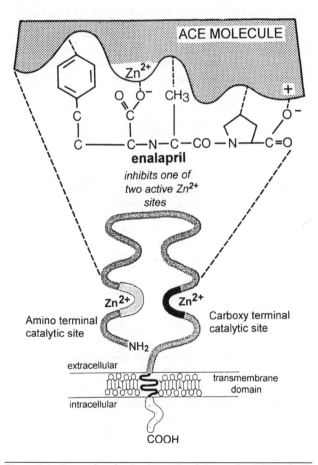

Figure 1-2. Proposed molecular interaction between the ACE molecule and an ACE inhibitor. Note that the zinc-containing inhibitory site lies within the vascular lumen. The structure of the ACE molecule is reproduced by kind permission of Johnston[33] and the American Heart Association. See also Soubrier et al.[70]

ultimate mobilization of calcium with a vasoconstrictor effect in vascular smooth muscle. These intervening steps constitute the *signaling system*. There are several interactions between the occupation of the receptor by angiotensin II and the stimulation of the enzyme phospholipase C that regulates one of the key steps of the phosphatidylinositol cycle (Fig 1-3).

The first component of the phosphatidylinositol system to be discovered was *inositol trisphosphate* (IP_3 or $InsP_3$) formed from the breakdown of inositol phospholipids.[7] The other component formed in this hydrolysis is diacylglycerol which initiates the activation of a specialized enzyme, called protein kinase C, that transfers a phosphate group from ATP to a target protein by the process of protein phosphorylation.[58] Diacylglycerol operates within the plane of the membrane to activate *protein kinase C* without entering the cytosolic space.[5] Thus it is thought that the ultimate messengers of the inositol signaling pathway are, first, IP_3 which liberates calcium from the intracellular sarcoplasmic reticulum by acting on its IP_3 receptor[6] and, second, protein kinase C which phosphorylates an as yet unknown target protein, possibly one of the contractile proteins (Fig 1-3).

In addition, angiotensin II enhances the activation of the voltage-dependent calcium channels, that is to say angiotensin II makes it easier for the channels to be in the open state in response to a wave of depolarization. This effect of

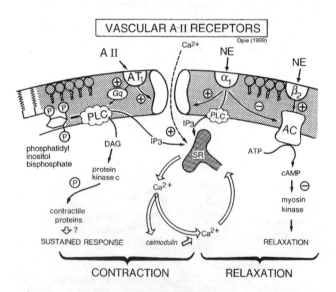

Figure 1-3. *Proposed messengers of vascular angiotensin II receptor stimulation, leading to vascular contraction. Activation of this receptor stimulates a phosphodiesterase to split phosphatidylinositol into two messengers: IP_3 (inositol trisphosphate) and DAG (1,2-diacylglycerol). IP_3 promotes the release of calcium from the sarcoplasmic reticulum (SR), and DAG activates protein kinase C, which is thought to act on the contractile apparatus to promote a sustained contractile response. Activity of the angiotensin II receptor also helps to open the calcium channel through an unknown mechanism possibly involving G-proteins, thereby further increasing vascular tone. Fig © LH Opie.*

angiotensin II is probably mediated by a GTP-binding protein. Such channels, whose opening probability is enhanced by G-proteins, are called *G-protein-gated channels*.[10] Alternatively, IP_3 can be changed into the closely related IP_4 (inositol tetraphosphate), which in turn can help open calcium channels.[40]

When the vascular angiotensin II receptors are stimulated, it is proposed that two mechanisms lead to an increased release of calcium from the sarcoplasmic reticulum: (1) the formation of IP_3 and (2) the direct G-protein-mediated stimulation of the calcium channel. Such increased release of calcium augments vascular contraction and tone. There is also some evidence for a hypothetical sequence whereby phosphorylation of the contractile proteins by protein kinase C leads to sustained contraction and maintenance of vascular tone.[54]

In the case of the myocardium, there are also angiotensin II receptors that again are thought to be coupled to the IP_3 system.[3] Protein kinase C activation by the nonphysiological experimental agents, the phorbol esters, leads to an increase of myocardial contractile force, supporting the proposal that there is an as yet ill-understood phosphorylation of the contractile proteins in response to activation of protein kinase C.

Phosphatidylinositol cycle. There are two limbs to the phosphatidylinositol cycle, the breakdown of phosphatidylinositol to inositol trisphosphate (IP_3) and thence to inositol, and the resynthesis of phosphatidylinositol from inositol (Fig 1-4). Phosphatidylinositol is a compound in which two fatty acid chains, the one predominantly stearic acid and the other predominantly arachidonic acid, are bound by a phosphate group to inositol. Hypothetically, phosphatidylinositol is regarded as the reservoir that supplies the precursor phosphatidylinositol monophosphate to maintain the small intracellular pool of phosphatidylinositol bisphosphate. According to the favored hypothesis,[7] it is the latter substance that responds to occupation of the angiotensin II receptor by undergoing hydrolysis when an enzyme, a phosphodiesterase, is activated (Fig 1-4). This enzyme is a phosphodiesterase called *phospholipase C*.[48] Just how occupation of the angiotensin II receptor is coupled to this phosphodiesterase is still not fully understood, but it probably involves a G-protein cycle.[5] Once IP_3 has formed, it can in turn undergo hydrolysis via inositol diphosphate and inositol monophosphate to inositol (Fig 1-4). The latter step is inhibited by lithium which may explain some of the antidepressant effects of that compound on the brain.

The next sequence is the phosphorylation of inositol to phosphatidylinositol phosphate. At this stage inositol interacts with a derivative of diacylglycerol.[7,58] Thereupon follows a further phosphorylation to phosphatidylinositol bisphosphate. Both of these phosphorylations take place under the action of a protein kinase and utilize ATP. Now the phosphatidyl inositol bisphosphate is again ready for

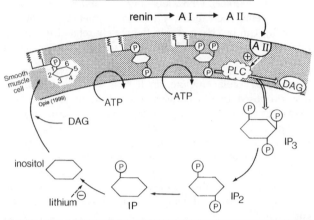

Figure 1-4. *The phosphatidylinositol cycle is shown using the model proposed by Berridge.[7] In vascular tissue, the reservoir compound is phosphatidylinositol, from which phosphatidylinositol bisphosphate is formed, the substrate for the phospholipase C (PLC), which is stimulated in response to occupation of the angiotensin II receptor. The resulting formation of inositol trisphosphate (IP₃), one of the intracellular messengers, precedes the formation of inositol bisphosphate (IP₂) and inositol monophosphate (IP). The latter compound is converted to inositol through a reaction inhibited by the antidepressant lithium. Inositol reacts with a derivative of diacylglycerol (DAG) to reform phosphatidylinositol (top left). Fig © LH Opie.*

hydrolysis in response to angiotensin II receptor occupation.

This phosphatidylinositol cycle is not confined to vascular tissue, rather it occurs in many different types of cells and has different functions including regulation of cell calcium and secretion.[6] An example of the ubiquitous nature of the system is that platelet-derived growth factor (PDGF) stimulates phospholipase C activity in fibroblasts[48] with mitogenic potential. It is, however, in vascular tissue that the cycling of phosphatidylinositol can clearly be linked to angiotensin II receptor stimulation and to contraction.

ANGIOTENSIN II RECEPTOR SUBTYPES: THE AT-1 AND AT-2 RECEPTORS

There is a family of angiotensin II receptor subtypes, including the AT_1 and AT_2 receptors (Fig 1-5). From the physiological point of view, it is the AT_1-receptors that mediate "all the principal responses" to angiotensin II.[76] The AT_1-receptors are further subdivided in types AT-1a and AT-1b. Subtype 1b occurs in trace amounts in the LV of the rat[31] so that subtype 1a knockout mice are used to assess the role of the AT-1 receptor in cardiovascular pathophysiology. For example, although the AT-1 receptors are involved in the growth response to A-II, yet in type 1a knockout mice, a pressure overload can induce acute hypertrophy, showing that AT-1 receptor stimulation is not

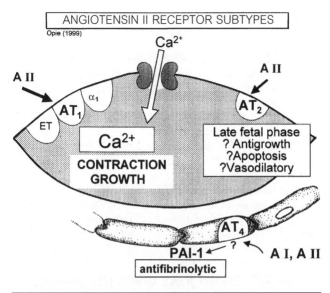

Figure 1-5. *Proposed roles of angiotensin II receptor subtypes, which are called AT-1, AT-2 and (putative) AT-4 subtypes. Most of the physiological effects in adult vascular smooth muscle cells are conveyed by the AT-1 receptor subtype. The AT-2 receptor is of substantial importance in late fetal vascular growth, exerting an antigrowth effect.[2] Hypothetically, these receptors may also play a role in various myocardial pathophysiological conditions (see text). AT-4 receptors are postulated to have an antifibrinolytic effect. Fig © LH Opie*

essential and suggesting an important role for pressure-induced hypertrophy.[29]

It is now often considered that the AT-2 receptors may become more relevant in pathophysiological conditions. Although of relatively little importance in the normal adult cardiovascular system, they are upregulated during hypertrophy in the rat[74] and upregulated relative to the AT-1 receptor in diseased human hearts.[30] The effects of A-II on the diseased heart and failing circulation are often regarded as adverse, such as stimulation of contraction, vasoconstriction, myocyte hypertrophy, and antinatriuresis. These effects are mediated by the AT-1 receptor. It is postulated by Dzau and others that the AT-2 receptors may reduce some of the adverse effects of AT-1 receptor stimulation by a Yin-Yang effect. Specifically, AT-2 receptor stimulation in certain experimental conditions has an antigrowth effect and may mediate apoptosis.[90] These postulated effects may hypothetically have mixed benefits. For example, anti-growth effects may lessen adverse postinfarct remodeling, whereas apoptosis promotion may increase the number of dying cells in the failing heart.

ANGIOTENSIN II AS VASOCONSTRICTOR

Release of norepinephrine via neuromodulation. In addition to the direct vasoconstrictory action of angiotensin II on the vascular AT-1 receptor, angiotensin also promotes the release of norepinephrine (NE) from the terminal neurons into the synaptic space. Norepinephrine in turn stimulates the postsynaptic vasoconstrictory alpha$_1$-receptors (Fig 1-3). By this process of *neuromodulation* that alters the rate of norepinephrine release, a large number of hormones and autonomic signals can achieve indirect control of the degree of vasoconstriction. For example, the parasympathetic autonomic messenger, acetylcholine, can decrease release of norepinephrine acting on the presynaptic muscarinic receptor on the terminal neuron (presynaptic receptor).

Angiotensin II and endothelin. Some of the vascular effects of angiotensin II are mediated by increased production of endothelin, a powerful vasoconstrictor and growth promoter.[41,53] (For role of endothelin, see Fig 3-4.)

ANGIOTENSIN II AS GROWTH SIGNAL

An interesting hypothesis can be constructed in relation to factors influencing blood vessel growth (angiogenesis). Both angiotensin II and alpha-receptor agonists have been shown to promote growth of vascular smooth muscle cells in certain conditions. Both types of stimulation are vasoconstrictory. Because calcium is involved in the regulation of muscle growth, a reasonable speculation would be that factors which act as vasoconstrictors in the short term, by temporarily increasing the level of cytosolic calcium, may during long continued stimulation of vascular smooth muscle lead to myointimal proliferation. Supporting this hypothesis is the finding that angiotensin II increases the turnover of the phosphatidylinositol cycle, and the expression of growth-stimulating proto-oncogenes.[42] Angiotensin II also promotes formation of endothelin, a powerful mitogen.[53] Furthermore, there is increasing evidence that angiotensin II may stimulate growth of the vascular matrix and in particular formation of collagen. Increased arteriolar growth induced by angiotensin II leads to a decreased ratio between the lumen and the media of the arterioles and an increased blood pressure.[53] The presumed mechanism is an increase in the systemic vascular resistance.

Myocardial growth. The signal systems underlying LV hypertrophy are shown in Fig 1-6.

RENAL AND ADRENAL INTERACTIONS

Renin release. The major factors stimulating release of renin from the juxtaglomerular cells of the kidney are: (1) increased beta$_1$-sympathetic activity, (2) a low arterial blood pressure, and (3) decreased sodium reabsorption in the distal tubule, as when dietary sodium is low or during diuretic therapy. On the other hand, renin release is inhibited by angiotensin II activity (Fig 1-7). The consequences of renin

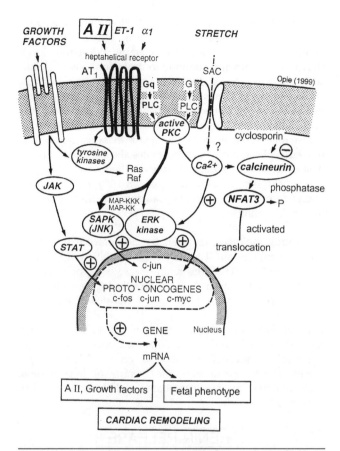

Figure 1-6. Cell signals in response to hypertrophic stimuli. Note highly active post-receptor cross-talk. For clarity some pathways are omitted, e.g. A II receptor linking to JAK. A II = angiotensin II; JAK = Janus Kinase (see Berk & Corson, Circ Res 80: 607, 1997); STAT = signal transducers and activators of transcription; JNK = SAPK, where JNK = c-JUN NH$_2$-terminal kinase; SAPK = stress-activated protein kinase (see Kudoh et al, Circ Res 80:139, 1997); ET-1 = endothelin-1; α_1 = α_1-adrenergic activity; SAC = stretch activated channel; PLC = phospholipase C; MAP = mitogen-activated protein; MAP kinase also includes ERK = extracellular signal related kinase; MAPKK = MAP kinase kinase, also includes MEK, where EK = ERK kinase. For calcineurin, see Sussman et al, Science 1998;281:1690. For NFAT$_3$, see Molketin et al, Cell 1998;93:215. Fig © LH Opie.

release are not limited to increased conversion of circulating angiotensinogen to angiotensin I, but probably exert an important intrarenal effect. Components of the renin-angiotensin system are present in the kidney and local formation of angiotensin II is thought to be the explanation for efferent arteriolar vasoconstriction following renin release (Fig 1-7). Thus, for example, during a state of arterial hypotension, the increased efferent arteriolar vasoconstriction resulting from increased angiotensin II will help to preserve renal function by maintaining the intraglomerular pressure.

Stimulation of aldosterone by angiotensin II. Besides acting as a vasoconstrictor, angiotensin II also stimulates the formation of the sodium-retaining hormone aldosterone. Hence ACE inhibition has potential indirect natriuretic effects. As angiotensin II levels fall during acute ACE inhibition, so do those of aldosterone.[45,86] However, aldosterone formation does not stay blocked during prolonged ACE inhibitor therapy. By 3 months of therapy, aldosterone levels start to rise again and continue to do so for 1 year.[72] While such *aldosterone escape* does not appear to compromise the antihypertensive effects achieved by ACE inhibitors, nonetheless it may detract from the benefit of ACE inhibition in heart failure. The proposed explanation for this late rise of aldosterone, resistant to ACE inhibitor therapy, may be that the early phase natriuresis promotes the production of aldosterone by the adrenal cortex.[61] Alternatively, the late rise in aldosterone formation may merely reflect the rebound formation of circulating angiotensin II, despite continued ACE inhibition.

Feedback inhibition of renin by angiotensin II. A third action of angiotensin II is a feedback inhibition of renin secretion (Fig 1-7). Therefore renin release is suppressed both directly by angiotensin II and indirectly by the sodium retention associated with the increased aldosterone levels.

Sodium loading. During conditions of sodium loading, renin secretion from the juxtaglomerular cells is suppressed. The result is that ACE inhibition, in general, has less hypotensive effect. Therefore in the therapy of hypertension, ACE inhibitors are often combined with a diuretic or low sodium diet or both.

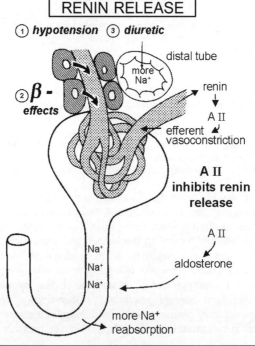

Figure 1-7. Mechanisms for release of renin from juxtaglomerular cells of kidney: (1) beta₁-sympathetic activity, (2) hypotension or decreased renal blood flow, and (3) decreased tubular reabsorption of sodium, as for example during a low-sodium diet or diuretic therapy. Note that renin, by forming angiotensin II, maintains efferent arteriolar vasoconstriction and, therefore, the intraglomerular pressure. Figure © LH Opie, 1999

AUTONOMIC INTERACTIONS

Permissive anti-adrenergic effects of ACE inhibitors. Angiotensin II promotes the release of norepinephrine from adrenergic terminal neurons, and also enhances adrenergic tone by central activation and by facilitation of ganglionic transmission.[4] Furthermore, angiotensin II amplifies the vasoconstriction achieved by alpha₁-receptor stimulation.[65] Thus, angiotensin II has facilitatory adrenergic actions leading to increased activity of vasoconstrictory norepinephrine (Fig 1-8). ACE inhibition has as substantial sympatholytic effect in the human forearm.[43] Direct inhibition of muscle sympathetic nerve activity occurs within 90 minutes of the oral administration of captopril, the prototype ACE inhibitor.[60] Furthermore angiotensin II releases vasoconstrictory endothelin from the endothelium.[53] These indirect effects of angiotensin II help to explain the vasodilatory action of ACE inhibitors.

Additional autonomic effects on the parasympathetic nervous system are possible, so that parasympathetic tone may

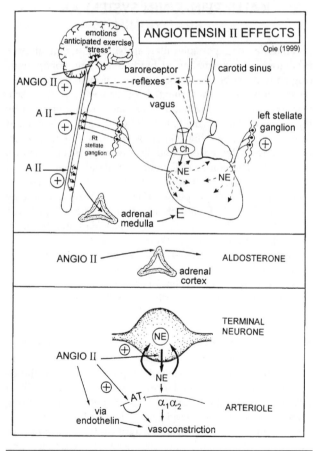

Figure 1-8. Multiple sites of action of angiotensin II (angio II) including central adrenergic activation facilitation of ganglionic transmission release of aldosterone from the adrenal medulla release of norepinephrine (NE) from terminal sympathetic varicosities with inhibition of re-uptake and direct stimulation of vascular angiotensin II receptors. Angiotensin II also releases vasoconstrictory endothelin from the endothelium. The major net effect is powerful vasoconstriction. Figure © LH Opie, 1999

be increased[1] suggesting a vagomimetic effect of ACE inhibition. There may also be changes in the activity of the baroreflexes, which serve to control the blood pressure. In response to ACE inhibition, downregulation of baroreflexes may develop, which means that the baroreceptors respond less well to incoming signals.[25] Such effects on baroreceptors and on the parasympathetic tone could explain why tachycardia is absent in response to peripheral vasodilation achieved by ACE inhibition.

Receptor cross-talk. Complex cross-talk is emerging. A-II downregulates α-adrenergic receptors as well as the proto-oncogenes that respond to α-adrenergic stimulation.[36] By promotion of bradykinin synthesis, ACE inhibition upregulates ß-adrenergic receptors in neonatal myocytes, a sequence which is postulated to benefit the situation in heart failure with downregulated ß-adrenergic receptors.[91] But the true role of such post-receptor cross talk is still unknown.

KALLIKREIN-KININ SYSTEM AND BRADYKININ

Foremost among possible alternate sites of action of ACE inhibitors is the formation of bradykinin. This nonapeptide originally described as causing slow contractions in the gut (*brady*, slow; *kinin*, movement) is of increasing cardiovascular importance.[41,68] Bradykinin is formed from kininogen by the action of the enzyme kallikrein, which in turn is derived from pre-kallikrein. Bradykinin is, in turn, inactivated by two *kininases*, kininase 1 and 2, the latter being identical with ACE. Therefore, ACE inhibition should logically lead to increased local formation of bradykinin,[26] which has major vasodilatory properties (Fig 1-1). There is emerging evidence that ACE inhibitors such as perindopril can directly stimulate the formation of vascular bradykinin at low concentrations, lower than those that give detectable changes in the A-II to A-I ratio.[13] The mechanism of this effect is unknown. Formation of bradykinin is often viewed as a cardioprotective mechanism[69] because it promotes the formation of protective nitric oxide by the endothelium (Fig 1-9).

Formation of bradykinin. There are two main stimuli to the formation of bradykinin, a process that occurs in the endothelium. Of prime physiologic importance may be the effect of an increased blood flow, probably acting by shear forces on the endothelium.[41] Thus, hypothetically, during exercise the increased blood flow achieved by an increased cardiac output can help promote local formation of bradykinin. The latter further increases arteriolar diameter and muscle blood flow. Second, when the endothelium is damaged, as by inflammation, tissue factor XIIA increases formation of kallikrein (Fig 1-1).

Properties of bradykinin. Bradykinin acts on bradykinin receptors in the vascular endothelium to promote the re-

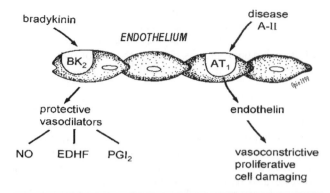

Figure 1-9. Protective vs harmful effects of products of vascular endothelium. BK_2 = bradykinin-2 receptor. NO = nitric oxide. EDHF = endothelial derived hyperpolarizing factor; see Nakashima et al.[56] PGI_2 = prostacyclin. Figure © LH Opie, 1999

lease of two vasodilators. First, there is increased formation of nitric oxide which may mediate vascular protection.[21] Second, there is increased conversion of arachidonic acid to vasodilatory prostaglandins, such as prostacyclin and PGE_2.[68]

Bradykinin receptors. Thus the concept is that bradykinin is formed locally in the vascular endothelium in response to specific stimuli.[21] The bradykinin acts locally on bradykinin receptors of the BK_2-subtype.[73] The result is increased formation in the endothelial cells of nitric oxide and prostaglandins.

Bradykinin inhibitors. Bradykinin does not contribute to the overall regulation of blood pressure, as shown by the injection of a BK_2-inhibitor to normotensive rats.[46] During ACE inhibition, however, the situation may change. The potential vasodilatory role of bradykinin during ACE inhibitor therapy could theoretically be followed by changes in blood bradykinin levels,[87] which, however, are unlikely to reflect changes in the local rates of formation and degradation of bradykinin. The hypotensive effect of ACE inhibition is reduced by the agent apoprotinin, which inhibits the conversion of prekallikrein to kallikrein.[50] In the specific situation of regional ischemia in the dog, bradykinin release into the coronary vein is increased many-fold after coronary occlusion; in addition, the release rate is further enhanced by captopril.[59] Thus, the current concept is that bradykinin formation, occurring locally and thus not easily measured, can participate in the hypotensive and vascular protective effects of ACE inhibitors.[82]

Prostaglandins and hypotensive effects of ACE inhibitors. During ACE inhibition there is increased local synthesis of the active bradykinin nonapeptide, bradykinin-(1-9), in the kidney.[12] Such bradykinin stimulates the conversion of arachidonic acid into vasodilatory prostacyclin (PGI_2) and PGE_2.[47,68] Indomethacin, which inhibits prostaglandin synthesis, reduces the vasodilatory effect of ACE inhibitors.[57] However, these studies do not give conclusive evidence for the role of vasodilatory prostaglandins in the effects of ACE inhibitors, because indomethacin has some additional actions such as blunting the rise of plasma renin activity after ACE inhibitor therapy.[88]

Bradykinin and anti-ischemic effect of ACE inhibitors.
In the heart, it is proposed that increased bradykinin during ACE inhibition protects against ischemic reperfusion damage at least in part by formation of protective nitric oxide and prostacyclin.[37,38] Lesser amounts of bradykinin might however also be formed by direct stimulation of the AT-2 receptor, as could occur during AT-1 receptor blockade.[23]

ENDOTHELIUM, NITRIC OXIDE AND ENDOTHELIN

Intuitively it might be supposed that because A-II potentially damages the endothelium and elicits the release of endothelin, that all A-II would inhibit the release of nitric oxide. This possibility is supported by the observation that in the heart ACEi decreased oxygen uptake, and increased nitrite production.[92] Furthermore these changes are annulled by the blocker of the bradykinin receptor, HOE 140, showing that the bradykinin-2 receptor is involved.

Yet there is apparently contradictory information, namely that A-II *increases* the release of nitric oxide, and that the symphathomimetic effect of A-II is most evident when NO formation is blocked.[39] This formation of NO could be regarded as a local inhibitory feedback modulator because NO in turn lessens sympathetic activity. In practice in almost all cardiovascular disease states, the endothelium is damaged and the release of NO is impaired. Thus ACE inhibition, both by formation of bradykinin, and by a decrease of the direct effects of A-II on the dysfunctional endothelium, would act to protect the endothelium.[82] A-II may at least in part exert its vasoconstrictory and growth promoting effects on vascular smooth muscle, via endothelin.[53] This provides another mechanism whereby ACE inhibitors and AT-1 blockers can exert beneficial vasodilatory and antigrowth effects.

TISSUE RENIN-ANGIOTENSIN SYSTEMS

Although the acute hypotensive effects of ACE inhibition can clearly be linked to decreased circulating levels of angiotensin II, during chronic ACE inhibition there is a reactive hyperreninemia linked to re-emergence of circulating angiotensin II.[44,52] Furthermore, ACE inhibition can be hypotensive even in low renin states.[15] Hence an important question is whether, as now increasingly thought, the tissue renin-angiotensin system, tissue ACE and tissue angiotensin

II are the major sites of action of the ACE inhibitors (see Table 3-1).

All the components of the renin-angiotensin system are found in vascular tissue (Fig 1-10) including the coronary vessels.[19] In a number of vascular beds, local production is the major source of angiotensin I and angiotensin II found in the veins.[11,67] Tissue ACE activity is found in the lungs, myocardium, brain, kidneys and testes.[44] An especially striking finding is the degree to which renal ACE activity is depressed to very low levels by ACE inhibitor therapy given to animals.[84] Furthermore, during chronic ACE inhibitor treatment when plasma ACE activity increases as a result of compensatory induction, there are still low levels of free tissue ACE in kidney, adrenals, and aorta of rats.[35] Evidence for an intracardiac renin-angiotensin system is reviewed by Dostal and Baker,[19] and by Dzau.[20]

The implication of the discovery of these tissue components of the renin-angiotensin system means that angiotensin II can be locally formed in or around blood vessels with possible vasoconstrictory and long-term atherogenic effects.[20] Local angiotensin II formation accounts for the autocrine-paracrine effects of the renin-angiotensin system (*autocrine,* local action on the same cells that produce the angiotensin II; *paracrine,* effects on neighboring cells). When an ACE inhibitor is given to spontaneously hypertensive rats (SH rats), the fall in blood pressure correlates better with the inhibition of the tissue than the circulating renin-angiotensin system.[16,77,85] According to the concept of local endothe-

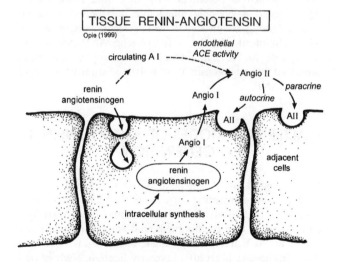

Figure 1-10. Proposed role of tissue renin-angiotensin systems. Renin and angiotensin from the extracellular space may enter the cell by means of receptor endocytosis. Intracellular renin-angiotensin can be derived either from such endocytosis or from local intracellular synthesis. Angiotensin I, thus formed, is released from the cell and converted to angiotensin II either by circulating ACE or by such enzyme attached externally to the cell. Extracellular angiotensin II can then act on the same cell from which the angiotensin I was derived, an autocrine effect. Alternatively, the angiotensin II can be conveyed to the circulation to other cells to exert effects on the angiotensin II receptor, a paracrine action. Fig © LH Opie

lial production of angiotensin II, there is "no need to postulate tissue penetration by ACE inhibitors to explain their inhibitory effect" on organs such as the heart or brain. Thus local tissue systems are important in the blood pressure lowering effects of ACE inhibitors, which would explain why antihypertensive effects can be maintained despite the later reactive increase of circulating angiotensin II and aldosterone.[44] Nonetheless, decisive studies to prove the significance of local tissue ACE inhibition in humans are still lacking.

Significance of local versus circulating renin-angiotensin systems. Ferrari[22] and others suggest that the circulating renin-angiotensin system has a short-term role in cardiovascular regulation, being activated for example by acute hypotension and heart failure. This system "aims to restore blood pressure and cardiac homeostasis". Thereafter, once compensation has been achieved, this system is suppressed as in the compensated phase of heart failure. In contrast, local ACE is remains continuously activated even during the compensated phase of heart failure. The continuous activation of tissue angiotensin II and the ongoing breakdown of bradykinin are thought to promote secondary structural changes of myocardial and vascular remodeling.

Interaction with atrial natriuretic peptide (atriopeptin-II). Natriuresis induced by atrial natriuretic peptide (ANP) occurs in two phases (peak and shoulder pattern), only the first of which is potentiated by ACE inhibition.[71] These data suggest a possible interactive link between the sodium-retaining renin-angiotensin system (susceptible to ACE inhibition) and the sodium-losing ANP system (not susceptible to ACE inhibition). For example, endothelin, produced by angiotensin II stimulation, stimulates the release of ANP.

ALTERNATE MODES OF ANGIOTENSIN II GENERATION

Not all angiotensin II is generated as a result of the activity of angiotensin-converting enzyme. *In the failing human heart*, it appears that most angiotensin II could be formed by a path sensitive to a membrane-bound serine proteinase and not to an ACE inhibitor.[79] Similar observations have been made in the dog heart after coronary ligation,[59] where both a serine and a cysteine protease are implicated. Other tissues in which angiotensin I can be converted to angiotensin II independently of the ACE activity are the renal arteries[62] and the lungs.[49]

A major controversy is the extent to which these independent pathways are of pathophysiological importance.[55,89,93] Whereas studies on cardiac homogenates are contradictory (compare Wolny with Zisman), in two good studies using whole heart preparations, including the human heart, only a low rate of non-ACE conversion was found.[55,93] In the isolated rat heart, the fall in coronary flow in response to renin was largely blocked by ACE inhibition.[55] In contrast, in the pig heart, most of the cardiac A-II is locally produced and such production is not inhibited by captopril.[80] Conflicting views are supported by claims of superior physiological conditions for the assays, though little could be more physiological than the intact human heart.

Vascular A-II. In the isolated coronary artery preparation, a chymase-like serine protease was responsible for most of the A-II production.[89] In humans with peripheral vascular disease, walking distance improved after treatment by NAF (nafamostat), an inhibitor of serine protease.[78] In rat aorta, only high dose perindopril decreased A-II levels, whereas even low doses increased bradykinin.[13]

Exercising humans. Most of the circulating A-II formed comes from a path not sensitive to inhibition by captopril.[51]

Renal A-II. In the intact rat, renal A-II levels decrease by 40% in response to relatively low doses of perindopril.[13]

Conclusions. It is evident that the role of non-ACE pathways is still the subject of controversy, although data from the intact healthy human heart favour a major role for ACE, and renal A-II may be especially sensitive to ACE inhibitors. Yet non-ACE paths may be of substantial importance in vascular smooth muscular tissue.

OTHER ANGIOTENSIN PEPTIDES

Vasodilatory angiotensin (1-7), or A-(1-7), is one of a number of biological active angiotensin peptides distinct from A-I and A-II. It is formed from A-I by neutral endopeptidases (NEP) and may be broken down by a path sensitive to ACE inhibition.[14] The increased antihypertensive effects found in spontaneously hypertensive rats during combined ACE inhibitor and AT-1 receptor blockade could in part be explained by increased levels of this peptide.[32]

Angiotensin (3-8), or A-IV, is derived from A-II by endothelial endopeptidases that split off two amino acids.[34] There is a specific binding site in heart cell membranes.[28] The proposal is that one of the actions of A-IV is on the fibrinolytic system (next section).

ANGIOTENSIN AND FIBRINOLYSIS - A ROLE FOR ANGIO IV RECEPTORS?

Plasminogen is converted by a plasminogen activator to active plasmin that has a thrombolytic action. A-II stimulates the synthesis of plasminogen activator inhibitor type 1 (PAI-1) in aortic cells,[81] possibly by the formation of bradykinin (Fig 1-11). This finding leads to the speculation that the apparent antithrombotic effect of ACE inhibitors could be due to decreased formation of PAI-1 by endothelial cells. A specific receptor, not yet cloned, appears to mediate the

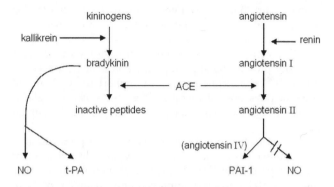

Figure 1-11. Proposed effects of ACE inhibition on thrombosis. Via bradykinin, formation of tissue plasminogen activator (t-PA) is encouraged. Via decreased simulation of the angiotensin IV receptor, formation of plasminogen activator inhibitor-1 (PAI-1) is decreased. Figure modified from Vaughan[83] by permission of author and the European Journal of Cardiology.

induction of PAI-1 expression by the hexapeptide angiotensin IV.[34] Thus, the overall proposal is that angiotensin I and II can be degraded to smaller fragments that stimulate the angiotensin IV receptors, thereby to stimulate the production of PAI-1. Of interest, these effects on PAI-1 are not blocked by specific blockers of either the AT-1 or the AT-2 receptors.[34] On the other hand, neointimal expression of PAI-1 is suppressed by captopril, showing the potential of ACE inhibitors to reduce pathological formation of PAI-1.[27]

SUMMARY

1. *Physiological role of angiotensin-II.* This octapeptide plays a crucial role in cardiovascular control. Physiologically, it is part of the system regulating blood pressure and blood volume. In response to a decreased circulating blood volume, renal release of renin leads via angiotensin-I to angiotensin-II, with strong peripheral vasoconstrictive and sodium retaining properties.

2. *Messenger systems for vasoconstriction.* Following occupation of the heptahelical angiotensin receptor, a membrane messenger system stimulates the enzyme phospholipase C, to break down inositol phospholipids with two main products: inositol trisphosphate that releases calcium from the sarcoplasmic reticulum, and diacyl glycerol that activates a key enzyme, protein kinase C (PKC). These changes lead through mechanism not yet well understood, to increased vascular tone, and an increased peripheral vascular resistance.

3. *Angiotensin receptor subtypes.* There are at least two, AT-1 and AT-2. Virtually all the principal physiological effects of angiotensin-II are mediated by the AT-1 receptors, with the AT-2 receptors playing an impor-

tant role in late fetal life and, it is proposed, in some pathophysiological conditions.

4. *Angiotensin-II as a neuromodulator.* It acts on the terminal sympathetic neurones to promote release of norepinephrine, thereby to reinforcing the direct vasoconstrictor activity.

5. *Angiotensin-II and growth.* It is also a powerful growth stimulator, acting at least in part as a component of the local tissue renin-angiotensin systems that, for example, respond to myocardial stretch.

6. *ACE inhibitor action.* These agents reduced blood pressure by decreasing the rate of formation of angiotensin-II and increasing that of vasodilator bradykinin and prostacyclin. ACE inhibitors also act as indirect anti-adrenergic agents.

7. *ACE-independent pathways.* There is evidence that angiotensin-II can form through such paths as a result, for example, of chymase activity. Such alternate paths might be of greatest importance in pathophysiological conditions, as in the failing human heart.

8. *Angiotensin-IV and fibrinolysis.* Angiotensin-IV or angiotensin (3-8), is derived from angiotensin-II. One of the actions of this peptide is inhibition of the blood fibrinolytic system.

REFERENCES

1. Ajayi AA, Campbell BC, Meredith PA, et al. The effect of captopril on the reflex control heart rate: possible mechanisms. Br J Clin Pharmacol 1985;20:17–25.

2. Akishita M, Ito M, Lehtonen JYA, et al. Expression of the AT2 receptor developmentally programs extracellular signal-regulated kinase activity and influences fetal vascular growth. J Clin Invest 1999;103:63–71.

3. Allen IS, Cohen NM, Dhallan RS, et al. Angiotensin-II increases spontaneous contractile frequency and stimulates calcium current in cultured neonatal rat heart myocytes: insights into the underlying biochemical mechanisms. Circ Res 1988;62:524–534.

4. Antonaccio MJ, Kerwin L. Pre- and postjunctional inhibition of vascular sympathetic function by captopril in SHR: implication of vascular angiotensin-II in hypertension and antihypertensive actions of captopril. Hypertension 1981;3 (Suppl 1):I-54 – I-62.

5. Berridge MJ. Inositol triphosphage, a novel second messenger in cellular signal transduction. Nature 1984;312:315–321.

6. Berridge MJ. Inositol triphosphate and calcium signalling. Nature 1993;361:315–325.

7. Berridge MJ. Rapid accumulation of inositol triphosphate reveals that agonists hydrolyse polyphosphoinositides instead of phosphatidylinositol. Biochem J 1983;212:849–858.

8. Braun-Menendez E, Fasciolo JC, Leloir LF, et al. The substance causing renal hypertension. J Physiol 1940;98:283–298.

9. Braun-Menendez E, Page IH. Suggested revision of nomenclature — angiotensin. Science 1958;127:242.

10. Brown AM, Birnbaumer L. Direct G-protein gating of ion channels. Am J Physiol 1988;254:H401–H410.

11. Campbell DJ. Circulating and tissue angiotensin systems. J Clin Invest 1987;79:1–6.

12. Campbell DJ, Kladis A, Duncan A-M. Bradykinin peptides in kidney, blood and other tissues of the rat. Hypertension 1993;21:155–165.

13. Campbell DJ, Kladis A, Duncan A-M. Effects of converting enzyme inhibitors on angiotensin and bradykinin peptides. Hypertension 1994;23:439–449.

14. Chappell MC, Pirro NT, Sykes A, et al. Metabolism of angiotensin-(1-7) by angiotensin-converting enzyme. Hypertension 1998;31 (part 2):362–367.

15. Chatterjee K, Opie LH. Angiotensin inhibitors and other vasodilators with special reference to congestive heart failure. Cardiovasc Drugs Ther 1987;1:1–18.

16. Cohen ML, Kurz KD. Angiotensin converting enzyme inhibition in tissues from spontaneously hypertensive rats after treatment with captopril or MK-421. Pharmacol Exp Ther 1982;220:63–69.

17. Cushman DW, Ondetti MA. History of the design of captopril and related inhibitors of angiotensin-converting enzyme. Hypertension 1991;17:589–592.

18. Derkx FHM, Tan-thong L, Wenting GJ, et al. Asynchronous changes in prorenin and renin secretion after captopril in patients with renal artery stenosis. Hypertension 1983;5:244–256.

19. Dostal DE, Baker KM. Evidence for a role of an intracardiac renin-angiotensin system in normal and failing hearts. Trends Cardiovasc Med 1993;3:67–74.

20. Dzau VJ. Mechanism of protective effects of ACE inhibition on coronary artery disease. Eur Heart J 1998;19 (Suppl J):J2–J6.

21. Farhy RD, Carretero OA, Ho K-L, et al. Role of kinins and nitric oxide in the effects of angiotensin-converting enzyme inhibitors on neointima formation. Circ Res 1993;72:1202–1210.

22. Ferrari R. Effect of ACE inhibition on myocardial ischaemia. Eur Heart J 1998;19 (Suppl J):J30–J35.

23. Gohlke P, Pees C, Unger T. AT_2 receptor stimulaiton increases aortic cyclic GMP in SHRSP by a kinin-dependent mechanism. Hypertension 1998;31 (part 2):349–355.

24. Goldblatt H, Lynch J, Hanzal RF, et al. Studies on experimental hypertension. I. The production of persistent elevation of systolic blood pressure by means of renal ischemia. J Exp Med 1934;59:347–349.

25. Guidicelli JF, Berdeaux A, Edouard A. The effect of enalapril on baroreceptor mediated reflex function in normotensive subjects. Br J Clin Pharmacol 1985;20:211–218.

26. Hajj-ali AF, Zimmerman BG. Kinin contribution to renal vasodilator effect of captopril in rabbit. Hypertension 1991;17:504–509.

27. Hamdan A, Quist WC, Gagne JB, et al. Angiotensin-converting enzyme inhibition suppresses plasminogen activator inhibitor-1 expression in the neointima of balloon-injured rat aorta. Circulation 1996;93:1073–1078.

28. Hanesworth JM, Sardinia MF, Krebls LT, et al. Elucidation of a specific binding site for angiotensin II(3-8), angiotensin IV, in mammalian heart membranes. J Pharmacol & Exp Therap 1993;268:1036–1042.

29. Harada K, Komuro I, Hayashi D, et al. Angiotensin II type 1a receptor is involved in the occurrence of reperfusion arrhythmias. Circulation 1998;97:315–317.

30. Haywood GA, Gullestad L, Katsuya T, et al. AT_1 and AT_2 angiotensin receptor gene expression in human heart failure. Circulation 1997;95:1201–1206.

31. Iwai N, Inagami T. Identificaiton of two subtypes in the rat type I angiotensin II receptor. FEBS 1992;298:257–260.

32. Iyer SN, Chappell MC, Averill DB, et al. Vasodepressor actions of angiotensin-(1-7) unmasked during combined treatment with lisinopril and losartan. Hypertension 1998;31:699–705.

33. Johnston CI. Tissue angiotensin-converting enzyme in cardiac and vascular hypertrophy, repair and remodeling. Hypertension 1994;23:258–268.

34. Kerins DM, Hao Q, Vaughan DE. Angiotensin induction of PAI-1 expression in endothelial cells is mediated by the hexapeptide angiotensin IV. J Clin Invest 1995;96:2515–2520.

35. Kohzuki M, Johnston CI, Chai SY, et al. Measurement of angiotensin converting enzyme induction and inhibition using quantative in vitro autoradiography: issue selective induction after chronic lisinopril treatment. J Hypertens 1991;9:579–587.

36. Li H-T, Long CS, Gray MO, et al. Cross talk between angiotensin AT_1 and alpha$_1$-adrenergic receptor subtype mRNA and density in neonatal rat cardiac myocytes. Circ Res 1997;81:396–403.

37. Linz W, Scholkens BA, Kaiser J, et al. Cardiac arrhythmias are ameliorated by local inhibition of angiotensin formation and bradykinin degradation with the converting-enzyme inhibitor ramipril. Cardiovasc Drugs Ther 1989;3:873–882.

38. Linz W, Wiemer G, Scholkens BA. ACE inhibition induces NO-formation in cultured bovine endothelial cells and protects isolated ischemic rat hearts. J Mol Cell Cardiol 1992;24:909–919.

39. Liu J-L, Murakami H, Zucker IH. Angiotensin II-nitric oxide interaction on sympathetic outflow in conscious rabbits. Circ Res 1998;82:496–502.

40. Luckhoff A, Clapham A. Inositol 1,2,3,4,5-tetrakisphosphate activates an endothelial Ca^{2+}-permeable channel. Nature 1992;355:356–358.

41. Luscher TF. Angiotensin, ACE inhibitors and endothelial control of vasomotor tone. Basic Res Cardiol 1993;88 (Suppl 1):15–24.

42. Lyall F, Dornan ES, McQueen J, et al. Angiotensin-II increases proto-oncogene expression and phosphoinositide turnover in vascular smooth muscle cells via the angiotensin-II AT_1 receptor. J Hypertens 1992; 10:1463–1469.

43. Lyons D, Roy S, O'Byrne S, et al. ACE Inhibition. Postsynaptic adrenergic sympatholytic action in men. Circulation 1997;96:911–915.

44. MacFadyen RJ, Lees KR, Reid JL. Tissue and plasma angiotensin converting enzyme and the response to ACE inhibitor drugs. Br J Clin Pharmacol 1991;31:1–13.

45. MacGregor GA, Markandu ND, Bayliss J, et al. Non-sulfydryl-containing angiotensin-converting enzyme inhibitor (MK421): evidence for role of renin system in normotensive subjects. Br Med J 1981;283:401–403.

46. Madeddu P, Anania V, Parpaglia PP, et al. Effects of HOE 140, a bradykinin B_2-receptor antagonist, on renal function in conscious normotensive rats. Br J Pharmacol 1992;106:380–386.

47. McGiff JC, Terragno NA, Malik KU, et al. Release of a prostaglandin E-like substance from canine kidney by bradykinin. Circ Res 1972;72:36-43.

48. Meisenhelder J, Suh P-G, Rhee S, et al. Phospholipase C-y is a substrate for the PDGF and EGF receptor protein-tyrosine kinases in vivo and in vitro. Cell 1989;57:1109-1122.

49. Mento PS, Wilkes BM. Plasma angiotensins and blood pressure during converting enzyme inhibition. Hypertension 1987;9 (Suppl III):32–48.

50. Mimran A, Targhetta R, Laroche B. The antihypertensive effect of captopril: evidence for an influence of kinins. Hypertension 1980;2:732–737.

51. Miura S, Ideishi M, Sakai T, et al. Angiotensin II formation by an alternative pathway during exercise in humans. J Hypertens 1994;12:1177–1181.

52. Mooser V, Nussberger J, Juillerat L, et al. Reactive hyperreninemia is a major determinant of plasma angiotensin-II during ACE inhibition. J Cardiovasc Pharmacol 1990;15:276–282.

53. Moreau P, d'Uscio LV, Shaw S, et al. Angiotensin II increases tissue endothelin and induces vascular hypertrophy. Circulation 1997;96:1593–1597.

54. Morgan KG. The role of calcium in the control of vascular tone as assessed by the Ca^{2+} indicator aequorin. Cardiovasc Drugs Ther 1990; 4:1355–1362.

55. Müller DN, Fischli W, Clozel J-P, et al. Local angiotensin II generation in the rat heart. Role of renin uptake. Circ Res 1998;82:13–20.

56. Nakashima M, Mombouli J-V, Taylor AA, et al. Endothelium-dependent hyperpolarization caused by bradykinin in human coronary arteries. J Clin Invest 1993;92:2867–2871.

57. Nishimura H, Kubo S, Ueyma M, et al. Peripheral hemodynamic effects of captopril in patients with congestive heart failure. Am Heart J 1989;117:100–105.

58. Nishizuka Y. Turnover of inositol phospholipids and signal transduction. Science 1984;222:1365.

59. Noda K, Sasaguri M, Ideishi M. Role of locally formed angiotensin-II and bradykinin in the reduction of myocardial infarct size in dogs. Cardiovasc Res 1993;27:334–340.

60. Noll G, Wenzel R, de Marchi S, et al. Differential effects of captopril and nitrates on muscle sympathetic nerve activity in volunteers. Circulation 1997;95:2286-2292.

61. Oelkers W, Brown JJ, Frazer R, et al. Sensitization of the adrenal cortex to angiotensin-II in sodium-deplete man. Circ Res 1974;34:69–77.

62. Okumura T, Okunishi H, Ayajiki K, et al. Conversion of angiotensin I to angiotensin II in dog isolated renal artery: Role of two different angiotensin II-generating enzymes. J Cardiovasc Pharmacol 1990;15:353–359.

63. Ondetti MA, Rubin B, Cushman DW. Design of specific inhibitors of angiotensin-converting enzyme: new class of orally active antihypertensive agents. Science 1977;196:441–444.

64. Page IH, Helmer OM. A crystalline pressor substance (agniotonin) resulting from the reaction between renin and renin-activator. J Exp Med 1940;71:29–42.

65. Purdy RE, Weber MA. Angiotensin-II amplification of alpha-adrenergic vasoconstriction: role of receptor reserve. Circ Res 1988;63:748–757.

66. Sadoshima J. Versatility of the angiotensin II type 1 receptor. Circ Res 1998;82:1352–1355.

67. Schalekamp MADH, Admiraal PJJ, Derkx FHM. Estimation of regional metabolism and production of angiotensins in hypertensive subjects. Br J Clin Pharmacol 1989;28:105S–113S.

68. Schror K. Role of prostaglandins in the cardiovascular effects of bradyki-
    nin and angiotensin-coverting enzyme inhibitors. J Cardiovasc Pharma-
    col 1992;20(Suppl 9):S68–S73.

69. Scicli AG. Increases in cardiac kinins as a new mechanism to protect the
    heart. Hypertension 1994; 23:419–421.

70. Soubrier F, Alhenc-Gelas F, Hubert C. Two putative active centers in hu-
    man angiotensin-I converting enzyme revealed by molecular cloning.
    Proc Natl Acad Sci 1988;85:9386–9390.

71. Spinelli F, Kamber B, Schnell C. Observations on the natriuretic response
    to intravenous infusions of atrial natriuretic factor in water-loaded anaes-
    thetized rats. J Hypertens 1986;4 (Suppl 2):S25–S29.

72. Staessen J, Lijnen P, Fagard R, et al. Rise in plasma concentration of al-
    dosterone during long-term angiotensin-II suppression. J Endocr
    1981;91:457–465.

73. Sung C-P, Arleth AJ, Shikano K, et al. Characterization and function of
    bradykinin receptors in vascular endothelial cells. J Pharmacol Exp Ther
    1988;247:8–13.

74. Suzuki J, Matsubara H, Urakami M, et al. Rat antiotensin II (Type 1A) re-
    ceptor mRNA regulation and subtype expression in myocardial growth
    and hypertrophy. Circ Res 1993;73:439–447.

75. Tigerstedt R, Bergman PG. Niere und Kreislauf. Skand Arch Physiol
    1898;8:223–271.

76. Timmermans P, Benfield P, Chiu AT. Angiotenin-II receptors and func-
    tional correlates. Am J Hypertens 1992;5:221S–235S.

77. Unger T, Ganten D, Lang RE, et al. Is tissue converting enzyme inhibi-
    tion a determinant of the antihypertensive efficacy of converting enzyme
    inhibitors? Studies with the two different compounds HOE 498 and MK
    421, in spontaneously hypertensive rats. J Cardiovasc Pharmacol
    1984;6:872-880.

78. Urabe Y, Ideishi M, Sasaguri M, et al. Beneficial effects of a serine pro-
    tease inhibitor in peripheral vascular disease. Am J Cardiol 1993;72:218–
    222.

79. Urata H, Healy B, Stewart RW, et al. Angiotensin-II-forming pathways in
    normal and failing human hearts. Circ Res 1990;66:883–890.

80. van Kats JP, Danser J, van Meegen JR, et al. Angiotensin production by
    the heart. A quantitative study in pigs with the use of radiolabeled an-
    giotensin infusions. Circulation 1998;98:73–81.

81. van Leeuwen RT, Kol A, Andreotti F, et al. Angiotensin II increases plas-
    minogen activator inhibitor type I and tissue-type plasminogen activator
    messenger RNA in cultured rate aortic smooth muscle cells. Circulation
    1994;90:362–368.

82. Vanhoutte PM. Endothelial dysfunction and inhibition of converting en-
    zyme. Eur Heart J 1998;19 (Suppl J):J7–J15.

83. Vaughan DE. Fibrinolytic balance, the renin-angiotensin system and
    atherosclerotic disease. Eur Heart J 1998;19 (Suppl G):G9–G12.

84. Veltmar A, Gohlke P, Unger T. From tissue angiotensin converting en-
    zyme inhibition to antihypertensive effect. Am J Hypertens 1991;4:263S–
    269S.

85. Weishaar RE, Panek RL, Major TC, et al. Evidence for a functional tissue
    renin-angiotensin system in the rat mesenteric vasculature and its invol-
    vement in regulating blood pressure. J Pharmacol Exp Ther 1991;
    256:568–574.

86. Wilkes BM. Evidence for a vasodepressor effect of the angiotensin-con-
    verting enzyme inhibitor, MK421 (enalapril), independent of blockade of
    angiotensin-II formation. J Cardiovasc Pharmacol 1984;6:1036–1042.

87. Williams GH. Converting-enzyme inhibitors in the treatment of hyper-
    tension. N Engl J Med 1988;319:1517–1525.

88. Witzgall H, Hirsch F, Scherer B, et al. Acute haemodynamic and hormo-
    nal effects of captopril are diminished by indomethacin. Clin Sci
    1982;62:611–615.

89. Wolny A, Clozel J-P, Rein J, et al. Functional and biochemical analysis of
    angiotensin II-forming pathways in the human heart. Circ Res 1997;
    80:219–227.

90. Yamada T, Horiuchi M, Dzau VJ. Angiotensin II type 2 receptor mediates
    programmed cell death. Proc Natl Acad Sci 1996;93:156–160.

91. Yonemochi H, Yasunaga S, Teshima Y, et al. Mechanism of beta adrener-
    gic receptor upregulation induced by ACE inhibition in cultured neona-
    tal rat cardiac myocytes. Roles of bradykinin and protein kinase C.
    Circulation 1998;97:2268–2273.

92. Zhang X, Xie Y-W, Nasjletti A, et al. ACE inhibitors promote nitric oxide
    accumulation to modulate myocardial oxygen consumption. Circulation
    1997;95:176–182.

93. Zisman LS, Abraham WT, Meixell GE, et al. Angiotensin II formation in
    the intact human heart. Predominance of the angiotensin-converting en-
    zyme pathway. J Clin Invest 1995;95:1490–1498.

CHAPTER 2

ACE Inhibitors, vascular structure and arterial disease

"Angiotensin II may directly contribute to the process of atherosclerosis" – Dzau (1998)[12]

There has been an exponential growth in our knowledge of vascular biology, which can now explain at least in part the multiple steps leading to coronary artery disease, still one of the major causes of death in Western societies. In hypertension, vascular disease and remodeling have come to the fore as a possible sites of action of anti-hypertensive drugs. Recent experiments have focused on the role of angiotensin II as an important factor either initiating or perpetuating arterial disease.

Among the many new concepts are the following. First, it is now recognized that the endothelium has an incredibly active role in controlling vascular tone of normal arterioles. Endothelial dysfunction occurs in the coronary system of hypertensives, and in the peripheral arterioles of patients with severe heart failure. Endothelial damage by hypertension could initiate and promote the process of atherosclerosis. Endothelial protection may be mediated by bradykinin, and/or by inhibition of the effects of angiotensin II. Second, the adverse consequences in hypertension of vascular smooth muscle hypertrophy and the associated increase in peripheral vascular resistance is now becoming well established. Third, processes leading to degeneration of the matrix of the vascular wall and especially the increase in fibrosis and the collagen/elastin ratio and consequent loss of elasticity lead to altered compliance and properties of the large vessels with, hypothetically, adverse consequences for the smaller arteriolar resistance vessels. Fourth, relatively non-specific arterial disease, such as that found in aging or in atherosclerosis, is intimately associated with the hypertensive process and the damages of hypertension on the vascular bed. Fifthly, and perhaps of greatest current interest, is the hypothesis that atherosclerosis is an inflammatory disease.[60] This chapter will first review arterial physiology, then the atherosclerotic process with special reference to the role of angiotensin II, and then the potential role of ACE inhibitors in controlling vascular disease will be critically assessed.

ARTERIAL PHYSIOLOGY

As arterial disease is the basis of ischemic heart disease and
hypertensive renal disease, and contributes to the deleterious influences of hypertension and ageing on the cerebral
circulation, the nature of such arterial disease must be
understood before considering the possible protective
effects of ACE inhibitors and other antihypertensive treat-
ments on vascular disease. Arterial disease adversely affects
the function of normal intima and media, and influences a
variety of cell types such as the endothelium, the smooth
muscle cells, and the elastin and collagen fibers of the
matrix. Hence it is necessary first to review vascular physiology as an introduction to an analysis of three types of
vascular damage: (1) endothelial and subintimal disease; (2)
medial hypertrophy in response to the increased intraluminal pressure of hypertension; and (3) end-stage arterial disease, which is the dilated stiff and often calcified arterial
wall, an end-product of ageing and accelerated by hypertension.

Endothelial structure and function. Arteries consist of
three basic layers: the intima, the media, and the adventitia
(Fig 2-1). Each of these can be adversely influenced by hypertension. The endothelium (Fig 2-2) is the crucial structure in the intimal layer; it consists of a monolayer of thin
cells, highly metabolically active in the control of the circulation which it achieves by the production of numerous vasoactive compounds including (1) endothelium-derived
relaxation factor (EDRF) now known to be nitric oxide; (2)
endothelin that acts to vasoconstrict; and (3) the synthesis
of angiotensin I and possibly angiotensin II.[69] Some of these
important functions are listed in Table 2-1.

The endothelium is a very active albeit very thin organ,
constantly synthesizing and releasing a variety of molecules
that can all contribute to the regulation of arterial tone.

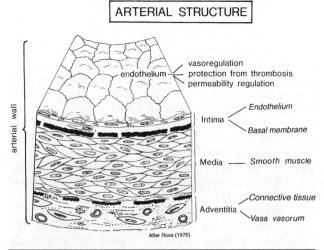

*Fig 2–1. Histological structure of normal muscular artery, emphasizing
different roles of endothelium, smooth muscle cells and fibrous tissue.
Modified with permission from Ross and Glomset (1976).[61]*

"The endothelium appears to serve as a mechanoreceptor within the vasculature that senses flow or pressure and modulates vascular tone accordingly".[20] Besides these functions, the endothelium protects the arterioles from a number of vasoconstrictory influences, such as serotonin released from damaged platelets. A classic Nobel-prize winning observation made by Furchgott and Zawadzki[18] was that endothelial integrity was required for acetylcholine, the messenger of parasympathetic activity, to exert its physiologic vasoconstrictory activity. When endothelial integrity was lost, then acetylcholine became vasoconstrictory. *Thus, endothelial damage can change a vasodilatory stimulus into a vasoconstrictory stimulus.*[68] Following this argument further, the endothelium can be damaged, for example by hypertensive mechanical stress when it is likely to lose its vasodilatory role and to become a vasoconstrictor organ. Speculatively, hypertensive damage to the endothelium could release vasoconstrictory endothelin or inhibit the release of vasodilatory nitric oxide that could, in turn, increase peripheral vascular resistance and exaggerate the severity of hypertension.

Subendothelial tissue. Endothelial cells rest on a basement membrane, separated from smooth muscle cells by the internal elastic lamina. This consists of sheets of elastic fibers with openings large enough to allow the permeation of metabolites, growth factors, and cells in either direction. In early vascular disease, the intima proliferates and

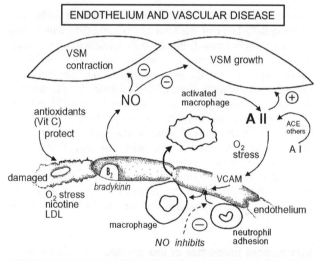

ENDOTHELIUM AND VASCULAR DISEASE

Fig 2–2. Role of healthy endothelium in producing protective nitric oxide (NO), in response to bradykinin and other stimuli. Endothelial integrity is maintained by antioxidants such as vitamin C, and damaged by oxidative stress, nicotine and low density lipoprotein (LDL). Angiotensin II (A-II) besides being a vasoconstrictor agent, promotes oxidative stress that in turn activates adhesion molecules such as VCAM (vascular cell adhesion molecule). The next step is increased adhesion to the endothelium of neutrophils and macrophages. After adhesion, macrophages penetrate the endothelium to become activated and able to take up LDL, thereby becoming foam cells. Activated macrophages also produce angiotensin II. ACE, angiotensin-converting enzyme; A–I, angiotensin I. Figure © LH Opie, 1999

TABLE 2-1: Proposed Functions of Vascular Endothelium

---

1. **Release of vasoactive agents**
   Nitric oxide, previously called EDRF (endothelium-derived relaxation factor)
   Endothelin
   Angiotensin I (and possibly angiotensin II)
   Prostacyclin
   Thromboxane
2. **Prevention of coagulation and fibrinolysis**
   Thromboresistant surface
   Formation of antiaggregant prostacyclin
   Formation of t-PA (tissue plasminogen activator)
   Formation of PAI-1 (plasminogen activator inhibitor-1)
3. **Immune function**
   Supply of antigens to immunocompetent cells
   Secretion of interleukin-I (a T-cell inducer)
4. **Enzymatic activity**
   Angiotensin converting enzyme (conversion of angiotensin I to angiotensin II)
5. **Growth signal to vascular smooth muscle**
   EDGF secretion (endothelium-derived growth factor)
   Heparin-like inhibitors of growth
6. **Protection of vascular smooth muscle from vasoconstrictory influences**
   Requirement of endothelial integrity for some vasodilator stimuli such as acetylcholine

---

smooth muscle cells from the tunica media move into the lesion to contribute to the developing plaque (Fig 2-3).

Tunica media and vascular smooth muscle cells. This is the middle layer of the arterial wall (Fig 2-1) which basically consists of smooth muscle cells lying within a connective tissue matrix. Thus, the two major components of the medial layer are (1) the smooth muscle cell that upon appropriate stimulation contracts to narrow the diameter of the arterial wall, and (2) the supporting matrix that binds the muscle cells into bundles and keeps them in the correct orientation in the arterial wall. In the *small muscular arterioles* ("small bore arteries", diameter less than 1 mm), it is these smooth muscle cells which respond to a rise of cytosolic calcium concentration by contracting and thereby decreasing the diameter of the arterioles, which increases the peripheral vascular resistance and causes the blood pressure to rise.

Mechanical properties of the arteries. The matrix of the medial layer is that component which determines to a major extent, together with the adventitia, the mechanical properties of the artery. First, the ratio of matrix to muscle cells varies. In the large conduit arteries, like the aorta and its major branches, elastin is the most important component of the matrix and in the largest vessels, such as the aorta, the major component of the arterial wall. It is the elastin in the aortic wall that allows the aorta to expand in systole as blood is rapidly ejected from the left ventricle, then in diastole the elastic recoil helps to propel the blood flow onwards and hence to maintain the diastolic blood pressure.

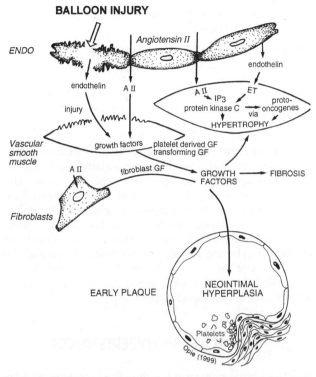

Fig 2–3. Proposed role of endothelium in response to vascular wall injury. Note role of growth factors (GF) which are also stimulated by angiotensin II (A-II). ET, endothelin; IP_3, inositol trisphosphate. Figure © LH Opie, 1999

This is the "pressure-equalizing" function of the elastic layer.

The elasticity of elastin is explained by its hydrophobic properties. When relaxed, crucial hydrophobic regions have minimal contact with the surrounding water of the extracellular space. When stretched, contact with water increases, and the hydrophobic area reacts in such a way that the fibers return to their original length. The synthesis of elastin from proelastin is triggered mechanically, whereas its breakdown by elastase is accelerated in old age.

Collagen is the other major connective tissue protein of the matrix and is closely related in structure to the collagen found in the myocardium. Collagen is an important component of the medial wall, helping it to keep its shape despite the high intraluminal pressure exerted by the blood. Hence collagen has extremely high tensile properties, and is distributed in such a way in the medial layer that the arteries are highly resistant to the intraluminal pressure. When, however, conduit arteries such as the external carotid or the common iliac are treated by collagenase, then segments of these arteries readily rupture when subjected to pressure.[11] Different types of collagen have different responses to mechanical stress. Types I and II collagen, the most common in the media, consist of fibrils about 20 to 90 nm in diameter. Groups of fibrils constitute fibers. Type III collagen is more elastic, while Type IV collagen is found chiefly in the intima and Type V in the basement membrane of the arterial wall.

Other matrix proteins are the glycoproteins which include *fibronectin*, a biological "glue", and the glycosaminoglycans (GAG) which are hydrophilic, forming aggregates that make up a gel containing electrolytes and small molecules in passage from blood to the various tissues through the vessel wall.

Adventitial layer. The adventitia, the external layer, separated from the media by the external elastic lamina, is essentially a vessel bearing and nerve conducting layer. The blood vessels running to the arterial wall are found here (vasa vasorum) as are lymphatics and the autonomic nerves. Histologically, this layer contains collagen, fibroblasts, and a few muscle cells besides the blood vessels. In the large conducting arteries, the adventitia is thin and the elastic layer of the media is dominant. In the small muscular arteries, the site of the peripheral vascular resistance, the adventitia is thicker especially its inner layer.

ARTERIOLES IN HYPERTENSION

It is the arterioles that are the site of the systemic vascular resistance and hence respond most to an increase in size of the medial wall. The reaction of the arterioles to hypertension can best be understood in terms of the Meerson hypothesis applied to the myocardium. This great Russian physiologist, currently still living in Moscow, described the well known three stages of myocardial adaptation. The first stage is the acute adaptation to the mechanical overload, a process involving the transduction of excess wall stress into protein synthesis, probably by stimulation of mechanoreceptors. The second stage is that of compensatory hypertrophy in which the enlarged hypertrophied myocardium has a wall stress that has reverted to normal. The third is the stage of decompensation and irreversible myocardial failure, when an excess prolonged load causes cardiac dilation. The transition from compensation to irreversible decompensation may be linked, hypothetically, to cellular ischemia and reactive stimulation of fibroblasts with collagen formation and fibrosis.

Similar principles may be applied to the arteries. In the first phase, an excess intraluminal pressure leads to compensatory protein synthesis, thereby establishing the second phase with the hypertrophied thickened medial wall, which restores normal wall tension despite the continued increase in the intraluminal pressure. In the third phase, the media degenerates and disorganization of the matrix leads to irreversible damage, often with calcinosis. The three crucial biological steps to understand are (1) the initiator of the complex process that changes a healthy to a damaged artery; (2) the trigger to smooth muscle growth; and (3) the nature of end-stage degeneration.

Endothelial morphology in hypertension. In hypertension, the subendothelial layer thickens with infiltrated cells derived from the media and with the growth of matrix cells. Morphologic changes include roughening of the intimal surface and discontinuity of the intercellular junctions.[4] The latter change may account for the increased permeability to macromolecules with risk of penetration of blood lipoprotein components and possible initiation of atheroma. The endothelium loses much of its vasodilator capacity and undergoes thickening.[20] These endothelial changes add to the risk of a reduction in luminal area of the arteriole. Although there is no direct proof of the role of an endothelial renin-angiotensin system in these changes, nonetheless it is of interest that vascular endothelial cells have the capacity for renin expression in culture.[56]

Endothelium, nitric oxide and hypertension. An increased peripheral (systemic) vascular resistance is one major cause of hypertension because

$$BP = CO \times PVR$$

where BP is blood pressure, CO is cardiac output and PVR is peripheral vascular resistance. Physiologically, the PVR increases with age. Another cause of an increased PVR in hypertension is an excess of vasoconstrictory stimuli, including angiotensin II whether circulating or locally formed. Other vasoconstrictory stimuli are increased alpha$_1$-adrenergic activity or endothelin. Alternatively, there could be a lack of vasodilatory stimulation, leading to a preponderance of vasoconstriction. Currently emphasized by Moncada, an "almost" Nobel prize winner in 1998, is the decreased capacity of the endothelium to form vasodilatory nitric oxide. In the salt-sensitive hypertensive rat there is unequivocal evidence of impaired ability to form nitric oxide.[57] Nitric oxide also decreases sodium excretion by the kidney. Such sodium retention can be linked to increased PVR by the proposed "natriuretic hormone" which inhibits the sodium pump in vascular smooth muscle, so that there is an increased cytosolic sodium, followed by activity of the sodium-calcium exchanger and increased vasoconstriction. Thus decreased production of nitric oxide can lead to an increased PVR by two different routes: (1) decreased peripheral vasodilation, and (2) decreased sodium excretion. Whether these mechanisms operate in salt sensitive humans remains to be shown.

Long term protective effects of nitric oxide. Nitric oxide has antiproliferative effects on vascular smooth muscle, which could theoretically lessen the long term development of atherosclerosis. The mechanism of this effect includes the formation of cyclic GMP, and possibly the inhibition of MAP kinase.[45] In addition, nitric oxide prevents the roll-on and adhesion of neutrophils to the endothelium, thought to be an important primary step in atherosclerosis (Fig 2-2).

ENDOTHELIAL DYSFUNCTION, VASCULAR INJURY AND DISEASE

Traditional risk factors for atherosclerosis. Currently the traditional risk factors are increasing suspected of initiating endothelial dysfunction, which in turn can impair dilation of small coronary arterioles.[27] Such damage may result from hypercholesterolemia,[29] nicotine and hypertension. Homocysteine may act here.[36] Hypertension might act by abnormal shear forces,[10] leading to increased formation of superoxide with endothelial damage. The result would be release of vasoconstrictory endothelin and/or less formation of vasodilatory nitric oxide. In hypertension, these endothelial changes allow the postulate of a vicious circle mechanism (Fig 3-8), whereby the increased arterial pressure damages the endothelium, to promote vasoconstriction and further to elevate the peripheral vascular resistance. The end result is an even higher arterial pressure.

Receptors for oxidized LDL (low density lipoproteins). Increasing evidence incriminates oxygen radical damage in atherosclerosis, and oxidized LDL is seen as one of the key culprits. Some of it forms in the circulation, to be taken up by the endothelium. Oxidized LDL also forms in the interstitial space as free radicals are produced by the macrophages. In general, anti-oxidants inhibit atherosclerosis.[66] The cell surface receptor that promotes uptake of oxidized LDL by the endothelium is a lectin-like molecule (LOX)

TABLE 2-2:   ANGIOTENSIN II AND ITS PROPOSED ROLE IN BLOOD VESSELS

---

1. **Evidence for local angiotensin II production**
   a. Induced coexpression of angiotensinogen renin and angiotensin-converting enzyme activity in medial layer[13]
   b. Induction of mRNA for angiotensinogen in media and neointima after balloon injury[55]
   c. Increase of aortic, mesenteric and renal artery renin levels despite normal circulating renin[52]
   d. Inhibition of angiotensin II release from perfused mesenteric artery by renin and ACE inhibitors[28]
2. **Effects of angiotensin II on growth factors and isolated myocytes**
   a. Increased growth of vascular smooth muscle cells stimulated by plasma factor[6]
   b. Hypertrophy of aortic smooth muscle cells[19]
   c. Induction of proto-oncogenes and platelet-derived growth factor (PDGF)[31, 42, 46]
   d. Receptor-mediated stimulation of collagen synthesis in cultured vascular smooth muscle cells[30]
3. **Effects on vascular hypertrophy in vivo**
   a. Angiotensin II infusion induces smooth muscle cell proliferation and DNA synthesis when infused into normotensive rats[8]
   b. AII promotes vascular hypertrophy via ET_A receptor[43]
4. **Calcification**
   a. Promotion of expression of osteopontin, that in turn leads to abnormal calcification (see text)
5. **Ischemic-reperfusion injury** – increased via AT-1 receptor[72]

---

which is upregulated in response to stimulation by inflammatory cytokines such tumor necrosis factor alpha (TNF-α).[34]

Inflammatory hypothesis for initial arterial damage: effect on smooth muscle cells. A current hypothesis is that atherosclerosis is a multifactorial disease involving at least in part an inflammatory response.[60] Besides influencing the endothelium (see above), inflammatory stimuli can alter the response of vascular smooth muscle cells (Table 2-3). A "stress" activated path, responding to cytokines, may be activated in vascular smooth muscle cells (VSM, where A-II can stimulate at least two paths.[65] The established path mediating growth signals involves the AT-1 receptor, phospholipid derived second messengers, protein kinase C (PKC), and leads via MAP kinase to stimulation of proto-oncogenes.[38] This path also functions in cardiac myocytes.[63] A more recently described path[65] is the JAK-STAT "stress" path that also responds to cytokines including TNF-α. This path may be involved in the growth response to cellular inflammatory reactions, to contribute to arterial damage and atherosclerosis. Formation of oxygen-derived free radicals may be another way in which A-II promotes arterial damage.

TABLE 2-3:   PROPOSED MECHANISMS WHEREBY INFLAMMATORY PROCESSES MAY CONTRIBUTE TO ATHEROSCLEROSIS*

1. Provision of leukocytes and macrophages, with production of reactive oxygen species
2. Inflammation promotes formation of cytokines that stimulate "inflammatory" type growth pathways that inhibit apoptosis[25] and, paradoxically, in some cases promote apoptosis
3. Increased cardiac synthesis of complement enhances formation of MAC (membrane attack complex)[73]
4. Indirect effect of tachycardia, acute phase proteins, inhibition of fibrinolysis

*For review see Kol and Libby.[33]

Angiotensin II and oxidative stress hypothesis. Oxygen derived free radicals that play an important part in arterial damage, are formed by macrophages. There are two other vascular sources of free radicals (Table 2-4). First, endothelial production of the superoxide anion (O_2^{-}).[15] This proposal is of interest because hypercholesterolemia can increase the production of superoxide by the endothelium.[50] Sec-

TABLE 2-4:   PROPOSED ROLE OF REACTIVE OXYGEN SPECIES (ROS) IN ATHEROSCLEROSIS

1. ROS promote oxidation of LDL cholesterol and endothelial damage[15]
2. Endothelial damage promotes entry of leukocytes to become macrophages and foam cells
3. Activated macrophages synthesize more ROS, with a vicious cycle
4. A-II promotes endothelial damage with greater formation of ROS

ondly, the vascular smooth muscle cells can make superoxide.[41] A potential mechanism is that A-II can stimulate NADH oxidase, and in the process superoxide is made.[21,53] Such increased hydrogen peroxide is an essential step in vascular smooth muscle hypertrophy, as shown in a novel cell line that overexpresses the enzyme catalase that mops up the peroxide.[74] If inflammatory cells in damaged vascular tissue can locally produce increased amounts of A-II[71] then a vicious circle is possible:[12]

> Hypercholesterolemia → endothelial superoxide → increased macrophage activation → increased LDL oxidation → increased tissue damage → increased local synthesis of A-II → increased superoxide → increased LDL oxidation, etc.

Upregulation of vascular A-II receptors. Hyperinsulinemia is linked to hypertension and obesity on the basis of epidemiological studies. Although the real mechanism is still obscure, an attractive proposal is that insulin can upregulate the vascular AT-1 receptors,[48] thereby increasing the sensitivity to circulating or locally generated A-II. Likewise, low density lipoprotein (LDL) can also upregulate the vascular AT-I receptor.[49] Thus, a further vicious circle is possible:

> Increased LDL → upregulation of A-II (AT-1) vascular receptors → increased peripheral resistance and increased hypertension → increased vascular damage → increased local A-II generation → greater upregulation of A-II vascular receptors → greater vascular damage.

Protection of endothelium by ACE inhibitors. These agents could theoretically protect the endothelium in one of three ways. First, they could diminish the amount of angiotensin II available to act on the endothelium; angiotensin II is one of the factors inducing release of the vasoconstrictory endothelin. Second, A-II is incriminated in the production of oxygen free radicals such as superoxide, which are thought to contribute to the atherosclerotic process by Dzau.[12] Thirdly, ACE inhibitors increase formation of bradykinin which, in turn, elicits the release of protective vasodilators such as nitric oxide from the endothelium. Although still hypothetical, these proposals suggest further mechanisms for vasoprotective effects of ACE inhibitors.[16,40]

VASCULAR REMODELING

In response to a sustained increased of arterial pressure, the structure of the vascular wall can undergo a complex series of structural changes known as vascular remodeling. Strictly speaking, some would limit the term "remodeling" to a rearrangement of otherwise normal material, thereby excluding the contribution of the growth process.[26] Others, including the present author, would by analogy with the established concept of postinfarct cardiac remodeling

(Fig 5-7), use the term vascular remodeling also to include cellular growth in response to increased intraluminal pressure and, hence, wall stress. Therefore, in the overall process of vascular remodeling, the VSM layer is increased in size, and there may be associated endothelial and/or intimal changes. Hypothetically, these vascular changes can contribute to the maintenance of hypertension (Fig 3-7).

Trigger to vascular smooth muscle growth. According to current concepts, the two major types of stimuli are (1) mechanical stretch, acting by deformation of the vascular cells, and (2) receptor agonists acting by intracellular signaling systems (Fig 2-4). The signals involved may overlap.[38]

Mechanical stimulation by stretch. Because stretch of isolated vascular myocytes leads to enhanced protein synthesis and cell hypertrophy,[39] hypertension could be acting at least in part through stretch-activated signals to cause medial hyperplasia and hypertrophy.[38] The role of pressure in vascular hypertrophy was proven by an ingenious experiment in which the pressure in the femoral artery was specifically reduced in spontaneously hypertensive rats by a partially occluding ligature.[5] In the distal artery protected from systemic hypertension, the following abnormalities reverted to normal: an increased medial wall thickness and cross-sectional area, and the increased media-lumen ratio.

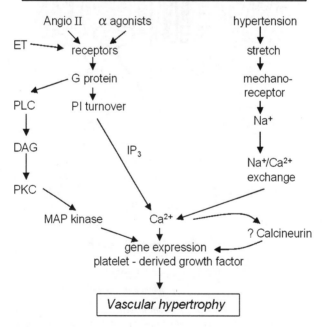

Fig 2–4. *Proposed mechanism whereby vasoconstrictive agents such as angiotensin II, alpha (α)-agonist stimulation and endothelin (ET) could lead to vascular growth. In addition, mechanical stretch can be the major or even sole factor causing vascular growth (Bund et al, 1991). IP₃, inositol trisphosphate. For role of PI and IP₃, see Fig 1-4. For other abbreviations see Figs 1-3 and 1-6. Figure © LH Opie, 1999*

Thus, in these experiments, it was not necessary to postulate the operation of any non-mechanical factor in achieving these improvements in vascular structure. Another way of dissociating the effects of angiotensin II and blood pressure is by infusing perindopril-treated hypertensive rats with saline.[23] The latter procedure restored the blood pressure to the previously elevated levels and once again increased wall media-lumen ratio.

Balloon injury of arteries. As already discussed, endothelial damage is an important initiator of atherosclerosis. Balloon injury (Fig 2-3) induces new growth of the intima to produce the *neointima*, with also medial hypertrophy.[55] Angiotensin II promotes such growth by the local production of growth factors.

Receptor stimulation as growth signal. An alternate hypothesis not involving mechanical effects is that receptor agonists acting as vasoconstrictors might also stimulate the signals to vascular smooth muscle growth (Fig 2-5). Among the potential agonists is the local vascular renin-angiotensin system (Table 2-2). The logical explanation would be that

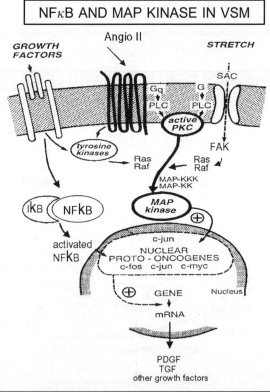

Figure 2–5 Growth in vascular smooth muscle cells. Two major paths for stimulation of nuclear proto-oncogenes: (1) growth factors acting via nuclear factor kappa B (NFκB); (2) angiotensin II and endothelin (ET) acting via mitogen activated protein kinase (MAP kinase). Stretch, as in hypertension, probably acts via the latter path, first acting via focal adhesion kinase (FAK). See Ymazaki et al (Circ Res 1998;82:430). For role of IκB (Inhibitor of kappa B), see Lee et al (Proc Natl Acad Sci 1998;95:9319). Figure © LH Opie, 1999

cytosolic calcium acts as the common factor with a short-lived calcium rise acting as a vasoconstrictor and a sustained calcium rise acting as a growth promoter. In particular, angiotensin II promotes both contraction and hypertrophy[19,20,32] and angiotensin II increases cytosolic calcium in vascular smooth muscle cells working in part by activation of voltage-dependent Ca^{2+} channels[51] and in part through stimulation of the phosphoinositol pathway.[64] Conversely, chronic ACE inhibitor therapy decreases arterial calcium content.[62] According to some current concepts, angiotensin II could be a stimulus to cell growth, acting in part by a sustained increase of cytosolic calcium which, in turn, stimulates gene expression and formation of proto-oncogenes which would lead to increased vascular growth (Figs 2–4, 2–5). Thus, it is not surprising that in animal models of hypertension captopril and perindopril not only prevent hypertension but lessen vascular hypertrophy with improved vascular function.[7,37]

Antihypertensive drugs and remodeling. An important issue is whether vascular remodeling during hypertension therapy is purely the result of pressure reduction or whether there is also a pressure-independent mechanism. Data with perindopril and enalapril suggest that not all of the benefit is mediated by the pressure drop.[59] This proposal leaves room for a specific adverse vascular effect of angiotensin II, or for specific benefits of bradykinin.

Consequences of arteriolar changes. Although the enlarged hypertrophied arteriole (compensated arteriolar hypertrophy, Stage II) is able to withstand the increased intraluminal pressure, there are inevitable disadvantages ("no gain without pain" as is said in sports medicine). There are two problems. First, the concentric hypertrophy not only increases the medial thickness but reduces the internal diameter of the lumen.[44] At this stage Poiseuille's law should be recalled. The vascular resistance (R) is:

$$R = P/Q = (8 \times viscosity \times length)/\pi.r^4$$

where Q is flow, r is radius, and P is pressure drop. Any given fall of radius leads to a much greater increase in resistance. Reduction of the diameter (or radius) of the arteriole by 5% increases the vascular resistance by 23%, whereas a 10% reduction increases the vascular resistance by as much as 70%.

The second disadvantage is that there is still a sustained sensitivity to vasoconstrictor agonists although in some experiments this response is muted.[37] Starting from a smaller arteriolar lumen, any vasoconstrictor stimulus such as angiotensin II or alpha$_1$-adrenergic activity will cause a greater rise in the systemic vascular resistance. For example, if the normal lumen is reduced by 5%, then the vascular resistance will increase by 23% as already calculated. However, if the lumen is already reduced, then an additional further reduction of another 5% will vastly increase the vascular resistance. Whether there is increased, decreased, or altered arteriolar response to the same degree of vasoconstrictor stimulation is still a matter of controversy.

A third point of note is that there is evidence for enhanced activity of the vasoconstrictor mechanisms in hypertension. For example, vascular renin activity appears to be increased in experimental hypertension.[13] In mildly hypertensive patients, there are increased circulating levels of catecholamines in response to psychologic stress such as mental arithmetic.[47] Furthermore, there may be alterations in the intracellular coupling systems. Thus, the alpha-receptor may be better coupled to its messenger system.[54] While the experimental vascular data largely relate to aorta and may not be applicable to arterioles, nonetheless the principle of a decreased resting lumen size and an increased reaction to vasoconstrictor stimulation would appear to be firmly established.

Enhanced arteriolar vasoconstriction may therefore perpetuate and exaggerate hypertension,[20] particularly in the presence of structural changes. Thus it is proposed that the arteriolar wall plays a crucial role in the continuation of the hypertensive process.

End-stage arterial disease. The genesis of end-stage arterial disease is not well understood and here the analogy with Meerson's Stage III is not exact. On the one hand, the arterial smooth muscle cells appear to undergo degeneration and to be replaced by an inflammatory infiltrate, as well as collagen fibrosis. This process corresponds reasonably well with Meerson's Stage III for the myocardium. In addition, however, there is marked intimal damage with fibrin deposition and often arteriolar occlusion. The latter process suggests that the hypertensive process has extensively damaged the endothelium and intima which, in turn, has resulted in fibrin deposition and arterial occlusion. The analogy with Meerson's Stage III for the heart can, however, be made by pointing out that end-stage arterial disease in the heart and in the arteriole are the result of unremitting intraluminal wall tension. In the one case the increased wall tension arises from left ventricular dilation and in the other case from sustained intraluminal hypertension.

Osteopontin. Calcification is still poorly understood. Angiotensin-II induces the expression of osteopontin in rat arteries.[9] Osteopontin is part of the non-collagenous protein matrix, and promotes calcification in atherosclerotic plaques.[17] Clearly the remedy for end-stage arterial disease is prevention, there being no cure.

EFFECTS OF ACE INHIBITORS ON ARTERIOLAR DISEASE

Both perindopril and captopril reduced the media/lumen ratio in arterioles of spontaneously hypertensive rats.[7,37] In stroke-prone spontaneously hypertensive rats, cilazapril inhibited the unfavorable remodeling of cerebral arterioles and improved their distensibility.[22] In the one model of hypertension (one kidney, one clip), captopril reduced the arterial wall density.[70]

During the active phase of treatment of hypertension in spontaneously hypertensive rats, ACE inhibition was more effective than other modalities of treatment in controlling the structural vascular abnormalities because the wall/ lumen ratio was lowest, particularly with perindopril.[7] Likewise, in the spontaneously hypertensive rat, captopril treatment reduced the abnormally increased wall/lumen ratio, the intima/lumen ratio, and the media/lumen ratio.[37]

Effects of withdrawal of therapy on arteriolar disease in experimental hypertension. If arteriolar structural changes are crucial to the development of hypertension, then the therapeutic improvement of the abnormalities involved should be followed by improvement in the blood pressure even when treatment is withdrawn. This proposal has been tested in spontaneously hypertensive rats treated by a variety of agents including the ACE inhibitors perindopril and captopril during the growth phase of the rats from 4 to 24 weeks.[7] During the phase of therapy withdrawal, from 24 to 36 weeks, the blood pressure remained controlled in those rats that had been treated by perindopril and captopril but not in those previously treated by the calcium antagonist isradipine, nor by the beta-blocker metoprolol, nor by the non-specific vasodilator hydralazine. The ACE inhibitors were better at normalizing the media/ lumen ratio, suggesting that therapeutic control of the arteriolar structural changes in these rats could have led to the sustained post-treatment normalization of blood pressure by the ACE inhibitors. The post-treatment hypotensive effect is found even at low doses of perindopril.[14]

In a particularly interesting study, Harrap et al[24] gave brief periods of ACE inhibitor therapy (perindopril 3 mg/kg/ day) from 6 to 10 weeks and found a reduction in the media/lumen ratio of mesenteric resistance vessels at 32 weeks of age. This reduction was reverted by infusion of angiotensin II with perindopril over the same time. Thus early perindopril therapy led to a late benefit in vascular structure.

It seems safe to conclude that in models of hypertension, ACE inhibition can have a post-treatment effect in lowering blood pressure and can maintain improvements in vascular structure that appear to exceed the effects achieved by representatives of other types of antihypertensive agents. Although these studies need confirmation in other models of animal hypertension, they do suggest that the hypertensive vicious circle outlined in Fig 3-7 could be interrupted therapeutically. While any application to human hypertension remains speculative, Gibbons and Dzau[20] have proposed that such reversion of vascular structure if found in humans could actually cure hypertension in a subset of patients.

Clinical vascular studies with ACE inhibitors. Doppler echocardiographic techniques have led to the establishment of non-invasive measurements of indices of vascular compliance and of blood flow velocity in the major arteries such as the carotids, the brachials, and the femorals. In normal volunteers, the ACE inhibitor perindopril markedly increased blood flow and decreased vascular resistance even when the changes in the blood pressure were slight.[58] Thus the suggestion is that vascular resistance decreased as the compliance increased.

In patients with ischemic heart disease, perindopril given chronically inhibits arterial converting enzyme acidity in both endothelium and adventitia.[75] Therefore this ACE inhibitor penetrates the vascular wall. In hypertensive subjects, in an acute study, intravenous perindoprilat (the active form of perindopril) increased brachial artery blood flow and diameter as well as compliance at a time when the blood pressure decreased.[3] These changes were especially evident at the higher dose used (2.5 μg/kg/min).

In a chronic study, oral perindopril also gave a similar increase in arterial compliance.[2] During chronic therapy over 1 year, the increase in compliance was maintained while cardiac mass decreased in those patients responding to perindopril monotherapy.[1] There was still some increase in brachial artery diameter even when wrist arterial occlusion had been used to reduce the brachial blood flow and hence to lessen any direct effect of the rate of blood flow on the diameter (flow-induced arterial dilation). When subcutaneous arteries are subject to biopsy, the increased media/lumen ratio of hypertensive subjects reverted to normal after 9 months of treatment by perindopril.[67] Vascular changes may also be induced by captopril. When compared with the hydralazine-like compound, cadralazine, there were comparable changes in blood pressure but only captopril increased arterial diameter and decreased pulse wave velocity.[35]

These human studies are still in their infancy. At present their importance is twofold. First, they show that the animal data can at least in part be extrapolated to human disease. Second, human data counter the argument that the high doses of all agents used in animal models might have induced vascular changes not achieved at the much lower doses used during chronic oral administration in humans. Although there is a more marked vascular response to a high dose of perindoprilat in humans,[3] vascular changes have been found even at standard oral doses. Overall, the basic and clinical data suggest that the *ACE inhibitors have multiple sites of action on the arterial tree*, including not only the pressure-induced changes resulting from a reduction of intraluminal pressure, but also specific changes dependent on inhibition of angiotensin II and formation of bradykinin, possibly independent of any effect on the blood pressure.

SUMMARY

1. *Endothelial dysfunction and nitric oxide.* That changes in vascular structure occur in hypertension is not a new concept, dating back at least to Folkow in 1973. The proposal has taken new meaning with the discovery of the prominent role of the vascular endothelium in producing vasoconstrictory endothelin and vasodilatory nitric oxide (previously called endothelium-derived relaxation factor). In 1998 the Nobel price for Medicine was awarded to Furchgott and co-workers for defining the role of the endothelium in producing nitric oxide, a molecule with vasodilator and vascular protector properties. The "almost winner" of the prize, Moncada, suggests that endothelial dysfunction with impaired production of nitric oxide, could perpetuate or even initiate hypertension.

2. *Role of inflammation and reactive oxygen species in initiating arterial damage.* Current hypotheses proposed by Dzau and others, propose that very early arterial damage can be caused by an inflammatory process, in which the generation of reactive oxygen species appears to play an important role. Locally produced A-II is hypothesized to make and important contribution to this process.

3. *Angiotensin II as growth signal.* Recent evidence from molecular biology of arterial tissue and morphimetric analysis of the structure of arteries that has shown the complex ways in which angiotensin II acts as a signal to vascular growth. For example, the AT-1 receptor is unregulated in response to hyperinsulinemia and in response to low-density lipoprotein. The other major signal to vascular growth is intraluminal stretch, resulting from the increased blood pressure. Experimental and clinical evidence with the use of ACE inhibitors shows that arterial and arteriolar changes associated with hypertension can at least in part be reverted toward normal. Of particular interest is a carry-over effect found when therapy has been stopped, which experimentally is found with the ACE inhibitors and not with the calcium antagonists, the beta-blockers, or hydralazine.

4. *Protective vascular effects of ACE-inhibitors.* The proposed specific role of angiotensin II in vascular damage and growth, leads to a new site of action of ACE inhibitors on the vascular tree. The protective effects of bradykinin, indirectly produced by ACE-inhibitors (Chapter 1), adds to the concept that these agents could interrupt a hypertensive vicious circle mechanism. Bradykinin generation may also help explain the reduction of myocardial infarction found in trials of heart failure.

5. The *clinical implications* of these proposals, well supported experimentally, will need careful evaluation in prospective trials.

REFERENCES

1. Asmar RG, Journo HJ, Lacolley PJ, et al. Treatment for one year with perindopril: effect on cardiac mass and arterial compliance in essential hypertension. J Hypertens 1988;6 (Suppl 3):S33–S39.

2. Asmar RG, Pannier B, Santoni JP, et al. Reversion of cardiac hypertrophy and reduced arterial compliance after converting enzyme inhibition in essential hypertension. Circulation 1988;78:941–950.

3. Benetos A, Santoni JP. Vascular effects of intravenous infusion of the angiotensin converting enzyme inhibitor perindopril. J Hypertens 1990;8:819–826.

4. Berry CL, Sosa-Melgarejo JA. Nexus junctions between vascular smooth muscle cells in the media of the thoracic aorta in normal and hypertensive rats. A freeze-fracture study. J Hypertens 1989;7:507–513.

5. Bund SJ, West KP, Heagerty AM. Effects of protection from pressure on resistance artery morphology and reactivity in spontaneously hypertensive and Wistar-Kyoto rats. Circ Res 1991;68:1230–1240.

6. Campbell-Boswell M, Robertson AL. Effects of angiotensin-II and vasopressin on human smooth muscle cells in vitro. Exp Mol Pathol 1981;35:265–276.

7. Christensen KL, Jespersen LT, Mulvany MJ. Development of blood pressure in spontaneously hypertensive rats after withdrawal of long-term treatment related to vascular structure. J Hypertens 1989;7:83–90.

8. Daemen MJAP, Lombardi DM, Bosman FT, et al. Angiotensin-II induces smooth muscle cell proliferation in the normal and injured rat arterial wall. Circ Res 1991;68:450–456.

9. de Blois D, Lombardi DM, Su EJ, et al. Angiotensin II induction of osteopontin expression and DNA replication in rat arteries. Hypertension 1996;28:1055–1063.

10. De Keulenaer GW, Chappell DC, Ishizaka N, et al. Oscillatory and steady laminar shear stress differentially affect human endothelias redox state. Circ Res 1998;82:1094–1101.

11. Dobrin PB, Baker WH, Gley WC. Elastolytic and collagenolytic studies of arteries. Arch Surg 1984;119:405–409.

12. Dzau VJ. Mechanism of protective effects of ACE inhibition on coronary artery disease. Eur Heart J 1998;19 (Suppl J):J2–J6.

13. Dzau VJ, Safar ME. Large conduit arteries in hypertension: role of the vascular renin-angiotensin system. Circulation 1988;77:947–954.

14. Eriksen S, Christensen KL, Thybo NK, et al. A negatie correlation between perindopril dose and persistent effects on blood pressure in spontaneously hypertensive rats. Acta Physiol Scand 1992;146 (Suppl 608):74.

15. Fang X, Weintraub NL, Rios CD, et al. Overexpression of human superoxide dismutase inhibits oxidation of low-density lipoprotein by endothelial cells. Circ Res 1998;82:1289–1297.

16. Farhy RD, Carretero OA, Ho K-L, et al. Role of kinins and nitric oxide in the effects of angiotensin-converting enzyme inhibitors on neointima formation. Circ Res 1993;72:1202–1210.

17. Fitzpatrick LA, Severson A, Edwards WD, et al. Diffuse calcification in human coronary arteries. J Clin Invest 1994;94:1597–1604.

18. Furchgott R, Zawadzki JV. The obligatory role of endothelial cells in the relaxation of arterial smooth muscle by acetylcholine. Nature 1980;288:373–376.

19. Geisterfer AAT, Peach MJ, Owens GK. Angiotensin II induces hypertrophy, not hyperplasia, of cultured rat aortic smooth muscle cells. Circ Res 1988;62:749–756.

20. Gibbons GH, Dzau VJ. Antiotensin converting enzyme inhibition and vascular hypertrophy in hypertension. Cardiovasc Drugs Therap 1990;4:237–242.

21. Griendling KK, Minieri CA, Ollenrenshaw JD, et al. Angiotensin II stimulates NADH and NADPH oxidase activity in cultured vascular smooth muscle cells. Circ Res 1994;74:1141–1148.

22. Hadju MA, Heistad DD, Baumbach GL. Effects of antihypertensive therapy on mechanics of cerebral arterioles in rats. Hypertension 1991;17:308–316.

23. Harrap SB, Mitchell GA, Casely DJ, et al. Angiotensin-II, sodium and cardiovascular hypertrophy in spontaneously hypertensive rats. Hypertension 1993;21:50–55.

24. Harrap SB, van der Merwe WM, Griffin SA, et al. Brief ACE inhibitor treatment in young spontaneously hypertensive rats reduces blood pressure long-term. Hypertension 1990;16:603–614.

25. Haunstetter A, Izumo S. Apoptosis. Basic mechanisms and implications for cardiovascular disease. Circ Res 1998;82:1111–1129.

26. Heagerty AM, Aalkjaer C, Bund SB, et al. Small artery structure in hypertension. Dual processes of remodeling and growth. Hypertension 1993;21:391–397.

27. Hein TW, Kuo L. LDLs impair vasomotor function of the coronary microcirculation. Role of superoxide anions. Circ Res 1998;83:404–414.

28. Higashimori K, Gante J, Holzemann G, et al. Significance of vascular renin for local generation of angiotensins. Hypertension 1991;17:270–277.

29. John S, Schlaich M, Langenfeld M, et al. Increased bioavailability of nitric oxide after lipid-lowering therapy in hypercholesterolemic patients. Circulation 1998;98:211–216.

30. Kato H, Suzuki H, Tajima S, et al. Angiotensin II stimulates collagen synthesis in cultured vascular smooth muscle cells. J Hypertens 1991;9:17–22.

31. Kawahara Y, Sunako M, Tsuda T, et al. Angiotensin-II induces expression of the c fos gene through protein kinase C activation and calcium ion metabilization in cultured vascular smooth muscle cells. Biochem Biophys Commun 1988;150:52–59.

32. Khairallah PA, Kanabus J. Angiotensin and myocardial protein synthesis. In: Tarazi RC, Dunbar JB, eds. Perspectives in Cardiovascular Research. New York: Raven Press, 1983 (vol 8) pp 337–347.

33. Kol A, Libby P. The mechanisms by which infectious agents may contribute to atherosclerosis and its clinical manifestations. Trends Cardiovasc Med 1998;8:191–199.

34. Kume N, Murase T, Moriwaki H, et al. Inducible expression of lectin-like oxidized LDL receptor-1 in vascular endothelial cells. Circ Res 1998;1998:322–327.

35. Lacolley PJ, Laurent ST, Billaud EB, et al. Carotid arterial hemodynamics in hypertension: acute administration of capropril or cadralazine. Cardiovasc Drugs Ther 1989;3:859–863.

36. Larkin M. Kilmer McCully: pioneer of the homocysteine theory. Lancet 1998;352:1364.

37. Lee RMKW, Rerecek KH, Tsoporis J, et al. Prevention of hypertension and vascular changes by captopril treatment. Hypertension 1991;17:141–150.

38. Lehoux S, Tedgui A. Signal transduction of mechanical stresses in vascular wall. Hypertension 1998;32:338–345.

39. Leung DYM, Glagov S, Mathews MB. Cyclic stretching stimulates synthesis of matrix components by arterial smooth muscle cells in vitro. Science 1976;191:475–477.

40. Luscher TF. Angiotensin, ACE inhibitors and endothelial control of vasomotor tone. Basic Res Cardiol 1993;88 (Suppl 1):15–24.

41. Miller Jr FJ, Gutterman DD, Rios CD, et al. Superoxide production in vascular smooth muscle contributes to oxidative stress and impaired relaxation in atherosclerosis. Circ Res 1998;82:1298–1305.

42. Moalic JM, Bauters C, Himbert D, et al. Phenylephrine, vasopressin and angiotensin-II as determinants of protooncogene and heat-shock protein gene expression in adult rat heart and aorta. J Hypertens 1989;7:195–201.

43. Moreau P, d'Uscio LV, Shaw S, et al. Angiotenin II increases tissue endothelin and induces vascular hypertrophy. Circulation 1997;96:1593–1597.

44. Mulvany MJ, Hansen PK, Aalkjaer C. Direct evidence that the greater contractility of resistance vessels in spontaneously hypertensive rats is associated with a narrowed lumen, a thickened media, and an increased number of smooth muscle. Circ Res 1978;43:854–864.

45. Murad F. What are the molecular mechanisms for the antiproliferative effects of nitric oxide and cGMP in vascular smooth muscle? Circulation 1997;95:1101–1103.

46. Naftilan AJ, Pratt RE, Dzau VJ. Induction of platelet-derived growth factor A-chain and c-myc gene expressions by angiotensin-II in cultured rat vascular smooth muscle cells. J Clin Invest 1989;83:1419–1424.

47. Nestel PJ. Blood pressure and catecholamine excretion after mental stress in labile hypertension. Lancet 1969;1:692–694.

48. Nickenig G, Roling J, Strehlow K, et al. Insulin induces upregulation of vascular AT_1 receptor gene expression by postranscriptional mechanisms. Circulation 1998;98:2543–2460.

49. Nickenig G, Sachinidis A, Michaelsen F, et al. Upregulation of vascular angiotensin II receptor gene expression by low-density lipoprotein in vascular smooth muscle cells. Circulation 1997;95:473-478.

50. O'Hara Y, Peterson TE, Harrison DG. Hypercholesterolaemia increases endothelial superoxide anion production. J Clin Invest 1993;91:2546–2551.

51. Ohya Y, Sperelakis N. Involvement of a GTP-binding protein in stimulating action of angiotensin-II on calcium channels in vascular smooth muscle cells. Circ Res 1991;68:763–771.

52. Okamura T, Myazaki M, Inagami T, et al. Vascular renin-angiotensin system in two-kidney, one clip hypertensive rats. Hypertension 1986;8:560–565.

53. Pagano PJ, Chanock SJ, Siwik DA, et al. Angiotensin II induces p67^{phox} mRNA expression and NADPH oxidase superoxide generation in rabbit aortic adventitial fibroblasts. Hypertension 1998;32:331–337.

54. Papageorgiou P, Morgan KG. Increased Ca^{2+} signaling after alpha-adrenoreceptor activation in vascular hypertrophy. Circ Res 1991;68:1080–1084.

55. Rakugi J, Jacob HJ, Kriger JH, et al. Vascular injury induces angiotensinogen gene expression in the media and neointima. Circulation 1993;87:283–290.

56. Re RN, Fallon TJ, Dzau VJ, et al. Renin synthesis by cultured arterial smooth muscle cells. Life Sci 1982;30:99–106.

57. Rees D, Ben-Ishay D, Moncada S. Nitric oxide and the regulation of blood pressure in the hypertension-prone and hypertension-resistant sabra rat. Hypertension 1996;28:367–371.

58. Richer C, Thuillez C, Giudicelli JF. Perindopril, converting enzyme blockade, and peripheral arterial hemodynamics in the healthy volunteer. J Cardiovasc Pharmacol 1987;9:94–102.

59. Rizzoni D, Porteri E, Piccoli A, et al. Effects of losartan and enalapril on small artery structure in hypertensive rats. Hypertension 1998;32:305–310.

60. Ross R. Atherosclerosis - an inflammatory disease. New Engl J Med 1999;340:115–126.

61. Ross R, Glomset J. The pathogenesis of atherosclerosis. N Engl J Med 1976;295:369–377.

62. Sada T, Hoike H, Ikeda M, et al. Cystolic free calcium of aorta in hypertensive rats. Chronic inhibition of angiotensin converting enzyme. Hypertension 1990;16:245–251.

63. Sadoshima J-I, Izumo S. Signal transduction pathways of angiotensin II-induced c-fos gene expression in cardiac myocytes in vitro. Roles of phospholipid-derived second messengers. Circ Res 1993;73:424–438.

64. Schelling P, Fischer H, Ganten D. Angiotensin and cell growth: a link to cardiovascular hypertrophy? J Hypertens 1991;9:3–15.

65. Schmitz U, Ishida T, Ishida M, et al. Angiotensin II stimulates p21-activated kinase in vascular smooth muscle cells. Role in activation of JNK. Circ Res 1998;82:1272–1278.

66. Schwenke D, Behr SR. Vitamin E combined with selenium inhibits atherosclerosis in hypercholesterolemic rabbits independently of effects on plasma cholesterol concentrations. Circ Res 1998;83:366–377.

67. Sihm I, Schroeder AP, Aalkjaer C, et al. Normalization of media to lumen ratio of human subcutaneous arteries during antihypertensive treatment with a perindopril based regimen (abstract). Eur Heart J 1993;14:63.

68. Vanhoutte PM. Endothelium and control of vascular function. State of the Art Lecture. Hypertension 1989;13:658–667.

69. Veltmar A, Gohlke P, Unger T. From tissue angiotensin converting enzyme inhibition to antihypertensive effect. Am J Hypertens 1991;4:263S–269S.

70. Wang D-H, Prewitt RL. Captopril reduces aortic and microvascular growth in hypertensive and normotensive rats. Hypertension 1990;15:68–77.

71. Weinstock JV, Kassab J. Chemotatic response of splenic mononuclear cells to angiotensin II in murine schistosoiasis. J Immunol 1986;137:2020–2024.

72. Yang BC, Phillips MI, Zhang YC, et al. Critical Role of AT_1 receptor expression after ischemia/reperfusion in isolated rat hearts. Beneficial effect of antisense oligodeoxynucleotides directed at AT_1 receptor mRNA. Circ Res 1998;83:552–559.

73. Yasojima K, Kilgore KS, Washington RA, et al. Complement gene expression by rabbit heart. Upregulation by ischemia and reperfusion. Circ Res 1998;82:1224–1230.

74. Zafari AM, Ushio-Fukai M, Akers M, et al. Role of NADH/NADPH oxidase-derived H_2O_2 in angiotensin II-induced vascular hypertrophy. Hypertension 1998;32:488–495.

75. Zhuo JL, Froomes P, Casley D, et al. Perindopril chronically inhibits angiotensin-converting enzyme in both the endothelium and adventitia of the internal mammary artery in patients with ischemic heart disease. Circulation 1997;96:174–182.

CHAPTER 3

ACE Inhibitors for hypertension, left ventricular hypertrophy and arterial disease

"ACE inhibitors once reserved for refractory hypertension, especially when renal in origin, have edged their way into a prime position" – Kaplan and Opie (1995)[85]

MECHANISMS OF HYPERTENSION. EFFECTS OF ACE INHIBITORS

Essential hypertension is often regarded as a multifactorial disease, resulting from a number of diverse genetic and environmental factors, whereby the vasoconstrictive influences exceed those that are vasodilator. Physiologically, the blood pressure (BP) is given by:

$$BP = CO \times SVR$$

where CO = cardiac output and SVR = systemic vascular resistance. When the cardiac output rises acutely, as during sympathetic adrenergic stimulation, baroreflex adjustments tend to decrease the systemic vascular resistance, so that normal blood pressure values are regained. However, in predisposed individuals, the baroreflex control is inadequate, or the tendency to peripheral vasoconstriction is excessive, so that temporary hypertension becomes permanent. In such circumstances, sustained hypertension will result (1) when the cardiac output is excessive, as in repetitive emotional stress, especially when associated with a tachycardia and (2) when the systemic vascular resistance is too high. The latter can result from increased activity of vasoconstrictive regulatory factors such as alpha-adrenergic drive, or renin-angiotensin overactivity, or there can be enhanced sensitivity of the peripheral arterioles to normally acting vasoconstrictive mechanisms (Fig 3–1).

Excess vasoconstriction may also be an important mechanism in salt-sensitive hypertension, in which it is thought that a relatively minor defect in the renal handling of sodium can lead to sodium retention in various cells of the body, including vascular smooth muscle.[20] Consequent on such intracellular sodium retention would follow increased activity of the sodium-calcium exchange, thereby leading to

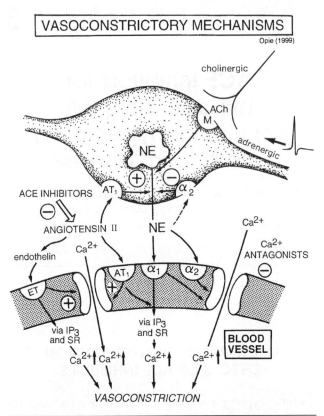

Figure 3-1. *Role of ACE inhibition in arterial control. Norepinephrine (NE), released from the storage granules of the terminal neurons, has predominantly vasoconstrictive effects acting via postsynaptic alpha-receptors. In addition, presynaptic alpha$_2$-receptors are stimulated to allow feedback inhibition of its release to modulate any excess release of NE. Parasympathetic cholinergic stimulation releases acetylcholine (ACh), which stimulates the muscarinic (m) receptors to inhibit the release of NE and thereby indirectly to cause vasodilation. Angiotensin-II, formed in response to renin released from the kidneys or locally formed, also is powerfully vasoconstrictive acting (1) to promote release of NE from the terminal neurons, (2) directly on the angiotensin II receptors, (3) to enhance calcium current influx, and (4) to release endothelin (ET) from the endothelium. The result is that ACE inhibitors cause vasodilation independently of mechanisms responsive to other therapeutic agents such as the alpha$_1$-blockers or the calcium antagonists. For IP$_3$ see Fig 1-3. Fig © LH Opie*

an increased cytosolic calcium ion concentration in the smooth muscle cell with vasoconstriction and elevation of the blood pressure. Abnormalities of cell membrane pumps and exchanges regulating sodium occur in black subjects, which may explain their greater tendency to a type of hypertension responding better to diuretic therapy. Furthermore, sodium retention inhibits renin secretion, which could help to explain why low-renin hypertension appears to be more common in black subjects.

Endothelium in hypertension. Role of endothelin. The normal endothelium produces vasodilatory and vasoconstrictor factors. Normal vasodilation is chiefly by the nitric oxide-cyclic GMP path (the description of this path achieved the Nobel prize in 1998). There is a lesser role for the *endothelial hyperpolarizing factor*, EDHF.[27] Hypothetically, the vascular endothelium is damaged in hypertension, perhaps as result of sustained excess shear stress, and the release of vasodilatory nitric oxide is less, and that of vasoconstrictory factors such as *endothelin* is increased. Endothelin may play a crucial role in the vasoconstriction resulting from A-II.[128] Thus endothelial damage may promote vasoconstriction which in turn could increased the blood pressure, thereby producing a hypertensive vicious circle.

Mechanisms of ACE inhibitors in hypertension. At least seven antihypertensive mechanisms may be involved (Fig 3-2). First, the major and self-evident effect of angiotensin-converting enzyme (ACE) inhibitors is to decrease circulating angiotensin II levels and thereby to have a vasodilatory and antihypertensive effect. A second and possibly major site of action is on the tissue renin-angiotensin system including ACE activity in vascular cells. A third potential antihypertensive mechanism is by modulation and down-regulation of the adrenergic activity and in particular the release of norepinephrine from terminal neurons. For example, intravenous perindoprilat decreased the vasoconstrictor effect of infused norepinephrine.[113] Central sympathetic outflow is however unchanged.[61] A fourth antihypertensive mechanism is by a lessened release of vasoconstrictory endothelin from the vascular endothelium. A fifth mechanism is by an increased formation of vasodilators such as bradykinin,[49] prostaglandins, and the newly emphasized angiotensin peptide, Ang (1-7). Sixth, natriuresis may be achieved or minor degrees of sodium retention countered by decreased release of aldosterone and increased renal blood flow. Finally, ACE inhibitors may have a particular role in hyperinsulinemia hypertension,[42] because of the inhibition of the sodium-retaining effect of in-

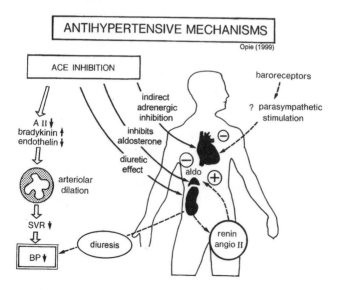

Figure 3-2. *Proposed mechanisms whereby ACE inhibitors as a class may exert their antihypertensive effects. Figure © LH Opie, 1999*

sulin,[126] and because insulin upregulates the vascular AT-1 receptor.[138]

Choice of first-line agent. Because it is not presently possible to predict which of the various mechanisms is the major one contributing to the blood pressure elevation in any given patient, there is no logical choice for first-line therapy. Accordingly, the initial choice of antihypertensive agent is often governed by the anticipated efficacy and side-effects of the agent concerned. When judged by hard outcome end-points, low dose diuretics are best documented for their benefit in reducing major outcome end-points such as stroke, coronary heart disease, heart failure, and cardiovascular and total mortality (JNC VI). Regarding ACE inhibitors, there is a general lack of hard-end point outcome studies with two exceptions: the CAPP study, and the UKPDS study (see later). Nonetheless certain recommendations have been made by JNC VI:[83]

1. *Compelling indications for ACE inhibitors* are diabetes mellitus type 1 with proteinuria, heart failure, and myocardial infarction with systolic dysfunction.
2. *"May benefit effects"* are those on co-morbid conditions, such as diabetes mellitus types 1 and 2 with proteinuria, or renal insufficiency.
3. *"May harm"* are ACE inhibitor effects on renovascular disease.
4. *Pregnancy* is a clear contraindication.

Although AT-1 blockers are not recognised as first-line therapy by the American Committee,[83] they are regarded as one of several options by the WHO-International Society of Hypertension.[205]

Treatment goals. First, the BP be should be adequately reduced. The criteria are dropping all the time. Trial data suggest optimal BP values of about 140/85 mmHg or lower.[76] In type 2 diabetics a decrease of the BP from means values of 154/87 mmHg to 144/82 mmHg reduced hard endpoints over 8.4 years.[189] Second, and closely related, adverse complications should be reduced to such an extent that the lifespan is not compromised by hypertension. Thirdly, the quality of life should also not be compromised.

SODIUM, RENIN, ALDOSTERONE AND HYPERTENSION

Sodium status. As sodium depletion is a major stimulus to the release of renin, it follows that variations in the sodium content of the diet have potentially a major effect on the efficacy of ACE inhibitors in antihypertensive therapy because of the high renin status following sodium depletion (Fig 3–3). In most studies, the sodium content of the diet has not been controlled. The ACE inhibitors have a natriuretic effect evident even in subjects on a moderate sodium intake of 80 mmol/day,[163] which is about 2 g sodium. Thus, the antihypertensive effect of ACE inhibitors

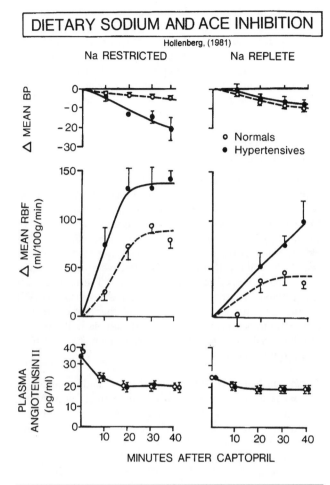

Figure 3-3. *The important effect of dietary sodium on the response of normotensive and hypertensive patients to acute administration of captopril. Despite an identical fall and time course of changes in plasma angiotensin II concentration in the normotensive and hypertensive patients, the renal vascular response (RBF, renal blood flow) is greater in the hypertensive patients than in the normal subjects. Note particularly that in sodium restriction, the fall in the blood pressure is much more marked in hypertensive patients than in states of sodium repletion. Part of the difference may be due to the greater increase in renal blood flow achieved in sodium-restricted hypertensive patients. Reproduced from Hollenberg et al,[74] with permission.*

could be expected to vary. In patients on a low-sodium intake and with high circulating renin levels, the antihypertensive effect is likely to be more evident because decreased peripheral vasoconstriction would follow decreased circulating levels of angiotensin II.[81] In contrast, patients on a high-sodium intake with low circulating renin levels are less likely to respond with an antihypertensive effect. An important additional beneficial mechanism could be the increased renal blood flow in salt-restricted subjects (Fig 3-3). Hence a low sodium diet should be standard advice to all patients receiving ACE inhibitor therapy for hypertension.[115,176] Alternatively or additionally, a low dose diuretic may be added.

Renin status. The plasma renin activity of the patient may also influence the response to ACE inhibition. In high-renin patients, for example those with renal artery stenosis, the response to ACE inhibition is consistent and often marked. In "average" patients with hypertension, the blood pressure fall after captopril could be related to the pretreatment plasma renin activity,[114] which in most patients was low. The concept of high versus low renin states is, however, more complex than just the level of plasma renin activity; the renin level should be related to the sodium intake to give the renin-sodium profile.[22]

Black patients and elderly patients are thought to be *low-renin hypertension groups,* which should theoretically not respond to ACE inhibitors. In the case of black patients, there are indeed several studies suggesting that ACE inhibitor therapy on its own is not likely to be effective.[118] In elderly white patients, however, increasing evidence shows that ACE inhibitor therapy can be effective as monotherapy, as will be discussed later in this chapter. The role of circulating renin activity in determining the response to ACE inhibitors is, therefore, not clear-cut. Rather, the mechanism of the antihypertensive effect of ACE inhibitors is probably multifactorial and only partially dependent on the renin and sodium status.

Renin profiling in hypertension. Circulating levels of plasma renin activity vary widely in patients with hypertension. On the one hand, as expected, high values are found in renovascular hypertension. On the other hand, much lower values are found in essential hypertension, with most falling within the normal range.[86] Certain population groups, such as black subjects or the elderly, are known to have relatively low renin levels for the group as a whole, although there are still marked individual variations. Logically, ACE inhibitors should work best in high-renin states[22] and diuretics should work best in low-renin states, as suggested by Laragh on the basis of his concept of renin-profiling.[93] These predictions work well for black subjects with their lower renin levels, and explain why they have a relatively poor response to ACE inhibitor therapy. In black elderly patients, ACE inhibition is almost totally ineffective.[118] Despite some defects, the concept of renin profiles explains ethnic differences. Also, high-renin values raise suspicion of renovascular hypertension and really low values suggest *primary aldosteronism.* In the individual patient with essential hypertension, the normal renin value usually found is not helpful in predicting whether or not there would be a therapeutic response to ACE inhibitor therapy.

Aldosterone-renin ratios. A more modern way of looking at the renin status is in relation to the aldosterone-renin ratio. The proposal is that an abnormally high ratio reflects either a Conn's syndrome of primary hyperaldosteronism, or bilateral adrenal hyperplasia. This ratio can be increased even when the plasma renin level is normal,[120] let alone low. A low plasma potassium, a classic sign of hyperaldosteronism, is often absent despite an increased aldosterone-renin ratio. The therapeutic implication of an increased ratio is that either an adrenal adenoma may need operative removal, or that hyperplasia may need indirect therapy by spironolactone. Theoretically there should be a poor response to ACE inhibitors in those with a high aldosterone-renin ratio, and (possibly) a good response to AT-1 receptor blockers. However, such logic may not hold, as shown by observations in anephric patients.

Observations in anephric patients. The basic observations of Man in't Veld et al[116] on an anephric patient drew attention to the potential effects of ACE inhibitors on systems other than the renin-angiotensin-aldosterone system activated by release of renin from the kidneys. One likely explanation is the existence of a tissue renin-angiotensin system. Additionally or alternatively, there may be other vasodilatory mechanisms, such as bradykinin,[49] or vasodilation via angiotensin (1-7).

Salt sensitivity and angiotensinogen genotype. Changes in the angiotensinogen gene may explain why certain individuals react adversely to a high salt intake by increasing the arterial blood pressure.[77] The AA angiotensinogen genotype predisposes to a higher than expected level of A-II.[77] Therefore the renal blood flow can not increase as it should in response to a sodium load.

ANGIOTENSIN-II AND LEFT VENTRICULAR HYPERTROPHY

Left ventricular hypertrophy (LVH) is currently regarded as one of the serious complications of hypertension, being an independent risk factor for coronary events according to the Framingham data.[103] Specifically, LVH gives an increased risk ratio for sudden death of 2.16 (CI, 1.22–3.81; $p = 0.008$).[66] ACE inhibitor therapy can reduce blood pressure, left ventricular mass, and improve early diastolic filling. The agents that have been used include captopril,[132] perindopril,[4,59] enalapril,[55,60] ramipril[150] and quinapril.[47] The mechanisms involved include, first, the reduction in blood pressure and thereby the reduction in intraluminal pressure; second, a specific anti-growth effect in the modification of the growth-stimulating properties of angiotensin II;[16,39] third, a reduction of angiotensin-mediated adrenergic outflow; fourth, decreased formation of endothelin-1;[78] and, fifth, increased formation of bradykinin.[153] Which of these is predominantly involved may depend on the model used (compare Harrap et al, 1993[69] with Baker et al, 1990[7]) but the overall evidence is that blood pressure reduction is most crucial.

Regulation of myocardial growth. Besides the mild inotropic effect of angiotensin II, a much more intriguing cardiac role for the renin-angiotensin system is as a growth regulator.[87,111,167] The idea that angiotensin II could help to regulate myocardial protein synthesis goes back to at least 1983.[88] Part of the stimulation results from the induction of a variety of complex growth regulating genes called proto-oncogenes[35] that play an important part in regulating the early processes leading to increased cell growth. Angiotensin-II acts on the AT-1 receptor to activate complex signal paths, mostly converging on MAP kinase, to promote growth (Fig 1-6). In addition, angiotensin II appears to up-regulate the cardiac hypertrophic response by inducing the angiotensinogen gene and the gene for transforming growth factor-β1.[158] Both myocyte and fibroblast growth are stimulated (Fig 3-4). The proposal that very low doses of an ACE inhibitor, too low to reduce the blood pressure, can regress left ventricular hypertrophy is controversial.[109,173] Recent experimental evidence is that ACE inhibition can limit both myocyte and interstitial remodeling despite continuing pressure overload. Clinically, sub-hypotensive doses of ramipril induced regression of left ventricular hypertrophy in one study.[108] Yet the dominant role of the effects of pressure overload is shown by the regression of LV hypertro-

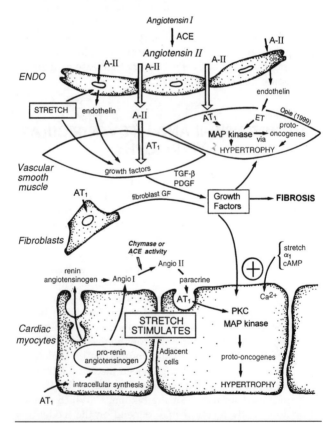

Figure 3-4. Some proposals for a multicellular interactive renin-angiotensin system involving cardiac myocytes, fibroblasts, vascular smooth muscle, and endothelium (for detailed evidence, see Dostal and Baker[35]). Although these systems are postulated to have an important function in regulating vascular and myocardial hypertrophy, proof of this significance is still awaited. For evidence favouring a myocardial renin-angiotensin system, see Table 3-1. For effects of angiotensin II on growth factors, see Table 3-2. Figure © LH Opie, 1999

TABLE 3-1:   EVIDENCE FOR CARDIAC AND MYOCARDIAL RENIN-
ANGIOTENSIN ACTIVITY

Angiotensinogen
1.   Angiotensinogen synthesis in isolated atria and in ventricles
after pressure-loading.
2.   Angiotensinogen release from perfused heart.
3.   Increased mRNA for angiotensinogen in non-infarcted left
ventricle in rat[110] and in left ventricle of aortic-banded rats.[7]
4.   Immunoreactive angiotensinogen in human heart especially
in atria-conducting system and subendocardial ventricle.[166]

*Renin**
1.   Renin gene expression in ventricles more than in atria.
2.   Cyclic AMP-responsive elements in 5′-flanking region of renin gene.
3.   Increased synthesis of renin in response to beta-agonist stimulation.

*Activity of angiotensin-converting enzyme (ACE)and/or
chymase*
1.   Evidence of occurrence in coronary vasculature and in neonatal myocytes.[34]
2.   Increased ACE activity in pressure-overloaded ventricle.[172]
3.   Increased mRNA for ACE in right ventricle of rat hearts with
post-infarct heart failure.[72]
4.   Note ACE-insensitive pathways for angiotensin generation in
volume-loaded ventricle.[157]
5.   Heart chymase cloned in human heart.[192]

Cardiac formation of angiotensin II
1.   Can be formed in perfused rat heart.
2.   Found in monkey ventricles.
3.   In nephrectomized rabbits with no renal source of renin,
ACE inhibition can decrease atrial content of angiotensin II.

Myocardial Angiotensin-II Receptors (AT-1)
1.   In sarcolemmal vesicle preparations, receptors are found
which meet kinetic requirements for receptor identification.
2.   In isolated rat neonatal myocytes, there are about 45,000
receptors per cell.
3.   In surviving ventricular myocytes from infarct hearts, A-II-
receptor density increased.[121]
4.   Autoradiographic identification in man shows receptors present in myocardial cells, coronary vessels, and in nerves.[191]
5.   Pathways for signal transduction are present chiefly involving phosphotidylinositol pathway, inositol triphosphate and
protein kinase C.[121]

* Controversial. See von Lutterotti et al[196] and Dzau and Re.[38]

phy achieved by long-term diuretic therapy,[56] which is
known to stimulate the renin-angiotensin system.

***Is there an essential role for A-II and the AT-1 receptor
in myocyte growth?*** Myocardial angiotensin II receptors,
now identified in isolated cardiac myocytes, have high affinity for angiotensin II with reversible binding and interact
with very low external concentrations of angiotensin II; in
technical terms, the Kd for angiotensin II is only about 1
nM.[6,155] The two receptor subtypes, AT-1 and AT-2 have already been alluded to (see Fig 1-5). There is controversy

about the dominant receptor type in cardiac tissue with one study suggesting that it is the AT-1 receptor that is dominant.[121] Regarding growth, in cultured adult rat heart cells, it is the AT-1 receptor that mediates growth, as all the effect is abolished by losartan, the AT-1 blocker, and none by an AT-2 blocker.[111] Furthermore, mechanical stress stimulates the secretion of A-II from cardiomyocytes.[159]

TABLE 3-2:   ANGIOTENSIN-II AND GROWTH FACTORS

---

1.   Angiotensin-II induces turnover of DNA and RNA, increases RNA content, and induces protein synthesis in chick heart cells.

2.   Angiotensin-II activates proto-oncogenes, including c-fos, c-jun, c-myc via protein kinase C and cell calcium.

3.   Angiotensin-II activates genes controlling growth factors (platelet-derived growth factor, transforming growth factor-ß; Kodama et al[89] and invokes release of growth factors from vascular smooth muscle cells.[35]

4.   Angiotensin-II activates JAK-STAT pathway, which also reacts to cytokines.[89]

Evidence from mice with AT-1 receptor knock-out. It might therefore be supposed that activation of the AT-1 receptor is a specific and essential step on the path to pressure-induced hypertrophy. Some clinical evidence supports this proposal.[68] But, that is not so. In a knock-out mouse with total deficiency of AT-1 receptors, an acute pressure overload could still induce a hypertrophic response as shown by an increase of proto-oncogene and mitogen activated protein (MAP) kinases as well as an increase in heart weight.[67] Therefore ultimately, it is the response to mechanical pressure, probably acting via stretch receptors that is fundamental (Fig 3-4). Superimposed on the stretch stimulus, A-II and the AT-1 receptor also play important roles in activating the signal systems that lead to growth.

Proposed protective role of AT-2 receptor in cardiac growth. In the hypertrophied rat heart, there is upregulation of the AT-2 receptor relative to the AT-1 receptor.[8] The hypothesis is that activity of the AT-2 receptor inhabits the cardiac growth in response to A-II assimilation. Thus, inhibition of the AT-2 receptors promotes the cardiac growth response to A-II infusion in isolated rat hearts.[8] In coronary endothelial cells, too, the AT-2 receptor appears to inhibit growth mediated by the AT-1 receptor.[178] In rats with heart failure following myocardial infarction, blockade of the AT-2 receptor removed most of the benefit of an AT-1 blocker.[112] The precise pathways involved in the protective effect of AT-2 receptor activity remain to be investigated, but putatively involve decreased activity of MAP kinase, or the formation of protective kinins such as bradykinin.[112] Nonetheless, not all studies are concordant. Almost all the growth affects of a long term infusion of angiotensin II into rats could be ascribed to the AT-1 receptor, with little role for the AT-2 receptor.[106] An important difference from the other studies with A-II exposure, is that Li et al[106] used long term infusion of A-II in the living rat, whereas the other studies were on cell cultures or perfused hearts.

FIBROSIS AND PATHOLOGICAL HYPERTROPHY

During the development of left ventricular hypertrophy and failure (Fig 3-5), there are important differences between the growth of myocytes (hypertrophy) and the collagen formation (fibrosis). Fibrous tissue helps to control the contractile behaviour of the heart, particularly diastolic relaxation.[199] Fibroblasts are stimulated to grow by angiotensin II and other promoters of tissue repair. In human cardiac fibroblasts, A-II is formed and acts locally.[65] As collagen accumulates in the interstitium of the myocardium, it becomes stiffer and relaxes less readily in diastole. Some phenotypes of cardiac fibroblasts, called *myofibroblasts* by Weber,[199] express smooth muscle α-actin, hence having contractile properties. Not all agents that cause regression of left ventricular hypertrophy also cause regression of fibrosis.[200] For example, verapamil reduced LVH in the spontaneously hypertensive rat without decreasing collagen content,[156] whereas minoxidil actually increased collagen concentration. The ACE inhibitors decreased collagen provided that therapy was sufficiently prolonged. Thus, prolonged therapy with captopril[79] or lisinopril[16] or perindopril[123] or enalapril[143] reduced myocardial fibrosis in

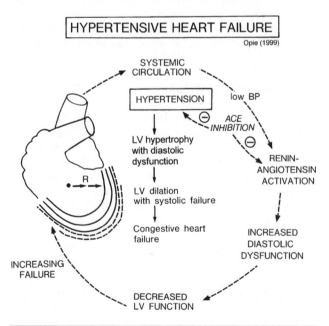

Figure 3-5. In established congestive heart failure due to hypertension, ACE inhibition may have two beneficial effects: first, reduction of the hypertension and, therefore, of the load on the heart and, second, inhibition of renin-angiotensin activation with relief of that component of the increased arteriolar resistance. Note the increased radius (R) associated with left ventricular dilation and poor left ventricular systolic function. Figure © LH Opie, 1999

the spontaneously hypertensive rat. In some studies, diastolic stiffness decreased, whereas in others chiefly systolic function improved.[55]

Collagen formation. Cardiac myofibroblasts elaborate collagen.[199] The exact way in which angiotensin II activity is related to fibroblasts and to collagen formation is not clear. Pressure overload is crucial, whereas volume overload does not increase collagen.[137] Indirect evidence suggests that A-II works at least in part by stimulation of secretion of aldosterone.[200, 201] and in part by promotion of the expression of the gene for transforming growth factor-β_1 (TGF-β_1).[199] In experimental LVH, there is more myocardial collagen formed, with an absolute increase in both types III and type I.[199] The collagen phenotype changes so that there is a relative increase in collagen type I, which may help increase myocardial stiffness. In rats, although both captopril and hydralazine could equally reduce blood pressure, only chronic captopril therapy could lessen the change in collagen phenotypes.[133]

Angiotensin II and AT-receptor subtypes in fibroblasts.
Angiotensin II receptors on cultured fibroblasts are of the AT-1 subtype.[65,136] Activation of the AT-1 receptor induces the formation of TGF-β_1, and may result in inhibition of the synthesis of nitric oxide.[186] In heart failure from dilated cardiomyopathy, the AT-1 receptors were downregulated, and the AT-2 receptors markedly upregulated.[188] The expression of the AT-2 subtype is associated with cardiac fibroblasts, and these receptors exert an inhibitory effect on A-II associated growth signals. Thus there is increasing evidence that the AT-I receptor in fibroblasts has its effects counteracted by the AT-2 receptor.[141,188]

Growth factors and fibroblasts. A number of growth factors stimulate the growth of cardiac fibroblasts, acting on growth receptors to give tyrosine phosphorylation. Such factors include transforming growth factor-β_1,[158] insulin-like growth factor-1 (ILGF-1) and growth hormone. Until recently it has been thought that angiotensin II acts only on its classical receptor system, linked by protein kinase C to growth and other signals. Now the unexpected information appears that there is post-receptor cross talk between the AT-1 receptor and at least one of the group of growth receptors. Thus stimulation of fibroblast growth by angiotensin II may be particularly powerful because of this additional path that is activated.[136]

Perivascular fibrosis in the hypertensive heart. During the development of left ventricular hypertrophy, the numerous complex structural changes include vascular changes. Just as increased myocardial collagen impairs mechanical properties of the heart, so does vascular remodeling impair vasodilation.[16] This is the one proposed explanation for the impaired coronary vasodilator reserve often observed in patients with LVH, the other being endothelial dysfunction. Collagen accumulates in the adventitial layer of the coronary arterioles. At least three factors are concerned: hypertensive pressure and stretch exerted on the vasculature, angiotensin II, and aldosterone. During the development of pressure overload in rats, vascular smooth muscle proliferation is AT-1 dependent, whereas endothelial cells are not.[119] Probably the AT-2 receptor lays a more important role in endothelial cells.[178]

Apoptosis. This process of programmed cell death can be detected in the hearts of spontaneously hypertensive rats (SHR), as well as in acute over-stretching of the heart secondary to aortic stenosis.[33] In the SHR model there is a tight relationship between the extent of apoptosis and the ACE activity of the LV.[33] Hypothetically, increased local A-II production decreases protective nitric oxide. This proposal is, however, still controversial, as is any possible role of apoptosis in the heart with LVH.

DIASTOLIC AND SYSTOLIC DYSFUNCTION IN LV HYPERTROPHY

Commonly, patients with hypertension and left ventricular failure present with exertional dyspnea, and such patients are regarded as having heart failure to be treated by digita-

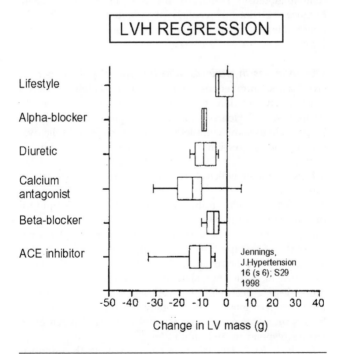

Figure 3-6. *Results of a meta-analysis of 32 studies of regression of left ventricular hypertrophy (LVH). 1896 subjects were involved, and the original data published between 1990 and 1995. Therefore further studies supporting the use of diuretics to achieve LVH regression, such as Gottdiener[56] would not be included. For overall role of modification of renin-angiotensin system in therapy of hypertension, see Table 3-3. Reprinted by permission of authors[82] and publishers (Lippincott, Williams and Wilkins).*

lis and diuretics. It is now becoming increasingly apparent, however, that many such patients have normal systolic function as assessed by the ejection fraction,[29,36] yet have diastolic dysfunction that is common in concentric left ventricular hypertrophy. In 37 hypertensive patients with radiological cardiomegaly, with none in clinical congestive heart failure, 28 had a normal or high ejection fraction.[82] For such patients, digitalis is inappropriate therapy. Rather, it may be supposed on first principles that treatment should be aimed at the regression of left ventricular hypertrophy by any agent consistently reducing the BP in other diuretics, by beta-blockers, by calcium antagonists, or by ACE inhibitors. Meta-analysis, of which there are many, consistently show regression of LV hypertrophy with ACE inhibitors (Fig 3–6). Beta-blockers come out rather unfavourably and have been inferior to ACE inhibitor or AT-1 blockers in direct comparisons. Of note are experimental data that infusion of angiotensin I to hypertrophied rat hearts impaired diastolic relaxation.[171] Excess diuretics are inappropriate because in diastolic dysfunction the atrial filling pressure needs to be maintained to achieve maximal left ventricular filling rates despite the diastolic dysfunction.

Experimental ischemia-induced diastolic dysfunction in LVH. When hypertrophic rat hearts are subject to acute ischemia, diastolic dysfunction develops.[41] Activation of the cardiac renin-angiotensin system is involved in the mechanism, because infusion of enalaprilat attenuated the diastolic abnormality in hypertrophic hearts but not in control hearts.

Observations in patients with hypertrophy. In hypertensive hearts, intravenous ACE inhibition acutely decreases diastolic dysfunction, possibly acting by relaxation of fibrous tissue.[199] Hence it might be supposed that it should be possible to show complete improvement in diastolic dysfunction as regression of left ventricular hypertrophy is achieved by ACE inhibition. This aim has not been achieved unless effective therapy is prolonged for up to three years.[47]

Mitral inflow pattern. In the study by Shahi et al,[174] captopril (mean daily dose 93 mg, usually with added diuretic) caused regression of left ventricular hypertrophy over 9 months of therapy but did not improve diastolic function as judged by echocardiographic patterns of mitral inflow. Enalapril also did not change the mitral inflow velocity ratios despite decreasing left ventricular mass.[55] The mitral inflow pattern may not be a totally reliable index of diastolic dysfunction since it may remain unchanged when other indices respond to ACE inhibition.[127]

Left ventricular systolic failure in hypertension. With continued left ventricular hypertrophy, eventual left ventricular dilation sets in. Once the radius of the left ventricle is unduly enlarged, wall stress augments, the ventricle stretches, and systolic power production is reduced (Fig 3-5). The result is diminished left ventricular ejection and a decreased systolic blood pressure. The resultant compensatory increase of adrenergic outflow leads to renin-angiotensin activation, an

TABLE 3-3:   Potential Cardiovascular Significance of
              Therapeutic Modification of Renin-
              Angiotensin System

Cardiac hypertrophy in hypertension

1. Therapy with small doses of ACE inhibitor not decreasing blood pressure can reduce left ventricular hypertrophy in aortic banded rats.[7]
2. However, in spontaneously hypertensive rats, blood pressure reduction rather than ACE inhibition is mechanism for regression of left ventricular hypertrophy with perindopril.[69]
3. ACE inhibition normalizes isomyosin profile in rats.[37]
4. Chronic ACE inhibitor therapy completely prevents interstitial fibrosis in genetic hypertension in rats.[16]

Sympathetic modulation

1. Less effect of sympathetic stimulation on heart rate and contractile activity after addition of ACE inhibitor.[152]
2. Captopril acutely decreases muscle sympathetic nerve activity in humans.[139]

Chronic congestive heart failure

1. ACE inhibitors have effects above and beyond those of conventional vasodilators (see Table 6-6).
2. Specific activation of cardiac mRNA for ACE and local synthesis of angiotensin II in experimental heart failure.[72]

Myocardial ischemia

1. Transient ischemia and fewer metabolic defects after addition of ramipril to isolated hearts.
2. Bradykinin inhibition appears to abolish effects.
3. In isolated rat hearts with left ventricular hypertrophy, enalaprilat lessens ischemia-induced diastolic dysfunction.[172]

Myocyte necrosis

1. Low-dose infusion of angiotensin II causes myocytolysis and subsequent fibrosis.[181] Captopril effective in preventing myocyte injury in renovascular hypertension.

Apoptosis

1. A-II mediates apoptosis in rat cardiac myocytes, acting on AT-1 not AT-2 receptors.[25]

Ischemic-reperfusion injury and stunning

1. Inhibitory effects of ACE inhibitors abolished by addition of angiotensin II and by bradykinin inhibition.
2. ACE inhibitor pretreatment lessens reperfusion ventricular fibrillation in pigs.[134]
3. AT-1 receptor upregulated; when inhibited by antisense therapy, improved post-ischemic recovery. No benefit from AT-1 block by losartan.[209]
4. Post-ischemic recovery in rat heart improved by AT-2 block, worsened by losartan.[45]
5. Enalapril better than hydralazine in preventing stunning in dogs, mechanism unknown.[149]

Postinfarct arrhythmias

1. Complete prevention of inducible ventricular tachycardia in pigs after acute administration of intravenous captopril.

Ventricular remodeling

1. Improved experimental and clinical remodeling by use of ACE inhibitors.[91]

Increased capillary density in LVH

1. Subhypertensive doses of rampipril.[190]

For other references, see Lindpaintner and Ganten.[109]
In the above situations, there is no proof that it is the cardiac myocyte renin-angiotensin system that is the target of drug action, as opposed to other cardiac systems such as the fibroblasts or vascular tissue, or circulating renin-angiotensin. See footnote to Table 3-1.

increased systemic vascular resistance, and a rise in the afterload. At this stage, ACE inhibition should be ideal therapy for the hypertensive patient, able to decrease blood pressure and to lessen the afterload. ACE inhibition should in these circumstances be accompanied by diuretic therapy to correct the volume and sodium retention characteristic of congestive heart failure.

REGRESSION OF LVH IN PATIENTS

Because an increased left ventricular mass is an independent risk factor for cardiovascular events, beyond the risk posed by the level of the blood pressure itself,[66,103] lessening the degree of LVH has become a major therapeutic aim (Fig 3–6). Indirect evidence from meta-analyses suggests that ACE inhibitors may be the best drug to achieve most regression of LVH.[31,82,168] Direct comparisons show that ACE inhibition is better than diuretic therapy,[31] and than the beta-blocker atenolol.[150] ACE inhibition is also better than minoxidil as part of triple therapy.[84] The predicted difference between ACE inhibitors and calcium antagonists on left ventricular regression is small.[31,168] Thus it is no surprise that perindopril and nifedipine were equi-effective in reducing both blood pressure and left ventricular mass.[170] Likewise, spirapril and isradipine gave equal reduction of LV mass.[117] Yet, over one year in another study, captopril gave regression, and diltiazem did not.[56] In the latter study, diuretics, often regarded as the agents least likely to induce regression, were among the most effective.

It is not easy to reconcile these differences, but the overall evidence shows that initial therapy by ACE inhibition is at least as effective as other treatment options in achieving regression (Fig 3–6). In reality, to reduce blood pressure to adequately low levels of systolic pressure[13] will often require several agents, among which should be an ACE inhibitor. Treatment of LVH should extend over several years, especially if monotherapy with an ACE inhibitor is used.[47] ACE inhibitors and diuretics may be an especially powerful combination. For example, low dose ramipril can induce regression independently of blood pressure in those also given a diuretic,[108] the latter stimulating the renin-angiotensin system and thereby enhancing the activity of the ACE inhibitor.

Combination of ACE inhibitor and AT-1 blockade. Theoretical reasons argue for the particular effectiveness of this combination, although thus far untested in LV hypertrophy in humans. For example, evidence for the formation of bradykinin is strongest with ACE inhibitors, and bradykinin might have a particular role in improving cardiac function in hypertrophic hearts.[53] On the other hand, evidence for complete blockade of the effects of A-II on the AT-1 receptor is strongest with AT-1 blockers, perhaps because non-ACE paths also form A-II. Therefore, combination therapy may be an important step forward, as found in spontaneously hypertensive rats.[140]

LARGE CONDUIT (CONDUCTING) ARTERIES IN HYPERTENSION

In hypertension, large conduit arteries, like the small bore arterioles, are exposed to increased intraluminal tension and also undergo an increase in mural thickness. Thus, there are two major sites of vascular damage in hypertension, the large conduit arteries (Fig 3–7) and the arterioles. Because there is relatively less muscle mass than matrix in these large arteries, an increase in the matrix mass becomes relatively more important. Of the two chief matrix components, elastin and collagen, it is the synthesis of collagen that responds to a greater extent, especially in male rats.[208] The net result is a fall in the ratio of elastin to collagen with a relative stiffening of the large arteries. Such changes may explain the *loss of arterial wall compliance*[161] found not only in the brachial arteries but also in the femoral arteries.[107]

Mechanism of collagen growth in conduit arteries. The two major proposed stimuli to growth of the elements of the arterial wall are (1) mechanical tension and (2) non-mechanical factors such as renin-angiotensin stimulation. In considering the whole aortic wall, one proposal is that an-

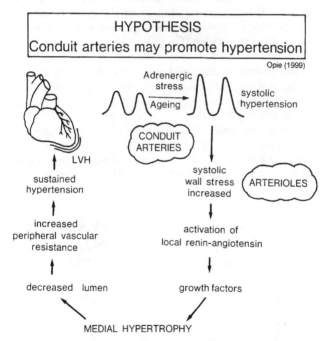

Figure 3-7. Hypothesis emphasizing possible role of conduit arteries in initiating hypertension in certain subsets of the population. For example, ageing by reducing aortic and conduit arterial elasticity causes a systolic hypertension which increases systolic wall stress and either mechanically or through activation of the local renin-angiotensin system causes medial hypertrophy with sustained hypertension. A similar sequence could be invoked to explain why catecholamine-inducing stress reactions can eventually cause sustained hypertension. It is not the intention of this figure to show that this mechanism operates in all patients with hypertension, but rather to point out a possible mechanism operating in some patients. LVH, left ventricular hypertrophy. Figure © LH Opie, 1999

giotensin II plays a specific role as a growth factor acting through the AT-1 receptor, with interactive control by the AT-2 receptor.[54] To assess the role of collagen production, Michel et al[124] transplanted the aortic wall of normotensive and hypertensive rats, thereby inducing arterial allograft rejection. Perindopril treatment reduced intimal thickening and collagen density. Other data suggest a selective enhancing effect of angiotensin II on growth signals for collagen growth, including the division of fibroblasts.[167]

Lumen size. Because of the large size of the lumen of the conduit arteries, it cannot be anticipated that any change in medial hypertrophy will impinge on the luminal diameter. Yet, the larger the vessel, the greater the matrix component of the composition of the wall. In patients with sustained uncomplicated essential hypertension, the unchanged internal diameter of the common carotid artery indicates a decreased compliance because there is an increased intraluminal pressure.[160] It is this decreased compliance that interferes with the buffering capacity of the large arteries.[40] In advanced arterial disease, a further factor reducing arterial compliance and increasing the stiffness is deposition of calcium. These changes in the mechanical properties of the conduit arteries lead to a hypothesis, here presented, that proposes that these arteries could be of crucial importance in the hypertensive process, at least in some subsets of the population (Fig 3-7).

Carotid intima-media thickness. In middle-aged hypertensive patients, ultrasound imaging using quantitative techniques allows measurement of the intima-media thickness of the carotid artery.[212] In such patients, over 80% have an intima-media thickness exceeding 1.3 mm, arbitrarily designated as plaque-formation in the protocol. Predisposing factors were age, systolic pressure, and pulse pressure. At least one current trial has this measure as endpoint.[212]

HYPOTHESIS : LARGE CONDUIT ARTERIES CAN PERPETUATE AND INCREASE THE SEVERITY OF HYPERTENSION

This hypothesis (Fig 3-7) rests upon the following proposals:

1. Large conduit arteries increase collagen[208] and lose elasticity in hypertension.[160]
2. Therefore, the pressure equalizing and buffering function of the large arteries is diminished.[40]
3. An increased systolic pressure is increasingly transmitted to the resistance arterioles, a self-evident proposition.
4. Pressure-induced stretch, acting as a growth stimulus in the arterioles, would cause medial hypertrophy and intimal damage.
5. Such arterioles have a reduced capacity to dilate maximally,[95] a decreased luminal diameter,[23] and a thicker

media[135] so that the systemic vascular resistance is increased.

6. An increased peripheral vascular resistance will perpetuate hypertension; this component of the hypothesis has previously been proposed by Lever.[97]

7. Therefore, a predominantly systolic hypertension, as found in conditions with an increased adrenergic drive in the young and during the ageing process, will be transmitted from the conduit to the resistance arteries and thereby converts systolic hypertension into sustained systolic and diastolic hypertension.

It is not proposed that this hypothesis would generally apply to all patients with hypertension. Rather two subsets of the hypertensive population may chiefly be involved. For example, this hypothesis would explain why hypertension in the young tends to be that of a high cardiac output type, whereas later it becomes a high vascular resistance type.[44] It would also explain why aged patients with systolic hypertension have diastolic values higher than could be expected solely from the changes in compliance.[151] The importance of this hypothesis is that a variety of agents interrupting the vicious circle whereby *"hypertension begets hypertension"* (Fig 3-8) or would be beneficial. The unexpected antihypertensive effects of heparin could thus be explained.[52] This agent which has no direct effect on vascular tone is able both to inhibit vascular smooth muscle cell growth and when given chronically to reduce the blood pressure,[207] apparently acting to inhibit renal glomerular fibrinoid lesions. The hypothesis would also explain why the pulsatile pressure (difference between systolic and diastolic values) is so closely linked to the mean arterial pressure[32] because increased pulsatile pressure would be followed by increased mean blood pressure. Furthermore, the hypothesis would explain the association between *an increased pulse pressure,* closely related to aortic stiffness, and coronary artery disease as well as left ventricular hypertrophy.[50] Also consonant with the hypothesis is the

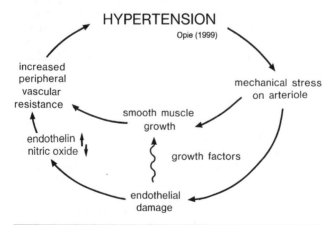

Figure 3-8. Role of mechanical stress on the arteriole both in causing endothelial damage and in stimulating smooth muscle growth. Note the possible release of endothelin during endothelial damage to increase peripheral vascular resistance. Figure © LH Opie, 1999

relationship between increased pulse pressure and cardio-vascular mortality in a French male population.[11]

The hypothesis would also accord special importance to those antihypertensive agents that act not only to reduce blood pressure but also to inhibit directly the growth process in the smooth muscle cells of the tunica media of arterioles. Such agents include the ACE inhibitors.

Therapeutic interruption of vascular vicious circle in hypertension. The vicious circle proposed could be interrupted at several points. First of all, any agent acting as a general non-specific antihypertensive will remove the major initial stimulus to the loss of compliance in the conduit arteries. Agents that reduce early episodes of increased cardiac output and systolic hypertension could likewise be expected eventually to diminish the cycle. Therefore, conventional antihypertensive therapy has a definite place. In addition, agents that specifically reduce systolic hypertension will help to decrease the propagation of the pressure wave to the resistance arterioles. There is provisional evidence that ACE inhibitors are better able to reduce the systolic component of hypertension than, for example, beta-blockers. Lisinopril and enalapril are better able than atenolol to achieve this aim.[10,70,144] A recent careful analysis of the comparative effects of perindopril on systolic and diastolic pressure by Safar's group supports the concept of a relatively greater reduction in the systolic component of the blood pressure.[4]

Conduit artery relaxation. The ACE inhibitors appear to maintain this. For example, captopril, enalapril and perindopril allow maintained increase in the arterial diameter during prolonged therapy, even when the blood pressure has fallen. In a particularly interesting study, Asmar et al[3] subjected patients with essential hypertension to 1 month of placebo therapy before administration of perindopril (mean dose 6 mg daily) for a period of 3 months and a subsequent placebo washout period also of 1 month. They compared the effects on brachial mechanical properties with the findings in two placebo periods, one before and one after the perindopril treatment. During the active treatment period, the brachial artery compliance increased as the blood pressure fell. Of specific interest is the increase in arterial diameter, the exact opposite of what would be expected from the decreased intraluminal pressure.

It is clear that the blood vessels must be regarded as a valid site for end-organ damage in hypertension, in addition to the conventional end-organs such as brain, retina, heart, and kidneys. Damage to blood vessels could play a crucial role in perpetuating hypertension, as already proposed by Folkow et al in 1973.[44] It is also clear that the experimental and clinical properties of the actions of ACE inhibitors on the blood vessels (Table 2-2) need careful appraisal for their potential role in lessening or even reversing hypertensive vascular disease.

EFFECTS OF ACE INHIBITORS ON ARTERIAL DISEASE

Two proposed mechanisms. An important question is the extent to which the changes found in the various studies with ACE inhibitors can be caused purely by intraluminal pressure reduction, or whether there is a more specific effect such as interference with the vascular tissue renin-angiotensin system. On the one hand, mechanical relief of pressure in the arterial tree induced simply by a local ligature can revert almost fully toward normal the abnormalities found in the resistance arterioles of spontaneously hypertensive rats.[19] On the other hand, there is another factor, independent of changes in intraluminal pressure. In a model of hypertension (one kidney, one clip) that is not renin-dependent, ACE inhibitor therapy decreases the severity of aortic wall hypertrophy. The mean blood pressure only fell from 193 ± 5 mmHg to 183 ± 5 mmHg in captopril treated rats and this small change was most unlikely to account for the decreased aortic wall thickness.[198] The most reasonable conclusion is that ACE inhibition in this model has a direct beneficial effect on the aortic wall. Thus, ACE inhibition potentially acts on arterial disease through both mechanisms, first reducing intraluminal pressure by the general blood pressure lowering effect and, second, by an additional effect independent of any pressure change, possibly related to the effects of angiotensin II in stimulating vascular growth.

Experimental effects on large arteries. In keeping with the basic data showing that angiotensin II is a specific stimulator of vascular growth (Table 2-2), it is not surprising that hypertension (renovascular model) leads to an increased thickness of the aorta and a fall in its compliance.[100] Treatment by the ACE inhibitor perindopril (1 mg/kg/day for 4 weeks) decreased the medial thickness of the arterial wall. In the spontaneously hypertensive rat model treated by perindopril, the elastin/collagen ratio fell and the thickness of the medial wall decreased.[98,99,101] Specifically, there were reductions in smooth muscle hypertrophy and in collagen density.[102]

In a second study, also in spontaneously hypertensive rats, the ACE inhibitor enalapril was given during the growth phase of rats with spontaneous hypertension.[15] Polyploidy is thought to contribute to the loss of compliance in large arteries in hypertension. Enalapril 25 to 30 mg/kg/day prevented the development of hypertension in this model and reduced the number of aortic smooth muscle cells that exhibited polyploidy (an increased number of nuclei in each cell).

Experimental effects on medium sized arteries. In *cerebral arteries* of spontaneously hypertensive rats, there is medial hypertrophy. When such rats were treated by cilazapril 10 mg/kg/day during the growth phase, then the medial hypertrophy diminished and the capacity of the cerebral arterial tree to undergo maximal vasodilation was increased toward normal.[26] In *mesenteric arteries* of spontaneously hypertensive rats treated by captopril, there was an increased lumen size at maximal relaxation and a decreased number of smooth muscle cell layers.[95] In another study, captopril treatment also reduced the wall/lumen ratio of the mesenteric arteries and had a greater effect than the non-specific vasodilator, dihydralazine.[48]

ACE INHIBITORS AS MONOTHERAPY IN HYPERTENSION

Captopril was the first ACE inhibitor clinically used in the therapy of hypertension. Initially its severe side-effects, including neutropenia and renal damage, led to its use only when other agents had failed. Gradually, as the dose given dropped, so did the side-effects, and it became evident that captopril could be effective even as initial monotherapy.[80] Thereupon, eminent leaders in the area of hypertension, such as Zanchetti,[211] mooted the possibility of using an ACE inhibitor as first-line monotherapy. In larger groups of patients, enalapril reduced blood pressure with a "flat" dose-response curve was confirmed, with a major antihypertensive effect at 10 mg daily.[162] More recently a host of ACE inhibitors have become available, including lisinopril, perindopril, ramipril, quinapril, cilazapril, trandolapril, fosinopril, and many others. They all have in common the capacity to reduce blood pressure when given as monotherapy in patients with mild to moderate hypertension (Fig 3–9). There is no reason to suppose that the mechanism of antihypertensive effect differs between these agents.

Response rates. Precisely because of the multifactorial causation of hypertension and the multi-mechanism mode of action of ACE inhibitors, it is not easy to predict whether or not ACE inhibitor monotherapy would be effective in a given patient, although an acute test may be useful.[122] In general, a good response to monotherapy can be obtained in only 35% to 70% of patients depending on the dose and criteria used.[206] In some series, even higher response rates are reported.[130] The concept of response rates is not easy to define, because generally the sodium status of the patients is not reported. The salt intake and the race of the patient may be crucial factors in determining the response to ACE inhibitors. For *genotypes and response rates,* see Chapter 8 (page 169).

Hard end-points in hypertension therapy. Increasingly, physicians are asking not whether a drug simply lowers blood pressure but a host of more sophisticated questions. What is the quality of life? Are there effects on organ damage, such as ventricular and vascular hypertrophy? What are the effects on renal function? Are the drugs metabolically neutral with reference to blood lipids and glucose, or even beneficial? Are there pharmacokinetic benefits to any

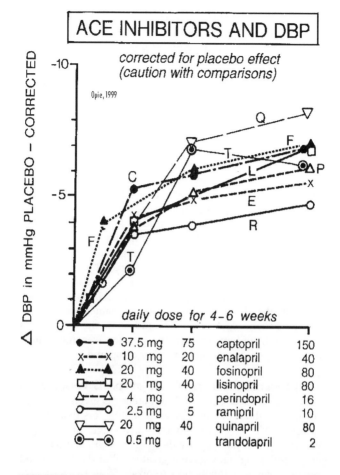

Figure 3-9. *By excluding concurrent placebo effect, the antihypertensive benefit of ACE inhibitors becomes less striking. A similar placebo effect could probably be found with every other class of antihypertensive agent. Note that in none of the studies is the salt intake stated, and some studies contain black patients. Hence, comparisons of dose-responses between agents are invalid. Figure © LH Opie, 1999*

particular drug (see Chapter 8)? Are there effects on hard end-points such as mortality, stroke, and heart attacks? While more and more of these questions can now be positively answered for the ACE inhibitors, it must be admitted that proof of reduction of hard end-points must still be obtained. This important aim has been addressed in the Captopril Prevention Project (CAPP).[21] Captopril was as effective as "conventional" therapy by β-blocker diuretic in reducing the blood pressure, yet with more strokes. Captopril was, however, given once or twice daily, so that 24 hour action was not sure. Captopril also prevented diabetes. In contrast, in the large UKPDS[189] over 8–9 years, tight control of hypertension in type two diabetics by either captopril twice daily or by atenolol equally reduced hard end points.[189] Another study of interest is STOP-2, in which mortality will be an end point, comparing conventional therapy (diuretic-β-blocker) versus "modern therapy" by an ACE inhibitor and/or calcium antagonist.

COMPARATIVE STUDIES WITH ACE INHIBITORS IN MILD TO MODERATE HYPERTENSION

ACE inhibitors versus placebo. The ideal protocol is that in which patients are randomized in a double-blinded manner to one of several doses of a drug and also to concurrent placebo therapy, in a parallel manner. The fall in blood pressure with ACE inhibitor therapy is much more marked when no allowance is made for the concurrent placebo effect than when allowance is made for the concurrent placebo effect In every case there is a relatively "flat" dose-response effect (Fig 3-9). Thus, some "average" antihypertensive doses can be suggested, such as captopril 37.5 to 75 mg daily, enalapril 10 to 20 mg daily, lisinopril 20 to 40 mg daily, perindopril 4 to 8 mg daily, and ramipril 2.5 to 5 mg daily. In attempting to compare these studies, it should be considered that several aspects were not standardized. For example, in *none was the salt intake stated.* Although the diastolic blood pressure values were taken with the patients supine in most studies, in one the subjects were seated, and in another the posture was not stated. Hence these studies cannot easily be compared.

Antihypertensive effects of ACE inhibitors versus each other. *Enalapril and captopril.* Equipotency is given by an enalapril dose about one-fifth or even slightly less than that of captopril.[24,105,182,197] An obvious advantage of enalapril over captopril is the longer half-life. *Perindopril and captopril.* Perindopril 4 mg daily gave a greater fall of diastolic blood pressure than 79 patients on captopril 25 mg twice daily.[96] Then the dose could be doubled and then a diuretic added. In the end, 75% of those initially receiving perindopril achieved satisfactory blood pressure reduction versus 57% of the captopril group. *Perindopril and enalapril.* Equivalent doses were perindopril 4 mg and enalapril 10 mg, or perindopril 8 mg and enalapril 20 mg.[129] Blood pressure control 24 hours after the dose was better with the longer-acting perindopril,[129] as were the trough/peak ratios of efficacy. *Ramipril and captopril* are approximately equieffective at daily doses of 10 mg and 100 mg respectively, as also are *ramipril and enalapril* with doses of 5 to 10 mg ramipril corresponding to 10 to 20 mg enalapril.[183] *Ramipril and lisinopril.* Lisinopril 10 mg daily was not quite as good as ramipril 2.5 mg.[90] *Lisinopril and enalapril.* In 110 patients randomized to either lisinopril 10 mg or enalapril 10 mg daily, the mean ambulatory blood pressure fell equally.[204] Lisinopril gave better control 24 hours after the dose. *Trandolapril and ramipril.* Trandolapril 2 mg was the equivalent of enalapril 20 mg, but after a missed dose the BP control persisted for longer with trandolapril.[193]

ACE inhibitors versus or combined with diuretic therapy. There have been numerous studies showing that ACE inhibitor therapy becomes more effective in the presence of concurrent diuretic therapy[148] (for earlier references

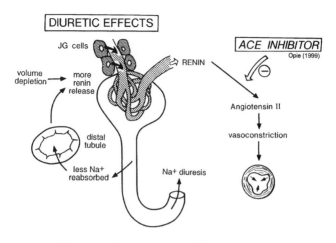

Figure 3-10. Rationale for combination of ACE inhibitors with diuretics. JG, juxtaglomerular. Figure © LH Opie, 1999

see second edition of this book), or sodium restriction.[129] Addition of a diuretic to a standard dose of ACE inhibitor gives a better response than increasing the dose of the ACE inhibitor.[164] The combination of captopril 50 mg daily and hydrochlorothiazide 25 mg daily reduced both blood pressure and plasma lipids.[92] The rationale for the combination is shown in Fig 3-10. In the case of hydrochlorothiazide, a low dose (12.5 mg daily) can be as effective as a standard dose (25 mg daily) in obtaining better blood pressure control when added to enalapril 20 mg daily.[30] The importance of the sodium status in the effect of ACE inhibitor therapy is shown by the added hypotensive effect of a low sodium diet added to treatment by captopril and a diuretic (Fig 3-11).

Ethnic effect. Compared with thiazide diuretics, ACE inhibitors are slightly more effective antihypertensive agents in white patients,[145] especially in younger patients.[118] Yet in black patients, whether younger or older groups are considered, diuretics are much better especially in the older age group.[118] To achieve a better response in black patients requires either (1) combination with a diuretic,[147,195] or (2) an increased dose of the ACE inhibitor.[203]

Comparison of metabolic effects of thiazide and captopril: insulin resistance. In an influential study, Pollare et al[146] achieved equal blood pressure reduction by using approximately a mean dose of captopril 80 mg daily and of hydrochlorothiazide 40 mg daily. Over the 4 month treatment period, captopril appeared to increase the sensitivity to infused insulin, whereas hydrochlorothiazide appeared to decrease it. Hydrochlorothiazide also increased serum cholesterol and triglyceride levels. No outcome data were presented to indicate that these adverse metabolic effects had effects on hard end-points such as a greater incidence of diabetes mellitus or coronary heart disease.

ACE inhibitor versus or combined with beta-blockade therapy. Review of 15 comparative studies on over 2,000 patients (Table 2-5 of second edition) reveals that ACE inhi-

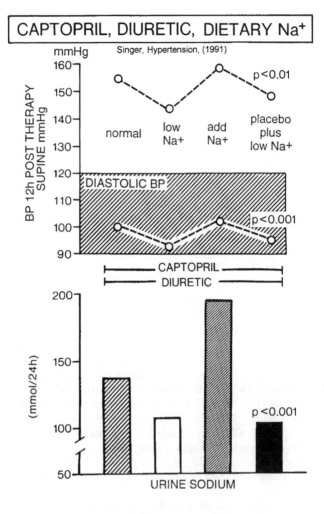

Figure 3-11. In patients already treated with captopril 50 mg twice daily and a diuretic, hydroclorothiazide 25 mg once daily, a low-salt diet further reduces the blood pressure and the urine sodium. When sodium is added in the form of Slow-Sodium tablets, blood pressure increases, and urine sodium rises. When Slow-Sodium placebo tablets are given, blood pressure reverts to that found with a low-sodium diet, as does urine sodium. Note highly significant fall in urine sodium and diastolic blood pressure with sodium restriction (right-hand column, Slow-Sodium placebo). These data, taken from Singer et al,[176] show that even in patients who are diuretic treated in addition to receiving an ACE inhibitor, a low sodium diet should be advised. The figure is redrawn from the data of Singer et al,[176] with permission.

bitor monotherapy is almost always as good as beta-blocker monotherapy and sometimes better, particularly in relation to reduction of systolic blood pressure. There are, however, few long-term outcome studies available with ACE inhibitors in hypertension when compared to beta-blockers.

Combination ACE inhibitor with beta-blocker. If ACE inhibitor therapy is most effective for hypertension that is associated with a high plasma renin level and if beta-blockade reduces plasma renin levels,[75] then it may follow that beta-blockade and ACE inhibition should not be a good antihypertensive combination. However, in a large multicenter parallel group study on 100 patients, the addition of lisinopril 10 to 20 mg daily was more effective than placebo in reducing the blood pressure of patients previously inadequately controlled on atenolol 50 mg daily.[177] These data suggest that combination therapy of an ACE inhibitor with a beta-blocker could be more promising than usually thought.

ACE inhibitors compared with or combined with calcium antagonists. Although ACE inhibitors have not been so well compared with calcium antagonists as with beta-blockers, a number of studies testify to the approximate equivalence of the antihypertensive effects of both types of agents (Table 2-6 of second edition).

Combination of ACE inhibitors and calcium antagonists. In several studies of both and captopril plus nifedipine gave better blood pressure reduction than either agent alone.[64,169,175] In 16 patients with moderately severe hypertension, monotherapy with a calcium antagonist (verapamil or nitrendipine) did not satisfactorily reduce the diastolic blood pressure, but combination with captopril was successful.[18] Isradipine monotherapy (1.25 or 2.5 mg twice daily) reduced diastolic BP from a mean of 100 mmHg to below 95 mmHg in 64% of patients,[210] whereupon addition of captopril increased the response rate to 90%. The combination of nitrendipine (10 mg once daily) and captopril (25 mg twice daily) reduced blood pressure more than double the dose of either agent alone.[51]

Evaluation of ACE inhibitor therapy compared with or combined with calcium antagonists. Compared with calcium antagonists, ACE inhibitors are approximately equieffective antihypertensive agents, often with fewer side-effects. The ACE inhibitors are more likely to be effective at lower blood pressure levels, with an estimated threshold of efficacy at 120/80 mmHg compared with that of calcium antagonists at 135/85 mmHg.[71] Yet an optimal response to ACE inhibitors requires a low sodium diet and, fairly frequently, the addition of a diuretic. ACE inhibitors are much less likely to be effective in black patients, and are virtually ineffective in elderly black subjects.[118] Regarding the calcium antagonist-ACE inhibitor combination, there are only a relatively small number of studies, as in regression of left ventricular hypertrophy.[117] Yet the attraction of these agents in combination is that neither has any negative central effects nor adverse effects on blood lipid profile nor on metabolic parameters, such as plasma potassium or uric acid. The only known defect of this combination, as far as is known, is cost. An additional problem that must be emphasized is that there are no formal long-term outcome studies in hypertension with this combination, nor for that matter with any other combinations.

ACE inhibitors vs or combined with AT-1 receptor blockers. In general, similar BP reduction is achieved by appropriate doses of both types of agents, with however less cough with the receptor blockers, and a tendency for better BP reduction with the ACE inhibitor.

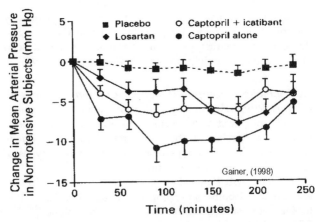

Figure 3-12. Proposed role of bradykinin in effect of captopril on blood pressure of normotensive, salt-depleted subjects. When given with icatibant, the specific bradykinin receptor blocker (BK block), the acute hypotensive effect is much less, and roughly corresponds to the values obtained with losartan alone. Therefore, in these experimental conditions, the superior hypotensive effect of the ACE inhibitor compared with the AT-1 blocker, can be ascribed to the effects of bradykinin. Reproduced with permission of the authors[49] and the publishers of the New England Journal of Medicine.

Captopril vs losartan (Fig 3-12). When given acutely to salt depleted hypertensives, captopril 25 mg gave a better BP reduction than did losartan 75 mg.[49] Urinary sodium excretion was, however, higher with losartan.

Enalapril vs or combined with losartan. These were approximately equally effective at doses of enalapril 20 mg and losartan 50 mg.[58] At eight weeks, however, lowest BP readings were found with enalapril. When combined (enalapril 10 mg, losartan 50 mg) the blood pressure fell more than with only enalapril 20 mg.[5]

Perindopril vs losartan. An unexpected finding was that, in obese hypertensives, *insulin resistance* was reduced by perindopril 4 mg daily, but not by losartan 50 mg daily, although BP reductions were equivalent.[43]

LARGE MULTIDRUG STUDIES

Two large studies on male subjects have compared an ACE inhibitor with a calcium antagonist, a beta-blocker, a diuretic and an alpha-blocker as first-line therapy (Table 2-7, previous edition). In very mildly hypertensive patients with a mean blood pressure of only 140/91 mmHg and all receiving lifestyle advice and a low salt diet, there was no difference in the hypotensive potencies of the various drugs used, all in low doses.[185] Metabolically, the diuretic increased the plasma total cholesterol at 1 year but not 4 years,[184] whereas the beta-blocker unexpectedly decreased LDL-cholesterol and, as expected, triglyceride levels. It should be recalled that acebutolol has specific qualities, namely cardioselectivity and intrinsic sympathomimetic activity (ISA). The diuretic also increased plasma uric acid and decreased potassium values. Most parameters judging the quality of life were unchanged in all groups, except that the "general functioning index" improved slightly with the beta-blocker and with the diuretic, whereas it fell with the alpha-blocker. Paradoxically, the diuretic *increased* the incidence of impotence, whereas the alpha-blocker gave the lowest incidence of impotence.[62] It follows that at least some of the male patients "functioned" better if they had impotence (sexual intercourse is a strain?). In virtually all aspects, the ACE inhibitor had similar side-effects to placebo.

Whereas the TOMH study was largely on whites (80%), the second had 42% blacks.[118] Although each of the five categories of drugs used in the TOHM report was also used, none of the drugs were the same. A sixth drug, clonidine, was also used and gave good antihypertensive results, yet with unacceptable side-effects. The hypotensive effects of the drugs differed according to race and age. In younger whites (mean age 50 years) the ACE inhibitor captopril was most effective, with 55% of patients responding. Next came the beta-blocker atenolol, then the alpha-blocker prazosin, then the calcium antagonist diltiazem, and lastly the diuretic. In older whites, the ACE inhibitor only came third. In younger blacks, the ACE inhibitor came last, and in older blacks, it was no better than placebo. There was no information on salt intake, which could have differed between the races and the age groups. The diuretic gave rise to most metabolic disturbances. This study shows the major impact of race and to a lesser extent of age on the use of ACE inhibitors.

Left ventricular hypertrophy. In the one year echocardiographic follow up study,[56] limited to those whose BP was controlled on the initially assigned monotherapy, the major decreases in LV mass were with hydrochlorothiazide (-66%), captopril (-45%), and atenolol (-37%). Clonidine and prazosin were ineffective and diltiazem actually increased LV mass, although initially it had been among the most effective in reducing BP. *Left atrial size.* Over two years, only the thiazide significantly reduced left atrial size, with the others including captopril and atenolol only showing a similar trend.[57]

Peripheral vascular resistance. In a unique invasive study, Omvik and Lund-Johansen[142] sequentially undertook hemodynamic studies on 171 white patients in non-matched groups, using nine different drugs, the tenth group receiving a low salt diet. Each patient was subject to outpatient drug titration for 6 to 12 months before the second hemodynamic study. Lisinopril (mean daily dose 25 mg) gave the second best pressure reduction at rest, exceeded only by the combined alpha-beta blocker carvedilol (mean daily dose 52 mg). Of importance is that, when lisinopril was accompanied by a low salt diet or by hydrochlorothiazide 12.5 to 25 mg daily, it reduced the total peripheral resistance as much as did carvedilol or the calcium antagonists.

ACE INHIBITOR THERAPY FOR SEVERE OR REFRACTORY HYPERTENSION

Acute therapy. Of the ACE inhibitors, captopril, which is not a prodrug, has one of the most rapid onsets of action and has been used in the therapy of acute severe hypertension.[169] In the study of Tschollar and Belz,[187] the initial mean blood pressure of 6 patients was 233/132 mmHg; 30 minutes after sublingual captopril the values were very much lower. In another small study by Biollaz et al,[14] the mean blood pressure decreased from 239/134 mmHg to 204/118 mmHg 30 minutes following captopril 25 mg. In this study and another,[169] the maximal hypotensive effect of captopril only occurred 4 hours after administration.

Captopril vs nifedipine capsules. Each agent has potential problems. Nifedipine can cause abrupt and excess blood pressure reduction, precipitating myocardial ischemia.[63] Captopril has the advantage of a smoother slower fall in blood pressure,[169] yet at 4 hours post-dose similar BP reductions are achieved. After the acute phase, when only one agent achieves a response, combination therapy both captopril and nifedipine, as well as other agents, is often required.[169]

Intravenous enalaprilat. In the USA, this is licensed for use in hypertension in a dose of 1.25 mg over 5 min every 6 hours, reduced to 0.625 mg initially for prior diuretic therapy, or in heat failure, or for renal impairment with a creatinine clearance of 30 ml/min or below, or a serum creatinine of 3 mg/dl or higher. A *caution* regarding the acute use of either captopril or enalaprilat in the emergency situation, is that it is difficult to exclude bilateral renal artery stenosis or severe unilateral renal artery stenosis. Either of these could result in an excess precipitous fall in blood pressure or even serious prolonged renal failure.

ACE inhibitor therapy combined with several other agents. Multi-drug therapy is becoming increasingly common, and the BP levels aimed at increasingly lower. Thus, in the HOT study, to achieve the diastolic BP values of below 90 mmHg, two or three drugs were often used.[76] An increasingly common combination is that of an ACE inhibitor with a calcium blocker. In such patients not achieving the target BP, the addition of a diuretic is better able to control BP than an added beta-blocker.[2]

ACE INHIBITORS IN SPECIAL GROUPS OF PATIENTS

In general, ACE inhibitors can be used in most clinical situations that are associated with hypertension. In the presence of aortic stenosis, caution is required to avoid excess blood pressure falls, thereby increasing the gradient across the valve, and in bilateral renal artery stenosis or pregnancy these drugs are contraindicated.

Hypertension in diabetics. Because of the neutral or possibly favorable effects of ACE inhibitors and carbohydrate metabolism[146] and the consistent reports showing a decrease in microalbuminuria,[9] ACE inhibitors may be preferential therapy for diabetic hypertensive patients.[145] Captopril improves hard endpoints in type 1 diabetic nephropathy.[104] In type 2 diabetics in the ABCD study, enalapril gave fewer adverse cardiovascular events than did the vascular selective calcium antagonist nisoldipine.[1] Also in type two diabetics, in a large study over a mean of 8.4 years, very tight BP control down to a mean of 144/82 mmHg by captopril or atenolol gave similar beneficial reduction of hard end-points such as diabetes-related mortality, strokes and microvascular end points.[189] However, in the atenolol group more patients dropped out, and glucose tolerance decreased as shown by an increased requirement for anti-diabetic therapy. Taking these data together with the benefits of prolonged ACE inhibitor therapy in non-diabetic chronic renal disease (Chapter 4), the present author's preference for initial ACE inhibitor therapy remains (Chapter 11). JNC VI regards diabetes mellitus type 1 with proteinuria as a compelling indication for the use of ACE inhibitors to treat the hypertension. Nonetheless it must be pointed out that combination antihypertensive therapy is often need to adequately reduce the diastolic BP to below 85 mmHg as recommended by JNC VI, or to a mean value of 82 mmHg as found in the UK study.

Chronic pulmonary disease. In some patients, ACE inhibitors may improve pulmonary function by decreasing hypoxic vasoconstriction;[12] nonetheless, the high incidence of cough as a side-effect is disturbing. Although it is reasonably well established that ACE inhibitors do not precipitate asthma and in this way differ from beta-blockers, an irritating cough in a patient with pulmonary disease can be disabling and distressing.

Hypertensive heart failure. In view of the great efficacy of ACE inhibitors in heart failure, the combination ACE inhibitor-diuretic should be prime therapy for such patients presenting with congestive heart failure. This situation is regarded as a compelling indication to treat by an ACE inhibitor, according to JNC VI.[83] There are, however, no formal trials to support this recommendation.

Hypertension and peripheral vascular disease. In a placebo-controlled cross-over study, continuing over 6 months, captopril 25 mg twice daily was compared with atenolol 100 mg once daily, labetalol 200 mg twice daily or pindolol 10 mg twice daily.[154] Beta-blockers, even those with added alpha-blockade or intrinsic sympathomimetic activity, were less effective than captopril in maintaining walking distance in patients with intermittent claudication.

Hypertension and coronary artery disease. In such patients ACE inhibitors can be expected to have beneficial effects. In contrast to beta-blockers, ACE inhibitors cannot be expected to have a consistent antianginal effect. Yet they are anti-ischemic (Chapter 5) and appear to lessen re-infarction. They also relieve the increased oxygen demand induced increased wall stress as in the left ventricular wall dilation in left ventricular failure and/or by their antihypertensive effect.

Postinfarct hypertension. There are no formal studies on such patients. Beta-blockers remain one of the agents of choice because of their known effect in improving postinfarct mortality. On the other hand, ACE inhibitors may be freely used, particularly in view of their beneficial effects on postinfarct prognosis in patients with left ventricular dysfunction. Therefore, it would be logical to combine ACE inhibitors with beta-blockers.

Hypertension and renal disease. Although ACE inhibitors are generally regarded as safe in patients with chronic renal failure, occasionally deterioration of renal function takes place. Evidence for the overall benefit of ACE inhibition even in non-diabetic renal disease is presented in Chapter 4. In patients with renovascular hypertension, ACE inhibitor therapy is the cornerstone of the medical management (taking care for excess first dose hypotension). Although renal failure is a risk in patients with bilateral renal artery stenosis or stenosis of a solitary kidney, Hollenberg[73] found only 6% of such patients developed renal failure.

Scleroderma crisis. In patients with scleroderma (progressive systemic sclerosis), there may be the combination of a rapid fall off in renal function together with malignant hypertension. At least some of these patients respond to captopril therapy, which may lessen severe renal impairment.[17]

The elderly. Current indications are that ACE inhibitors can be almost as effective as monotherapy in the elderly as in younger whites, despite the low renin status of most elderly patients. In a large multicenter study, lisinopril (mean daily dose 50 mg) was as effective in elderly patients as in those whose age was below 65 years.[144] In 12 elderly patients, with chiefly systolic hypertension (initial blood pressure 189/89 mmHg sitting), a mean dose of captopril of 50 mg twice daily reduced the blood pressure to 172/83 mmHg.[28] In 34 elderly patients, perindopril reduced blood pressure from a mean of 185/95 mmHg to 164/87 mmHg.[46] In the study on six possible first-line antihypertensive drugs, captopril was the best for younger whites (mean age 50), third best in older whites (mean age 66), but strikingly ineffective in older blacks.[118]

Hypertension in black patients. Here ACE inhibitors are not as effective as in white patients, so that concurrent diuretic therapy is often required to achieve a benefit.[194] After administration of hydrochlorothiazide, equal blood pressure decreases were found in the two ethnic groups.[195] Alternatively, the dose of the ACE inhibitor can be doubled as recommended in the USA package insert for trandolapril. In the case of lisinopril, there were similar racial differences in the response,[144] and even the addition of hydro-chlorothiazide did not achieve as great a blood pressure fall in black patients as in white patients.[147] In the recent VA study, older black males did not respond at all to capto-pril.[118] In a much smaller study on South African blacks aged 18 to 65 (no mean given), enalapril was partially effec-tive.[125]

As a group, black patients are thought to have low-renin hypertension,[165] which logically should respond less well to ACE inhibitors. Logically too, a low-salt diet and/or diure-tic therapy should increase renin levels and make the patients more susceptible to ACE inhibitor therapy. It should be recalled, though, that despite the general trend to lower renin values in black patients, in one large series on 371 subjects, 42% had low-renin hypertension, 46% had normal renin values, and 12% had high values.[131]

High blood uric acid. Diuretics may cause hyperuricemia and predispose to gout by inducing renal retention of urate. In contrast, ACE inhibitors increase renal urate excretion in normal volunteers and in hypertensive patients.[94] The me-chanism of this uricosuric effect is not known, but it does indicate that ACE inhibitor therapy could be a choice for patients with gout and hypertension or for hypertensive hy-peruricemic patients. However caution is required in that a vigorous uricosuric effect may precipitate gouty stones so that the ACE inhibitors should be instituted gradually.[94]

Pregnancy. Since the initial reports linking captopril usage to possible skull defects and oligohydramnios, and the find-ing of toxicity in animal studies, captopril has been re-garded as an embryopathic drug that should be avoided or used with great caution in pregnancy. By analogy, other ACE inhibitors have the same restriction, and recently the Food and Drugs Administration in the United States has re-quired a prominent warning against the use of all ACE in-hibitors during the second and third trimesters of pregnancy. A similar warning relates to the use of the AT-receptor blockers.

ACUTE TESTING OF ACE INHIBITORS

Not all patients respond to one specific type of drug given as first-line monotherapy. In the case of ACE inhibitors, an acute test may predict long-term response.[122] Unfortunately, a full therapeutic dose cannot be routinely used as a test dose because patients with high-renin hypertension are at risk of excessively decreasing the blood pressure when given standard doses of the ACE inhibitor.[202] A reasonable practical policy might be to give a low initial test dose of captopril (6.25 mg) and to wait for 30 minutes. If there is no excessive response sensitivity to the ACE inhibitor, 25 mg of captopril can be given. If the blood pressure comes down within another hour, then the patient is poten-tially responsive to ACE inhibition and the agent of choice can then be given long-term. This approach does not, how-ever, exclude a placebo response. Although this policy has no documentation in the literature, it seems reasonable and practicable.

COMPARATIVE EVALUATION OF ACE INHIBITORS AS ANTIHYPERTENSIVE AGENTS

General comparison. The data available show that ACE inhibitors are acceptable first-line antihypertensive agents, albeit largely lacking the solid outcome data available for low-dose diuretics. There are relatively few contraindica-tions. ACE inhibitors can be used in a variety of co-existing disease states.[83,179] Although expensive, they do not precipi-tate diseases, such as diabetes or gout as in the case of high-dose diuretics, nor do they pose respiratory problems nor decrease the heart rate or cause heart block as in the case of beta-blockers. They do not cause impotence as may even low dose diuretics or beta-blockers. As a group, white males with a mean age of about 50 years respond very well to the ACE inhibitor captopril[118] as do patients with high-renin hypertension or low-renin hypertension on a low salt diet. Certain *co-existing disease* states favor the use of ACE inhibitor therapy, including large vessel vascular disease, left ventricular hypertrophy, diabetic nephropathy, and the presence of left ventricular failure. The latter two situations are regarded as compelling indications for ACE inhibition by JNC VI.

On the other hand, there are a number of situations sug-gesting caution or reserve in the use of ACE inhibitors as first-line antihypertensive agents (Table 2-8, previous edi-tion). These include patients on a high salt diet, black patients, when expense is crucial, and when there is a pre-existing dry cough. In addition, there are a number of uncommon *absolute or relative contraindications* including bilateral renal artery stenosis, stenosis in a single kidney, unilateral renal artery stenosis in the presence of excess diuresis, and sodium-depleted patients with severe conges-tive heart failure.

Comparison of ACE inhibitors with diuretic therapy. The following factors favor ACE inhibitors as first choice agents (Table 2-8, previous edition): type-II diabetes or family his-tory of diabetes, gout or family history of gout, hyperlipide-mia or a borderline lipid profile, or when the salt intake is low. On the other hand, diuretics should be considered as first-line agents when cost is crucial, when the salt intake is high and cannot easily be reduced, when there is renal dis-ease with sodium retention, or when the patient is black. In obese hypertensives, there is evidence favoring diuretics and also ACE inhibitors.[43] Both types of agents are used for heart failure, but only in the case of ACE inhibitors is there evidence for mortality reduction. In hypertension, low dose diuretics remain the best tested for reduction of hard end points,[83] but the response in younger white males is poor[118] and the risk of impotence relatively high.[62] These factors may swing the argument in favour of ACE inhibitors as first line agents.

Comparison of ACE inhibitors with beta-blockers. As first-line therapy, the initial use of ACE inhibitors may be favored when there is unstable left ventricular failure, when peak physical and mental activity is required, when there is hyperlipidemia or a borderline lipid profile, when there is borderline glucose tolerance, in the presence of diabetes mellitus especially with nephropathy, when there is peripheral vascular disease, when the hypertension is predominantly systolic, and when there are contraindications to beta-blockade therapy (Table 2-9, previous edition). On the other hand, favoring the use of beta-blockers is the co-existence of ischemic heart disease, angina or the postinfarct state unaccompanied by left ventricular dilation; co-existing anxiety or tachycardia; pre-existing dry cough; and pregnant hypertensive patients. Neither type of agent is suited for first-line therapy of black hypertensive patients.

Comparison of ACE inhibitors with calcium antagonists. Both agents have positive arguments for first-line therapy (Table 2-10, previous edition). For example, both ACE inhibitors and calcium antagonists are claimed to maintain optimal physical and mental activity, to be lipid neutral, not to alter insulin tolerance, to revert left ventricular hypertrophy, to inhibit experimental atherosclerosis, to improve arterial compliance, to treat diabetic nephropathy, and to benefit Raynaud's phenomenon. ACE inhibitors are preferred therapy in the presence of left ventricular systolic failure when calcium antagonists are contraindicated, or when there is combination therapy with diuretics (because calcium antagonists have some diuretic properties of their own). Calcium antagonists are preferred in combination with beta-blockers where the evidence is that, at least some studies, ACE inhibitors do not show a fully additive antihypertensive effect when combined with beta-blockers. Calcium antagonists are preferred in black patients and when there is co-existing angina especially on a vasospastic basis. Calcium antagonists (longer acting dihydropyridines) have positive outcome evidence in their favour in elderly hypertensives with systolic hypertension.[180] In severe urgent hypertension, both agents can be shown to work, but there are risks attached to nifedipine capsules. There must always be at least some risk of occult renal artery stenosis, which is a relative contraindication to ACE inhibitors. There is a strong contraindication to ACE inhbitors when the stenosis is bilateral.

Comparison of ACE inhibitors with AT-1 receptor blockers. At present there are no outcome studies in hypertension with either type of agent. There is general agreement that both inhibit the renin-angiotensin system, acting at least in part through different mechanisms. In hypertension with heart failure or LV dysfunction, there is good evi-

dence favouring the use of ACE inhibitors, as strongly
supported by JNC VI.[83] But again, comparative data are
lacking.

SUMMARY

1. *Left ventricular hypertrophy.* LVH is increasing recog-
    nized an independent risk factor for cardiovascular
    disease, and particularly for sudden death. There are
    numerous basic studies showing that angiotensin II
    acting on the AT-1 receptor, is a powerful promoter of
    the growth both of myocytes and of fibroblasts. The
    latter effect is mediated by transforming growth fac-
    tor-β_1. Yet a pressure load can induce hypertrophy in
    an AT-1 receptor knock-out mouse model. Therefore
    pressure overload rather than stimulation of the angio-
    tensin cardiac receptor is the fundamental initiating
    factor. Clinical evidence suggests that ACE inhibitors
    are at least as good as other antihypertensive agents in
    achieving regression of LV mass, but prolonged ther-
    apy even with the humble diuretic is also effective.
    Whether, in addition, ACE inhibitors have a superior
    capacity to normalize vascular abnormalities in hyper-
    tension still remains to be proven although this is an
    intriguing possibility.

2. *Vascular vicious circle: role of large conduit arteries.* The
    hypothesis is proposed that ageing of the large arteries
    such as the aorta and others, not only causes systolic
    hypertension, but promotes diastolic hypertension. The
    latter in turn causes arterial remodelling, so that there
    is a vascular vicious circle in hypertension. Therapy
    directed towards vascular disease may therefore have
    prophylactic importance. Some evidence favours a spe-
    cial role for ACE inhibitors in protecting from vascular
    remodelling in hypertension.

3. *ACE inhibitors as anti-hypertensive agents.* The picture
    that emerges is that ACE inhibitors are a group of
    agents effective in blood pressure reduction in most
    patient groups except when given as monotherapy to
    blacks. There is a relatively low cost in terms of side-
    effects and contraindications. Although ACE inhibitors
    are highly effective in high-renin patients, yet in
    elderly whites, a low-renin group, these agents work
    well as monotherapy. In general, they are about as
    effective as other potential first-line agents, such as the
    diuretics, beta-blockers, and calcium antagonists. There
    are, as yet, few outcome studies.

4. *Combination therapy.* A particularly attractive combina-
    tion is that with diuretics, because diuretics increase
    circulating renin activity and angiotensin II levels,
    which ACE inhibitors counter-regulate by inhibiting
    the conversion of angiotensin I to angiotensin II. Add-
    ing a low dose diuretic to a standard dose of ACE
    inhibitor seems more effective than increasing the ACE
    inhibitor dose, and sensitizes black patients to the anti-

hypertensive effects of ACE inhibitors. In addition, an oft neglected point is that dietary sodium restriction should be advised for all patients receiving ACE inhibitor monotherapy or ACE inhibitor plus diuretic therapy. Two drug combinations now receiving increasing attention are: (1) an ACE inhibitor with calcium antagonist, and (2) an ACE inhibitor with an AT-1 receptor blocker. Both combinations involve agents that have complementary actions.

5. *Choice of first-line therapy: diuretics vs ACE inhibitors.* The particular properties of a given patient can define whether that patient is a strong candidate for first-line ACE inhibitor therapy or whether there should be caution or reserve. Low dose diuretics remain the best tested group of drugs for reduction of hard end points, but the response in younger white males may be poor, and the risk of impotence relatively high when compared to ACE inhibitors and other agents. Factors promoting the increasing use of ACE inhibitors include the following: minimal side-effects (often limited to cough), simplicity of use, a flat dose-response curve, and ready combination with other modalities of treatment, as well as acceptability by the elderly. In addition, there is the virtual absence of contraindications except for pregnancy, bilateral renal artery stenosis and some related types of renal impairment. Specific arguments exist for the use of ACE inhibitors in hypertensives with diabetes or heart failure.

REFERENCES

1. ABCD Study. Estacio RO, Jeffers BW, W Hiatt, et al. The effect of nisoldipine as compared with enalapril on cardiovascular outcomes in patients with non-insulin-dependent diabetes and hypertension. N Engl J Med 1998;338:645–652.
2. Antonios T, Cappuccio F, Markandu N, et al. A diuretic is more effective than a ß-blocker in hypertensive patients not controlled on amlodipine and lisinopril. Hypertension 1996;27:1325–1328.
3. Asmar RG, Pannier B, Santoni JP, et al. Reversion of cardiac hypertrophy and reduced arterial compliance after converting enzyme inhibition in essential hypertension. Circulation 1988;78:941–950.
4. Asmar RG, Pannier B, Santoni JP, et al. Angiotensin converting enzyme inhibition decreases systolic blood pressure more than diastolic pressure as shown by ambulatory blood pressure monitoring. J Hypertens 1988;6 (Suppl 3):S79–S81.
5. Azizi M, Guyene T-T, Chatellier G, et al. Additive effects of losartan and enalapril on blood pressure and plasma active renin. Hypertension 1997;29:634–640.
6. Baker KM, Campanile CP, Trachte GJ, et al. Identification and characterization of the rabbit angiotensin II myocardial receptor. Circ Res 1984;54:286–293.
7. Baker KM, Cherin MI, Wixon SK, et al. Renin angiotensin system involvement in pressure-overload cardiac hypertrophy in rats. Am J Physiol 1990;259:H324–H332.
8. Bartunek J, Weinberg EO, Tajima M, et al. Angiotensin II type 2 receptor blockade amplifies the early signals of cardiac growth response to angiotensin II in hypertrophied hearts. Circulation 1999;99:22–25.
9. Bauduceau B, Genes N, Chamontin B, et al. Ambulatory blood pressure and urnary albumin excretion in diabetic (non-insulin-dependent and insulin-dependent) hypertensive patients: relationships at baseline and after treatment by the angiotensin converting enzyme inhibitor trandolapril. Am J Hypertens 1998;11:1065–1073.
10. Beevers DG, Blackwood RA, Garnham S, et al. Comparison of lisinopril vs atenolol for mild to moderate essential hypertension. Am J Cardiol 1991;67:59–62.

11. Benetos A, Safar M, Rudnichi A, et al. Pulse pressure: a predictor of long-term cardiovascular mortality in a French male population. Hypertension 1997; 30:1410–1415.

12. Bertoli L, Cicero SL, Busnardo I, et al. Effects of captopril on hemodynamics and blood gases in chronic obstructive lung disease with pulmonary hypertension. Respiration 1986;49:251–256.

13. Bielen EC, Fagard RH, Lijnen PJ, et al. Comparison of the effects of isradipine and lisinopril on left ventricular structure and function in essential hypertension. Am J Cardiol 1992;69:1200–1206.

14. Biollaz J, Waeber B, Brunner H. Hypertensive crisis treated with orally administered captopril. Eur J Clin Pharmacol 1983;25:145–149.

15. Black MJ, Adams MA, Bobik A, et al. Effects of enalapril on aortic smooth muscle cell polyploidy in the spontaneously hypertensive rat. J Hypertens 1989;7:997—1003.

16. Brilla CG, Janicki JS, Weber KT. Cardioreparative effects of lisinopril in rats with genetic hypertension and left ventricular hypertrophy. Circulation 1991;83:1771–1779.

17. Brogden R, Todd P, Sorkin E. Captopril. An update of its pharmacodynamic and pharmacokinetic properties, and therapeutic use in hypertension and congestive heart failure. Drugs 1988;36:540–600.

18. Brouwer R, Bolli P, Erne P, et al. Antihypertensive treatment using calcium antagonists in combination with captopril rather than diuretics. J Cardiovasc Pharmacol 1985;7:S88–S91.

19. Bund SJ, West KP, Heagerty AM. Effects of protection from pressure on resistance artery morphology and reactivity in spontaneously hypertensive and Wistar-Kyoto rats. Circ Res 1991;68:1230–1240.

20. Campese VM. Salt senstivity in hypertension. Renal and cardiovascular implications. Hypertension 1994;23:531–550.

21. CAPP Study Group. Hansson L, Lindholm LH, Niskanen L, et al. Effect of angiotensin-converting-enzyme inhibition compared with conventional therapy on cardiovascular morbidity and mortality in hypertension: the Captopril Prevention Project (CAPPP) randomised trial. Lancet 1999;353:611–616.

22. Case DB, Wallace JM, Keim HJ, et al. Possible role of renin in hypertension as suggested by renin-sodium profiling and inhibition of converting enzyme. N Engl J Med 1977;296:641–646.

23. Christensen KL, Jespersen LT, Mulvany MJ. Development of blood pressure in spontaneously hypertensive rats after withdrawal of long-term treatment related to vascular structure. J Hypertens 1989;7:83–90.

24. Chrysant SG, Singh BI, Johnson B, et al. A comparative study of captopril and enalapril in patients with severe hypertension. J Clin Pharmacol 1985;25:149–151.

25. Cigola E, Kajstura J, Li B, et al. Angiotensin II activates programmed myocyte cell death in vitro. Exp Cell Res 1997;231:363–371.

26. Clozel JP, Kuhn J, Hefti F. Effects of cilazapril on the cerebral circulation in spontaneously hypertensive rats. Hypertension 1989;14:645–651.

27. Cohen RA, Vanhoutte PM. Endothelium-dependent hyperpolarization. Beyond nitric oxide and cyclic GMP. Circulation 1995;92:3337–3349.

28. Cox J, Duggan J, O'Boyle C, et al. A double-blind evaluation of captopril in elderly hypertensives. J Hypertens 1989;7:299–303.

29. Cuocolo A, Sax FL, Brush JE, et al. Left ventricular hypertrophy and impaired diastolic filling in essential hypertension. Diastolic mechanisms for systolic dysfunction during exercise. Circulation 1990;81:978–986.

30. Dahlof B, Andren L, Eggertsen R, et al. Potentiation of the antihypertensive effect of enalapril by randomised addition of different doses of hydrochlorothiazide. J Hypertens 1985;3:S483–S486.

31. Dahlof B, Pennert K, Hansson L. Reversal of left ventricular hypertrophy in hypertensive patients. A meta-analysis of 109 treatment studies. Am J Hypertens 1992;5:95–110.

32. Darne B, Girerd X, Safar M, et al. Pulsatile versus steady component of blood pressure: a cross-sectional analysis and a prospective analysis on cardiovascular mortality. Hypertension 1989;13:392–400.

33. Diez J, Panizo A, Hernandez M, et al. Cardiomyocyte apoptosis and cardiac angiotensin-converting enzyme in spontaneously hypertensive rats. Hypertension 1997;30:1029–1034.

34. Dostal D, Rothblum K, Conrad K, et al. Detection of angiotensin-I and II in cultured rat cardiac myocytes and fibroblasts. Am J Physiol 1992;263:C851–C863.

35. Dostal DE, Baker KM. Evidence for a role of an intracardiac renin-angiotensin system in normal and failing hearts. Trends Cardiovasc Med 1993;3:67–74.

36. Dougherty AH, Naccarekku GV, Gray EL, et al. Congestive heart failure with normal systolic function. Am J Cardiol 1984;54:778–782.

37. Dussaule J-C, Michel J-B, Auzan C, et al. Effect of antihypertensive treat-
    ment on the left ventricular isomyosin profile in one-clip, two-kidney hy-
    pertensive rats. J Pharmacol Exp Ther 1986;236:512–518.

38. Dzau V, Re R. Tissue angiotensin system in cardiovascular medicine. A
    paradigm shift? Circulation 1994;89:493–498.

39. Dzau VJ. Mechanism of protective effects of ACE inhibition on coronary
    artery disease. Eur Heart J 1998;19 (Suppl J):J2–J6.

40. Dzau VJ, Safar ME. Large conduit arteries in hypertension: role of the
    vascular renin-angiotensin system. Circulation 1988;77:947–954.

41. Eberli FR, Apstein CS, Ngoy S, et al. Exacerbation of left ventricular is-
    chemic diastolic dysfunction by pressure-overload hypertrophy. Modifi-
    caiton by specific inhibition of cardiac angiotensin converting enzyme.
    Circ Res 1992;70:931–943.

42. Fang T-C, Huang W-C. Role of angiotensin II in hyperinsulinemia-in-
    duced hypertension in rats. J Hypertens 1998;16:1767–1774.

43. Fogari R, Zoppi A, Lazzari P, et al. ACE inhibition but not angiotensin II
    antagonism reduces plasma fibrinogen and insulin resistance in over-
    weight hypertensive patients. J Cardiovasc Pharmacol 1998;32:616–620.

44. Folkow B, Hallback M, Lundgren Y. Importance of adaptive changes in
    vascular design for establishment of primary hypertension, studied in
    man and in spontaneously hypertensive rats. Circ Res 1973;32 & 33
    (Suppl I):I-2 – I-16.

45. Ford WR, Clanachan AS, Jugdutt BI. Opposite effects of angiotensin AT_1
    and AT_2 receptor antagonists on recovery of mechanical function after
    ischemia-reperfusion in isolated working rat hearts. Circulation
    1996;94:3087–3089.

46. Forette F, Claran JM, Delesalle M, et al. Value of angiotensin converting
    enzyme inhibitors in the elderly: the example of perindopril. Clin Exper
    Theory Pract 1989;All (Suppl 2):507–603.

47. Franz I-W, Tonnesmann U, Muller JFM. Time course of complete normal-
    ization of left ventricular hypertrophy during long-term antihypertensive
    therapy with angiotensin converting enzyme inhibitors. Am J Hypert
    1998;11:631–639.

48. Freslon JL, Guidicelli JF. Compared myocardial and vascular effects of
    captopril and dihydralazine during hypertension in spontaneously hy-
    pertensive rats. Br J Pharmacol 1983;80:533–543.

49. Gainer JV, Morrow JD, Loveland A, et al. Effect of bradykinin-receptor
    blockade on the response to angiotensin-converting-enzyme inhibitor in
    normotensive and hypertensive subjects. N Engl J Med 1998;339:1285–
    1292.

50. Gatzka CD, Cameron JD, Kingwell BA, et al. Relation between coronary
    artery disease, aortic stiffness and left ventricular structure in a popula-
    tion sample. Hypertension 1998;32:575–578.

51. Gennari C, Nami R, Pavese G, et al. Calcium-channel blockade (nitrendi-
    pine) in combination with ACE inhibition (captopril) in the treatment of
    mild to moderate hypertension. Cardiovasc Drugs Ther 1989;3:319–325.

52. Gibbons GH, Dzau VJ. Angiotensin converting enzyme inhibition and
    vascular hypertrophy in hypertension. Cardiovasc Drugs Therap
    1990;4:237–242.

53. Gohlke P, Linz W, Scholkens BA, et al. Angiotensin-converting enzyme
    inhibition improves cardiac function. Hypertension 1994;23:411–418.

54. Gohlke P, Pees C, Unger T. AT_2 receptor stimulation increases aortic cyc-
    lic GMP in SHRSP rats by a kinin-dependent mechanism. Hypertension
    1998;31 (part 2):349–355.

55. Gosse P, Roudaut R, Herrero G, et al. Beta-blockers vs angiotensin-con-
    verting enzyme inhibitors in hypertension: effects on left ventricular hy-
    pertrophy. J Cardiovasc Pharmacol 1990;16:S145–S150.

56. Gottdiener JS, Reda DJ, Massie BM, et al. Effect of single-drug therapy
    on reduction of left ventricular mass in mild to moderate hypertension.
    Circulation 1997;95:2007–2014.

57. Gottdiener JS, Reda DJ, Williams DW, et al. For the VA Cooperative
    Study Group on Antihypertensive Agents. Effect of single-drug therapy
    on reduction of left ventricular size in mild to moderate hypertension.
    Comparison of six antihypertensive agents. Circulation 1998;98:140–148.

58. Gradman AH, Arcuri KE, Goldberg AI, et al. A randomized, placebo-
    controlled, double-blind, parallel study of various doses of losartan po-
    tassium compared with enalpril maleate in patients with essential hyper-
    tension. Hypertension 1995;25:1345–1350.

59. Grandi AM, Venco A, Barzizza A, et al. Double-blind comparison of
    perindopril and captopril in hypetension. Effects on left ventricular mor-
    phology and function. Am J Hypertens 1991;4:516–520.

60. Grandi AM, Venco A, Barzizza F, et al. Effect of enalapril on left ventri-
    cular mass and performance in essential hypertension. Am J Cardiol
    1989;63:1093–1097.

61. Grassi G, Turri C, Dell'Oro R, et al. Effect of chronic angiotensin convert-
    ing enzyme inhibition on sympathetic nerve traffic and baroreflex control

of the circulation in essential hypertension. J Hypertens 1998;16:1789–1796.

62. Grimm RH, Grandits GA, Prineas RJ, et al. Long-term effects on sexual function of five antihypertensive drugs and nutritional hygienic treatment in hypertensive men and women. Treatment of Mild Hypertension Study (TOMHS). Hypertension 1997;29:8-14.

63. Grossman E, Messerli FH, Grodzicki T, et al. Should a moratorium be placed on sublingual nifedipine capsules given for hypertensive emergencies and pseudoemergencies. JAMA 1996;276:1328–1331.

64. Guazzi MD, Cesare ND, Galli C. Calcium-channel blockade with nifedipine and angiotensin converting enzyme inhibition with captopril in the therapy of patients with severe primary hypertension. Circulation 1984;70:279–284.

65. Hafizi S, Wharton J, Morgan K, et al. Expression of functional angiotensin-converting enzyme and AT_1 receptors in cultured human cardiac fibroblasts. Circulation 1998;98:2553–2559.

66. Haider AW, Larson MG, Benjamin EJ, et al. Increased left ventricular mass and hypertrophy are associated with increased risk for sudden death. J Am Coll Cardiol 1998;32:1454–1459.

67. Harada K, Komuro I, Hayashi D, et al. Angiotensin II type 1a receptor is involved in the occurrence of reperfusion arrhythmias. Cirulation 1998;97:315–317.

68. Harrap SB, Dominiczak AF, Fraser R, et al. Plasma angiotensin II, predispostion to hypertension, and left ventricular size in healthy young adults. Circulation 1996;93:1148–1154.

69. Harrap SB, Mitchell GA, Casely DJ, et al. Angiotensin-II, sodium and cardiovascular hypertrophy in spontaneously hypertensive rats. Hypertension 1993;21:50–55.

70. Helgeland A, Strommen R, Hagelund CH, et al. Enalapril, atenolol and hydrochlorothiazide in mild to moderate hypertension. A comparative multicentre study in general practice in Norway. Lancet 1986;1986:872–875.

71. Herpin D, Vaisse B, Pitiot M, et al. Comparison of angiotensin-converting enzyme inhibitors and calcium antagonists in the treatment of mild to moderate systemic hypertension, according to baseline ambulatory blood pressure level. Am J Cardiol 1992;69:923–926.

72. Hirsch A, Talsness C, Schunkert H, et al. Tissue-specific activation of cardiac angiotensin converting enzyme in experimental heart failure. Circ Res 1991;69:475–482.

73. Hollenberg N. Medical therapy of renovascular hypertension: efficacy and safety of captopril in 269 patients. Cardiovasc Rev Rep 1983;4:852–876.

74. Hollenberg NK, Meggs LG, Williams GH, et al. Sodium intake and renal responses to captopril in normal man and in essential hypertension. Kidney Int 1981;20:240–245.

75. Holmer SR, Hense H-W, Danser AHJ, et al. ß-adrenergic blockers lower renin in patients treated with ACE inhibitors and diuretics. Heart 1998;80:45–48.

76. HOT Study. Hansson L, Zanchetti A, Carruthers SG, et al. Effects of intensive blood-pressure lowering and low-dose aspirin in patients with hypertension: principal results of the Hypertension Optimal Treatment (HOT) randomised trial. Lancet 1998;351:1755–1762.

77. Hunt SC, Cook NR, Oberman A, et al. Angiotensinogen genotype, sodium reduction, weight loss, and prevention of hypertension. Trials of hypertension prevention, phase II. Hypertension 1998;32:393–401.

78. Ito H, Hirata Y, Adachi M, et al. Endothelin-1 is an autocrine/paracrine factor in the mechanism of angiotensin II-induced hypertrophy in cultured rat cardiomyocytes. J Clin Invest 1993;92:398–403.

79. Jalil JE, Janicki JS, Weber KT. Coronary vascular remodeling and myocardial bribrosis in the rat with renovascular hypertension. Response to captopril. Am J Hypertens 1991;4:51–55.

80. Jenkins AC, Deslinski GR, Tadross SS, et al. Captopril in hypertension: seven years later. J Cardiovasc Pharmacol 1985;7:S96—S101.

81. Jenkins AC, McKinstry DN. Review of clinical studies of hypertensive patients treated with captopril. Med J Aust 1979;2:32–37.

82. Jennings G, Wong J. Regression of left ventricular hypertrophy in hypertension: changing patterns with successive meta-analyses. J Hypertens 1998;16 (suppl 6):S29–S34.

83. JNC VI. Joint National Committee on Prevention, Detection, Evaluation and Treatment of High Blood Pressure. The Sixth Report of the Joint National Committee on Prevention, Detection, Evaluation and Treatment of High Blood Pressure. Arch Intern Med 1997;157:2413–2446.

84. Julien J, Dufluoux M-A, Prasquier R, et al. Effects of captopril and minoxidil on left ventricular hypertrophy in resistant hypertensive patients: A 6-month double-blind comparison. Am Coll Cardiol 1990;16:137–142.

85. Kaplan N, Opie L. Antihypertensive Drugs. In: Opie L, ed. Drugs for the Heart. Philadelphia: W B Saunders Co, 1995.

86. Kaplan NM. Renin profiles. The unfulfilled promises. JAMA 1977;238:611–613.

87. Katz AM. Cardiomyopathy of overload. A major determinant of prognosis in congestive heart failure. N Eng J Med 1990;322:100–110.

88. Khairallah PA, Kanabus J. Angiotensin and myocardial protein synthesis. In: Tarazi RC, Dunbar JB, eds. Perspectives in Cardiovascular Research. New York: Raven Press, 1983 (vol 8) pp 337–347.

89. Kodama H, Fukuda K, Pan J, et al. Biphasic activation of the JAK/STAT pathway by angiotensin II in rat cardiomyocytes. Circ Res 1998;82:244–250.

90. Koenig W. On behalf of the Multicentre Study Group. Ramipril vs lisinopril in the treatment of mild to moderate primary hypertension – a randomised double-blind multicentre trial. Drug Invest 1992:450–457.

91. Konstam MA, Kronenberg MW, Rousseau MF, et al. SOLVD Investigators. Effects of the angiotensin-converting enzyme inhibitor enalapril on the long-term progression of left ventricular dilatation in patients with asymptomatic systolic dysfunction. Circulation 1993;88:2227–2283.

92. Lacourciere Y, Gagne C. Influence of combination of captopril and hydrochlorothiazide on plasma lipids, lipoproteins and apolipoproteins in primary hypertension. J Human Hypertens 1993;7:149–152.

93. Laragh JH. Issues, goals and guidelines in selecting first-line drug therapy for hypertension. Hypertension 1989;13 (Suppl 1):I-103 – I-112.

94. Leary W, Reyes A. Angiotensin-I converting enzyme inhibitors and the renal excretion of urate. Cardiovasc Drugs Ther 1987;1:29–38.

95. Lee RMKW, Rerecek KH, Tsoporis J, et al. Prevention of hypertension and vascular changes by captopril treatment. Hypertension 1991;17:141–150.

96. Lees KR, Reid JC, Scott MG, et al. Captopril versus perindopril: a double-blind study in essential hypertension. J Human Hypertens 1989;3:17–22.

97. Lever AF. Slow pressor mechanisms in hypertension: a role for hypertrophy of resistance vessels? J Hypertension 1986;4:515–524.

98. Levy BI, Michel JB, Salzmann JL, et al. Arterial effects of angiotensin converting enzyme inhibition in renovascular and spontaneously hypertensive rats. J Hypertens 1988;6 (Suppl 3):S23–S25.

99. Levy BI, Michel JB, Salzmann JL, et al. Effects of chronic converting enzyme inhibition on the structure and function of large arteries in the rat. Clin Exper Ther Prac 1989;All (Suppl 2):487–498.

100. Levy BI, Michel JB, Salzmann JL, et al. Effects of chronic inhibition of converting enzyme on mechanical and structural properties of arteries in rat renovascular hypertension. Cir Res 1988;63:2227–2239.

101. Levy BI, Michel JB, Salzmann JL, et al. Remodeling of heart and arteries by chronic converting enzyme inhibition in spontaneously hypertensive rats. Am J Hypertens 1991;4:240S–245S.

102. Levy BI, Michel JB, Sazmann JL, et al. Long-term effects of angiotensin-converting enzyme inhibition on the arterial wall of adult spontaneously hypertensive rats. Am J Cardiol 1993;71:8E–16E.

103. Levy D, Garrison RJ, Savage DD, et al. Prognostic implications of echocardiographically determined left ventricular mass in the Framingham heart study. N Engl J Med 1990;322:1561–1566.

104. Lewis E, Hunsicker L, Bain R, et al. For the Collaborative Study Group. The effect of angiotensin-converting enzyme inhibition on diabetic nephropathy. N Engl J Med 1993;329:1456–1462.

105. Lewis RA, Baker KM, Ayers CR, et al. Captopril versus enalapril maleate: a comparison of antihypertensive and hormonal effects. J Cardiovasc Pharmacol 1985;7 (Suppl 1):S12–S15.

106. Li JS, Touyz RH, Schiffrin E. Effects of AT_1 and AT_2 angiotensin receptor antagonists in angiotensin II-infused rats. Hypertension 1998;31 (part 2):487–492.

107. Liao JK, Bettmann MA, Sandor T, et al. Differential impairment of vasodilator responsiveness of peripheral resistance and conduit vessels in humans with atherosclerosis. Circ Res 1991;68:1027–1034.

108. Lievre M, Gueret P, Gayet C, et al. On behalf of the HYCAR Study Group. Ramipril-induced regression of left ventricular hypertrophy in treated hypertensive idividuals. Hypertension 1995;25:92–97.

109. Lindpainter K, Ganten D. The cardiac renin-angiotensin system. An appraisal of present experimental and clinical evidence. Circ Res 1991;68:905–921.

110. Lindpainter K, Lu W, Niedermajer N, et al. Distribution and functional significance of cardiac angiotensin converting enzyme in hypertrophied rat hearts. J Moll Cell Cardiol 1993;25:133–143.

111. Liu J-L, Murakami H, Zucker IH. Angiotensin II-nitric oxide interaction on sympathetic outflow in conscious rabbits. Circ Res 1998;82:496–502.

112. Liu Y-H, Yang Z-P, Sharov VG, et al. Effects of angiotensin-converting enzyme inhibitors and angiotensin II type I receptor antagonists in rats with heart failure. J Clin Invest 1997;99:1926–1935.

113. Lyons D, Roy S, O'Byrne S, et al. ACE Inhibition. Postsynaptic adrenergic sympatholytic action in men. Circulation 1997;96:911–915.

114. MacGregor G, Markandu N, Banks R, et al. Captopril in essential hypertension; contrasting effects of adding hydrochlorothiazide or propranolol. Br Med J 1982;284:693–696.

115. MacGregor GA, Markandu ND, Singer DA, et al. Moderate sodium restriction with angiotensin converting enzyme inhibitor in essential hypertension: a double blind study. Br Med J 1987;294:531–534.

116. Man in't Veld AJ, J WG, H SMAD. Does captopril lower blood pressure in anephric patients? Br Med J 1979;ii:1110.

117. Manolis AJ, Beldekos D, Handanis S, et al. Comparison of spirapril, isradipine, or combination in hypertensive patients with left ventricular hypertrophy. Am J Hypertens 1998;11:640–648.

118. Materson BJ, Reda DJ, Cushman WC, et al. Single-drug therapy for hypertension in men. A comparison of six antihypertensive agents with placebo. N Engl J Med 1993;328:914–469.

119. McEwan PE, Gray GA, Sherry L, et al. Differential effects of angiotensin II on cardiac cell proliferation and intramyocardial perivascular fibrosis in vivo. Circulation 1998;98:2765–2773.

120. McKenna TJ, Sequeira SJ, Heffernan A, et al. Diagnosis under random conditions of all disorders of the renin-angiotensin-aldosterone axis, including primary hyperaldosteronism. J Clin Endocrinol Metab 1991;73:952–957.

121. Meggs LG, Coupet J, Huang H, et al. Regulation of angiotensin II receptors on ventricular myocytes after myocardial infarction in rats. Circ Res 1993;72:1149–1162.

122. Meredith PA, Donnelly R, Elliott HL. Prediction of the antihypertensive response to enalapril. J Hypertens 1990;8:1085–1090.

123. Michel J-B. Relationship between decrease in afterload and beneficial effects of ACE inhibitors in experimental cardiac hypertrophy and congestive heart failure. Eur Heart J 1990;11 (Suppl D):17–26.

124. Michel JB, Plissonier D, Bruneval P. Effect of perindopril on the immune arterial wall remodeling in the rat model of arterial graft rejection. Am J Med 1992;92 (Suppl 4B):39S–46S.

125. Middlemost SJ, Sack M, Davis J. Effects of long acting nifedipine on casual office blood pressure measurements, 24 hour ambulatory blood pressure profiles, exercise parameters and left ventricular mass and funciton in black patients with mild to moderate systemic hypertension. Am J Cardiol 1992;70:474–478.

126. Miyazaki Y, Hirata A, Murakami H, et al. Effects of aging on the insulin actions for the glucose metabolism and renal function in normotensives and essential hypertensives. Am J Hypertens 1998;11:1056–1064.

127. Modena MG, Mattioli AV, Parato VM, et al. effectiveness of the antihypertensive action of lisinopril on left ventricular mass and diastolic filling. Eur Heart J 1992;13:1540–1544.

128. Moreau P, d'Uscio LV, Shaw S, et al. Angiotenin II increases tissue endothelin and induces vascular hypertrophy. Circulation 1997;96:1593–1597.

129. Morgan T, Anderson A. Clinical efficacy of perindopril in hypertension. Pharmacol Physiol 1992;19:61–65.

130. Morlin C, Baglivo H, Boeijinga JK, et al. Comparative trial of lisinopril and nifedipine in mild to severe essential hypertension. J Cardiovasc Pharmacol 1987;9:S48–S52.

131. Mroczek W, Finnerty F, Catt K. Lack of association between plasmarenin and history of heart attack or stroke in patients with essential hypertension. Lancet 1973;2:464–469.

132. Muiesan ML, Ababiti-Rosei E, Romanelli G, et al. Beneficial effects of one year's treatment with captopril on left ventricular anatomy and function in hypertensive patients with left ventricular hypertrophy. Am J Med 1988;84 (Suppl 3A):129.

133. Mukherjee D, Sen S. Alteration of cardiac collagen phenotypes in hypertensive hypertrophy: role of blood pressure. J Moll Cell Cardiol 1993;25:185–196.

134. Muller G, Weid S. The sulfonylurea drug, glimepiride, stimulates glucose transport, glucose transporter translocation, and dephosphorylation in insulin-resistant rat adipocytes in vivo. Diabetes 1993;42:1852–1867.

135. Mulvany MJ, Hansen PK, Aalkjaer C. Direct evidence that the greater contractility of resistance vessels in spontaneously hypertensive rats is associated with a narrowed lumen, a thickened media, and an increased number of smooth muscle. Circ Res 1978;43:854–864.

136. Murasawa S, Mori Y, Nozawa Y, et al. Angiotensin II type 1 receptor-induced extracellular signal-regulated protein kinase activation is

mediated by Ca^{2+}/calmodulin-dependent transactivation of epidermal growth factor receptor. Circ Res 1998;82:1338–1348.

137. Namba T, Tsutsui H, Tagawa H, et al. Regulation of fibrillar collagen gene expression and protein accumulation in volume-overloaded cardiac hypertrophy. Circulation 1997;95:2448–2454.

138. Nickenig G, Roling J, Strehlow K, et al. Insulin induces upregulation of vascular AT_1 receptor gene expression by postranscriptional mechanisms. Circulation 1998;98:2543–2460.

139. Noll G, Wenzel R, de Marchi S, et al. Differential effects of captopril and nitrates on muscle sympathetic nerve activity in volunteers. Circulation 1997;95:2286–2292.

140. Nunez E, Hosoya K, Susic D, et al. Enalapril and losartan reduced cardiac mass and improved coronary hemodynamics in SHR. Hypertension 1997;29:519–524.

141. Ohkubo N, Matsubara H, Nozawa Y, et al. Angiotensin type II receptors are reexpressed by cardiac fibroblasts from failing myopathic hamster hearts and inhibit cell growth and fibrillar collagen metabolism. Circulation 1997;96:3954–3962.

142. Omvik P, Lund-Johansen P. Long-term hemodynamic effects at rest and during exercise of newer antihypertensive agents and salt restriction in essential hypertension: review of epanolol, doxazosin, amlodipine, felodipine, diltiazem, lisinopril, dilevalol, carvedilol, and ketanserin. Cardiovasc Drugs Ther 1993;7:191–206.

143. Pahor M, Bernabei R, Sgadari A, et al. Enalapril prevents cardiac fibrosis and arrhythmias in hypertensive rats. Hypertension 1991;18:148–157.

144. Pannier B, Garabedian V, Madonna O, et al. Lisinopril versus atenolol: decrease in systolic versus diastolic blood pressure with converting enzyme inhibition. Cardiovasc Drugs Ther 1991;5:775–782.

145. Perry I, Beevers D. ACE inhibitors compared with thiazide diuretics as first-step antihypertensive therapy. Cardiovasc Drugs Ther 1989;3:815–819.

146. Pollare T, Lithell H, Berne C. A comparison of the effects of hydrochlorothiazide and captopril on glucose and lipid metabolism in patients with hypertension. N Eng J Med 1989;321:868–873.

147. Pool J, Gennari J, Goldstein R, et al. Controlled multicentre study of antihypertensive effects of lisinopril, hydrochlorothiazide and lisinopril plus hydrochlorothiazide in the treatment of 394 patients with mild to moderate essential hypertension. J Cardiovasc Pharmacol 1987;9:S36–S42.

148. Pool JL, Cushman WC, Saini RK, et al. Use of the factorial design and quadratic response surface models to evaluate the fosinopril and hydrochlorothiazide combination therapy in hypertension. Am J Hypertens 1997;10:117–123.

149. Przyklenk K, Kloner R. Acute effects of hydralazine and enalapril on contractile function of postischemic "stunned" myocardium. Am J Cardiol 1987;60:934–936.

150. RACE Study, Agabati-Rosei E, Ambrosioni E, Palu CD, et al. On behalf of the RACE Study Group. ACE inhibitor ramipril is more effective than the β-blocker atenolol in reducing left ventricular mass in hypertension. Results of the RACE (Ramipril Cardioprotective Evaluation) study. J Hypertens 1995;13:1325–1334.

151. Randall OS, Bos GCvd, Westerhof N. Systemic compliance: does it play a role in the genesis of essential hypertension? Cardiovasc Res 1984; 18:455–462.

152. Remme WJ, Kruyssen DA, Look MP, et al. Systemic and cardiac neuroendocrine activation and severity of myocardial ischemia in humans. J Am Coll Cardiol 1994;23:82–91.

153. Ritchie RH, Marsh JD, Lancaster WD, et al. Bradykinin blocks angiotensin II-induced hypertrophy in the presence of endothelial cells. Hypertension 1998;31 (part 1):39–44.

154. Roberts D, Tsao Y, McLoughlin G, et al. Placebo-controlled comparison of captopril, atenolol, labetalol, and pindolol in hypertension complicated by intermittent claudication. Lancet 1987;2:650–653.

155. Rogers TB. High affinity angiotensin-II receptors in myocardial sarcolemmal membranes. Characterization of receptors and covalent linkage of[125]I-angiotensin-II to a membrane component of 116,000 daltons. J Biol Chem 1984;259:8106–8114.

156. Ruskoaho HJ, Savolainen E-R. Effects of long-term verapamil treatment on blood pressure, cardiac hypertrophy and collagen metabolism in spontaneously hypertensive rats. Cardiovasc Res 1985;19:355–362.

157. Ruzicka M, Yuan B, Harmsen E, et al. The renin-angiotensin system and volume overload-induced cardiac hypertrophy in rats. Effects of angiotensin-converting enzyme inhibitor versus angiotensin-II receptor blocker. Circulation 1993;87:921–930.

158. Sadoshima J-I, Izumo S. Signal transduction pathways of angiotensin II-induced c-fos gene expression in cardiac mycytes in vitor. Roles of phospholipid-derived second messengers. Circ Res 1993;73:424–438.

159. Sadoshima K, Xu Y, Slayter HS, et al. Autocrine release of angiotensin-II mediates stretch-induced hypertrophy of cardiac myocytes in vitro of cardiac myoctyes in vitro. Cell 1993;75:977–984.

160. Safar M. Therapeutic trials and large arteries in hypertension. Am Heart J 1988;115:702–710.

161. Safar ME, London GM. Arterial and venous compliance in sustained essential hypertension. Hypertension 1987;10:133–139.

162. Salvetti A, Arzilli F. Chronic dose-response curve of enalapril in essential hypertensives. An Italian multicenter study. Am J Hypertens 1989;2:352–354.

163. Sanchez RA, Marco E, Gilbert HB, et al. Natriuretic effect and changes in renal haemodymics induced by enalapril in essential hypertension. Drugs 1985;30 (Suppl 1):49–58.

164. Sassano P, Chatellier G, Billaud E, et al. Comparison of increase in the enalapril dose and addition of hydrochlorothiazide as second-step treatment of hypertensive patients not controlled by analapril alone. J Cardiovasc Pharmacol 1989;13:314–319.

165. Savage D, Watkins L, Grim C, et al. Hypertension in black populations. In: Laragh J, Brenner B, eds. Hypertension, Pathophysiology, Diagnosis, and Management. New York: Raven Press, 1990.

166. Sawa H, Tokuchi F, Mochizuki N. Expression of the angiotensinogen gene and localization of its protein in the human heart. Circulation 1992;86:138–146.

167. Schelling P, Fischer H, Ganten D. Angiotensin and cell growth: a link to cardiovascular hypertrophy? J Hypertens 1991;9:3-15.

168. Schmieder RE, Martus P, Klingbeil A. Reversal of left ventricular hypertrophy in essential hypertension. JAMA 1996;275:1507–1513.

169. Schneider E, Jennings AA, Opie LH. Captopril, nifedipine and their combination for therapy of hypertensive urgencies. S Afr Med J 1991;80:265–270.

170. Schulte K-L, Meyer-Sabellek W, Liederwald K, et al. Relation of regression of left ventricular hypertrophy to changes in ambulatory blood pressure after long-term therapy with perindopril versus nifedipine. Am J Cardiol 1992;70:468–473.

171. Schunkert H, Dzau VJ, Tang SS, et al. Increased rat cardiac angiotensin-converting enzyme activity and mRNA expression in pressure overload left ventricular hypertrophy. J Clin Invest 1990;86:1913–1920.

172. Schunkert H, Jackson B, Tang S, et al. Distribution and functional significance of cardiac angiotensin converting enzyme in hypertrophied rat hearts. Circulation 1993;87:1328–1339.

173. Scicli AG. Increases in cardiac kinins as a new mechanism to protect the heart. Hypertension 1994; 23:419–421.

174. Shahi M, Thom S, Poulter N, et al. Regression of hypertensive function. Lancet 1990;336:458–461.

175. Singer D, Markandu N, Shore A, et al. Captopril and nifedipine in combination for moderate to severe essential hypertension. Hypertension 1987;9:629–633.

176. Singer D, Markandu N, Sugden A, et al. Sodium restriction in hypertensive patients treated with a converting enzyme inhibitor and a thiazide. Hypertension 1991;17:798–803.

177. Soininen K, Gerlin-Piira L, Suihkonen J, et al. A study of the effects of lisinopril when used in addition to atenolol. J Human Hypertens 1992;6:321–324.

178. Stoll M, Steckelings UM, Paul M, et al. The angiotensin AT_2-receptor mediates inhibition of cell proliferation in coronary endothelial cells. J Clin Invest 1995;95:651–657.

179. Stumpe KO. Overlack A on behalf of the Perindopril Therapeutic Safety Study Groups (PLUTS). A new trial of the efficacy, tolerability and safety of angiotensin-converting enzyme inhibition in mild systemic hypertension with concomitant diseases and therapies. Am J Cardiol 1993;71:32E–37E.

180. Syst-Eur Trial. Staessen JA, Fagard R, Thijs L, et al. Randomised double-blind comparison of placebo and active treatment for older patients with isolated systolic hypertension (Syst-Eur Trial). Lancet 1997;350:754–764.

181. Tan L-B, Jalil JE, Pick R, et al. Cardiac myocyte necrosis induced by angiotensin-II. Circ Res 1991;69:1185–1195.

182. Thind GS, Johnson A, Bhatnagar D, et al. A parallel study of enalapril and captopril and 1 year of experience with enalapril treatment in moderate-to-severe essential hypertension. Am Heart J 1985;109:852–858.

183. Todd PA, Benfield P. Ramipril. A review of its pharmacological properties and therapeutic efficacy in cardiovascular disorders. Drugs 1990;1:110–135.

184. TOMH Study. Treatment of Mild Hypertension Research Group (TOMH). The treatment of mild hypertension study. A randomized, pla-

cebo-controlled trial of a nutritional-hygenic regimen along with various drug monotherapies. Arch Intern Med 1991;151:1413–1423.

185. TOMH Study, Neaton JD, Grimm RH, Prineas RJ, et al. Treatment of Mild Hypertension study (TOMH). Final results. JAMA 1993;270:713–724.

186. Tomita H, Egashira K, Ohara Y, et al. Early induction of transforming growth factor-ß via angiotensin II type 1 receptors contributes to cardiac fibrosis induced by long-term blockade of nitric oxide synthesis in rats. Hypertension 1998;32:273–279.

187. Tschollar W, Belz G. Sublingual captopril in hypertensive crises (Letter). Lancet 1985;2:34–35.

188. Tsutsumi Y, Mtasubara H, Ohkubo N, et al. Angiotensin II type 2 receptor is upregulated in human heart with interstitial fibrosis, and cardiac fibroblasts are the major cell type for its expression. Circ Res 1998;83:1035–1046.

189. UKPDS Study. UK Prospective Diabetes Study Group. Efficacy of atenolol and captopril in reducing risk of macrovascular and microvascular complications in type 2 diabetes: UKPDS 39. BMJ 1998;317:713–20.

190. Unger T, Mattfeldt T, Lamberty V, et al. Effect of early onset angiotensin-converting enzyme inhibition on myocardial capillaries. Hypertension 1992;20:478–482.

191. Urata H, Healy B, Stewart R, et al. Angiotensin-II receptors in normal and failing human hearts. J Clin Endocrinol Metab 1989;69:54–66.

192. Urata H, Kinoshita A, Perez DM. Cloning of the gene and cDNA for human heart chymase. J Biol Chem 1991;266:17173-17179.

193. Vaur L, Dutrey-Dupagne C, Boussac J, et al. Differential effects of a missed dose of trandolapril and enalapril on blood pressure control in hypertensive patients. J Cardiovasc Pharmacol 1995;26:127–131.

194. Veterans Administration Cooperative Study Group on Antihypertensive Agents. Captopril: evaluation of low doses, twice-daily doses and the addition of diuretic for the treatment of mild to moderate hypertension. Clin Sci 1982;14:127–131.

195. Vidt D. A controlled multiclinic study to compare the antihypertensive effects of MK-421, hydrochlorothiazide, and MK-421 combined with hydrochlorothiazide in patients with mild to moderate essential hypertension. J Hypertens 1984;2:227–233.

196. von Lutterotti N, Catanzaro DF, Sealey JE, et al. Renin is not synthesized by cardiac and extrarenal vascular tissues. A review of experimental evidence. Circulation 1994;89:458–470.

197. Walker JF, Kulaga SF, Kramsch DM. The efficacy and safety of enalapril in moderate to severe essentila hypertension. J Hypertens 1984;2 (Suppl 2):107–111.

198. Wang D-H, Prewitt RL. Captopril reduces aortic and microvascular growth in hypertensive and normotensive rats. Hypertension 1990;15:68–77.

199. Weber KT. Extracellular matrix remodeling in heart failure. A role for de novo angiotensin II generation. Circulation 1997;96:4065–4082.

200. Weber KT, Brilla CG. Pathological hypertrophy and cardiac interstitium. Fibrosis and renin-angiotensin-aldosterone system. Circulation 1991;83:1849–1865.

201. Weber KT, Sun Y, Tyagi SC, et al. Collagen network of the myocardium: function, structural remodeling and regulatory mechanisms. J Mol Cell Cardiol 1994;26:279–292.

202. Webster J. Interactions of NSAIDs with diuretics and β-blockers: mechanism and clinical implications. Drugs 1985;30:32–41.

203. Weir MR, Gray JM, Paster R, et al. Differing mechanisms of action of angiotensin-converting enzyme inhibition in black and white hypertensive patients. Hypertension 1995;25:124–130.

204. Whelton A, Dunne B, Glazer N, et al. Twenty-four hour blood pressure effect of once-daily lisinopril, enalapril, and placebo in patients with mild to moderate hypertension. J Human Hypertens 1992;6:325–331.

205. WHO-ISH Committee. World Health Organization-International Society of Hypertension Guidelines for the Management of Hypertension. J Hypertens 1999;17:151–183.

206. Williams GH. Converting-enzyme inhibitors in the treatment of hypertension. N Engl J Med 1988;319:1517–1525.

207. Wilson SK, Solez K, Boitnott JK, et al. The effects of heparin treatment on hypertension and vascular lesions in stroke-prone spontaneously hypertensive rats. Am J Pathol 1981;102:62–71.

208. Wolinsky H. Effects of hypertension and its reversal on the thoracic aorta of male and female rats. Circ Res 1971;28:622–637.

209. Yang BC, Phillips MI, Zhang YC, et al. Critical Role of AT$_1$ receptor expression after ischemia/reperfusion in isolated rat hearts. Beneficial effect of antisense oligodeoxynucleotides directed at AT$_1$ receptor mRNA. Circ Res 1998;83:552–559.

210. Yodfat Y, Cristal N. On behalf of the LOMIR^R-MCT-IL research group. A multicenter, double-blind, randomized, placebo-controlled study of isradipine and methyldopa as monotherapy or in combination with captopril in the treatment of hypertension. Am J Hypertens 1993;6:57S–61S.
211. Zanchetti A. A re-examination of stepped-care: a retrospective and a prospective. J Cardiovasc Pharmacol 1985;1:S126–S131.
212. Zanchetti A, Bond MG, Hennig M, et al. Risk factors associated with alterations in carotid intima-media thickness in hypertension: baseline data from the European Lacidipine Study on Atherosclerosis. J Hypertens 1998;16:949–961.

CHAPTER 4

ACE Inhibitors
and the kidney

*''Microalbuminuria predicts cardiovascular events and
renal insufficiency in patients with essential hypertension''
– Bigazzi et al (1998)[4]*

ANGIOTENSIN II AND RENAL PHYSIOLOGY

Localization of Angiotensin (AT) receptors. Autoradiography shows that the *AT-I receptor* is localized in (1) vascular tissue, in the afferent and efferent glomerular arterioles;
(2) in the proximal tubular epithelium; (3) in the mesangial
cells of the glomerulus; and (4) in the medullary interstitial
cells.[56] The first two locations are thought to relate to the
role of A-II in controlling sodium balance and blood volume. The later two sites may have a common function, in
that both types of cells are capable of secreting extracellular
matrix in response to A-II, which could result in the formation of fibrosis in chronic renal disease.[56] The *AT-2 receptor*
is abundant in human preglomerular blood vessels and of
unknown function.

Renal hemodynamic effects of angiotensin II. The importance of the renal circulation as a potential site of action
of angiotensin-converting enzyme (ACE) inhibitors is now
established. These agents can potentially modulate intraglomerular pressure because it is the angiotensin II receptors
in the proximal part of the renal afferent arterioles that help
to control the intraglomerular filtration pressure, as shown
by Edwards[15] who infused angiotensin II into isolated renal
microvessels. The glomerular filtration pressure is the result
of the balance between the preglomerular and postglomerular arterial tone (Fig 4-1). Thus, the relative degree of constriction or relaxation of efferent and afferent arterioles
regulates the filtration pressure and the amount of protein
excreted.[1] Experimental evidence favoring differential regulation of preglomerular and postglomerular arterial tone is
provided by measurements of renal vascular resistance in
dogs.[41] This normal balance between afferent and efferent
arteriolar control can be altered in diseased states. The crucial event leading to microalbuminuria is an increase of the
intraglomerular filtration pressure, and the long term threat
is glomerular closure (Fig 4-2).

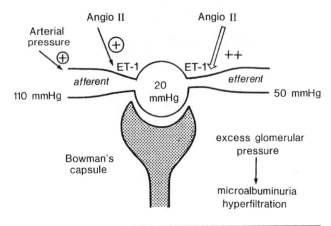

Figure 4-1. Schema for control of intraglomerular pressure by relative degrees of afferent and efferent arteriolar constriction. ET-1 = endothelin-1 Figure © LH Opie, 1999

In experimental hypertension, an increase in the preglomerular capillary resistance can protect the glomerulus from the increased systemic pressure.[1] This mechanism should lessen hypertensive microalbuminuria, which however occurs very early in the disease.[4] Presumably the hypertensive process causes glomerular damage. In renal disease, including diabetic nephropathy, there is also an increase in intraglomerular pressure with microalbuminuria or even proteinuria. A major effect of angiotensin II is promotion of efferent arteriolar vasoconstriction, so that therapy by ACE inhibition could be expected to benefit those conditions in which there is intraglomerular hypertension or glomerular damage, as in diabetes mellitus (Chapter 11).

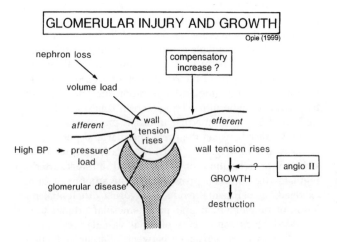

Figure 4-2. Glomerular injury with an increased intraglomerular pressure can evoke mesanginal growth with threat of complete glomerular closure. Angiotensin II may be an important growth signal. Figure © LH Opie, 1999

Effect of angiotensin II on sodium balance and potential natriuretic effect of ACE inhibitors. The effects of angiotensin II on the handling of sodium by the kidney can ultimately be traced to three different mechanisms (Fig 4-3). First, there is the relatively well-known stimulation of the release of aldosterone by angiotensin II. Second, there is an important effect of angiotensin II on the renal sodium pump; angiotensin II is thought to stimulate this pump to enhance the reabsorption of sodium by the kidney and, hence, to promote sodium retention.[52] Third, there may be an interaction with insulin-induced reabsorption.

First, in conditions in which aldosterone is thought to contribute to sodium retention, such as congestive heart failure, inhibition of its formation following ACE inhibition should lead to a diuretic effect. Nonetheless, various studies with captopril and other ACE inhibitors have not shown a consistent diuretic effect either in hypertensives or in those with heart failure. In contrast, the addition of an aldosterone antagonist can produce remarkable benefit, as shown in the RALES trial (page 141). It may, therefore, be proposed that ACE inhibitors do not consistently exhibit a net natriuretic effect, because of incomplete inhibition of aldosterone secretion. Furthermore, *the potential natriuretic effect of the ACE inhibitor is dependent on the state of sodium loading.* When there is a low sodium load, which calls forth a compensatory stimulation of renin secretion and, hence, formation of angiotensin II and aldosterone, then ACE inhibitors are more likely to have a diuretic effect.

Second, angiotensin II at physiological levels has an anti-

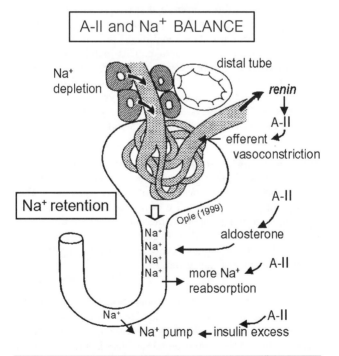

Figure 4-3. Mechanisms whereby angiotensin II (A-II) promotes sodium retention. The physiological role is to retain sodium in responsive to sodium depletion. Figure © LH Opie, 1999

natriuretic effect by increasing sodium reabsorption in the proximal tubules.[32] Third, an interaction with insulin is suggested, because ACE inhibition lessens the sodium-retaining effect of hyperinsulinemia.[40] This effect of insulin on sodium reabsorption may in part mediated by increased activity of the renal sodium pump. Besides the effects on efferent arterioles and sodium balance, angiotensin II has vasoconstrictive effects on the blood vessels and vasa recta.[8] Decreased plasma flow will decrease sodium reabsorption. It also causes contraction of the mesangial cells of the glomerulus[8] with risk of fibrosis and permanent renal damage.[56] Thus, acting by all these mechanisms, secretion of angiotensin II helps maintain normal renal function, but with potential for adverse effects with excess activity.

Formation of renin and angiotensin II by the kidney. Although a considerable amount of conversion of angiotensin I to angiotensin II occurs in the vascular endothelium of the lung, nonetheless there is also an intrarenal renin system. In the kidney, ACE is found in the vascular endothelium of the juxtaglomerular apparatus and the efferent arterioles, where angiotensin has a prominent vascular effect.[15] Phylogenetic evidence suggests that the intrarenal renin system existed for millions of years before the appearance of amphibia with their lung tissue. The natural question, asked by Hollenberg and Williams,[27] is what the physiological role of this primitive renin-angiotensin system might be. They propose that the intrarenal system is the "original, primitive volume-control apparatus, acting through its strategic intrarenal location to control renal perfusion". These authors propose that people in whom there is a tendency to excess local production of angiotensin II would fail to increase their renal blood flow in response to a large increase in sodium intake. This inability to change the renal vascular responsiveness to angiotensin II has been termed non-modulation (see Fig 1–9, previous edition, page 12) and is thought to correspond to the group of salt-sensitive hypertensive subjects. In such subjects, ACE inhibition restores the renal capacity to handle a sodium load.[27]

Angiotensinogen formation by kidney. The renal tissue content of mRNA for angiotensinogen is increased by a low sodium diet, both in cortical and medullary fractions.[28] This finding supports the existence of a local renal renin-angiotensin system and provides a mechanism for upgrading of the renin-angiotensin system in response to a low salt diet, because the level of angiotensinogen appears to be the rate limiting substrate of the system.

Renal autoregulation and maintenance of glomerular filtration rate. In response to a low perfusion pressure, angiotensin II maintains efferent arteriolar tone.[7] It follows that ACE inhibitors should be administered with caution to those patients who already have a low level of renal perfusion as in severe congestive heart failure or those with bilateral renal artery stenosis (Figs 4-4 to 4-7).

INTRAGLOMERULAR HYPERTENSION AND ACE INHIBITION

Hypertensive renal damage. The prototype experiments for hypertensive renal damage consist of experimental hypertension in which part of one kidney has been removed. There is a corresponding strain on the remaining nephrons, which coupled with the systemic hypertension leads to a intraglomerular hypertension that in turn leads to protein loss, i.e. microalbuminuria. Logically, therefore, it should be possible to lessen renal complications of hypertension in humans by ACE inhibition therapy. Nonetheless, it should be considered that renal end-points have never been studied in large trials of antihypertensive agents, i.e. the only end-points have been stroke and cardiac disease. It seems likely that mild to moderate hypertension is seldom complicated by overt renal failure. Some current studies are using microalbuminuria as a trial end-point. In one study over 36 months, the glomerular filtration rate fell less in patients with essential hypertension treated by an ACE inhibitor than a β-blocker.[24] Thus, the real relation between hypertension and renal glomerular vascular disease is not known. It is possible that the association between renal disease and hypertension frequently found is noted in patients in whom the renal disease had first developed. In contrast, in malignant hypertension, deterioration of renal function follows in the wake of excess accelerated hypertension with fibrinoid necrosis of the renal arterioles.

Pathogenic mechanisms in renal vascular disease. On first principles it might be expected that there could be two major mechanisms for inducing glomerular damage. First, an excess intraluminal pressure could both damage the vessel wall and also induce excess vascular growth (Fig 4–2), thereby endothelium and the setting in train a sequence of events that could end with obliteration of the glomerulus. Second, disease of the glomerular blood vessel wall, even in the presence of a normal intraluminal pressure, could sensitize the glomerulus to what would otherwise be an acceptable intraluminal pressure. An example of the first type of glomerular injury would be one dependent on hypertension. An example of the second type of glomerular injury would be one caused by diabetes mellitus. The combination of the two, as in patients with diabetic nephropathy with hypertension, is particularly likely to cause severe glomerular injury and irreversible damage (Chapter 11).

GLOMERULAR INJURY IN HYPERTENSION

The effects of chronic hypertension on the kidney have been reviewed by Reams and Bauer,[44] and Bauer.[1] In hypertensive renal disease, the renal vascular resistance undergoes a progressive rise as the renal plasma flow falls. On the whole, the glomerular filtration rate is relatively well maintained but falls in about 20% of patients with essential hypertension. Hypertension is a strong risk factor for end-stage renal disease in men.[31] Initially the changes are potentially reversible, presumably reflecting vasocon-striction in response to norepinephrine and angiotensin II. Once structural changes occur, then the process becomes irreversible. A decreased blood flow means that the glomeruli will suffer from ischemia, which brings in its wake the risk of hyaline formation in the capsular space, which is irreversible. There are a number of secondary changes such as tubular atrophy and interstitial fibrosis. Only when changes are severe and generalized does the entire kidney undergo ischemic atrophy.

Experimental glomerular injury and hyperfiltration. The normal adaptation to operative removal of renal mass in rats with spontaneous hypertension is dilation of the afferent arterioles to allow a greater filtration in the remaining glomeruli. Such hyperfiltration is accompanied by glomerular changes that can persist even if the systemic blood pressure is apparently well controlled. Experimentally, ACE inhibitor therapy is better than some other modalities in decreasing the hyperfiltration and the injury score of the glomeruli.[43] In rats with salt-sensitive hypertension, subject also to 5/6 nephrectomy, captopril and a calcium antagonist were equally able to decrease blood pressure but only captopril reduced proteinuria and the glomerular injury score.[51] These data suggest, but of course do not prove, that ACE inhibitor therapy may play a specific role in normalizing intraglomerular hypertension. Thus, the concept would be that ACE inhibitors have a protective effect in averting the hypertrophied hypertensive glomerulus.[14] Even in normotensive rats with renal ablation, ACE inhibitor therapy by perindopril can avert hyperfiltration.[10]

Angiotensin II, endothelin-1 (ET-1), and hyperfiltration. A recent hypothesis is that the hyperfiltration of chronic renal failure may, in part, be due to increased formation of the powerful vasoconstrictor, endothelin-1 (Fig 4–1). In rats with subtotal 5/6 nephrectomy, both captopril and the A-I receptor blocker losartan could prevent the development of proteinuria and lessened the content of ET-1 in the thoracic aorta and preglomerular arteries.[33] Only losartan reduced the content of ET-1 in the glomeruli and in the urine. Thus the ACE inhibitor and the A-I blocker both decreased proteinuria with, however, different effects on endothelin and therefore presumably acting through different mechanisms.

MICROALBUMINURIA

Microalbuminuria in hypertension. The incidence of microalbuminuria in hypertension must vary according to the population studied and the duration and severity of the hypertension. Thus the reported incidence varies from 7% in a relatively large study involving 787 untreated patients[42] to 40% in a smaller series.[3] Such microalbuminuria (Table 4-1) is eventually, over years, associated with a greater risk of

TABLE 4-1. LIMITS OF ALBUMINURIA (PROTEINURIA)

Descriptive Entity	Limits of urinary albumin excretion
Normoalbuminuria	<30 mg per 24 h
Microalbuminuria	30 – 299 mg per 24 h
Macroalbuminuria = proteinuria	300 or more mg per 24 h

cardiovascular events and faster decline in renal function.[4] Tight blood pressure control is needed[18] although there is no proof that decreasing microproteinuria is of specific benefit in avoiding overt renal disease.[45] Several studies suggest that ACE inhibitors have a greater capacity to reduce microalbuminuria than other groups of drugs, despite similar reductions in blood pressure.[3,5,12,23,37]

Microalbuminuria in renal failure. In chronic renal failure, from whatever cause, there is a progressive rise in serum creatinine and fall in glomerular function. An index of the severity of the disease is the degree of proteinuria (Table 4–1). Besides dietary protein restriction, a variety of drugs have been used with apparent benefit: ACE inhibitors, calcium antagonists, and combination drug therapy.[34] Experimentally, ACE inhibitors and calcium antagonists both reduce renal injury by different and possibly additive mechanisms.[14] Clinically, lisinopril but not amlodipine reduced proteinuria, a benefit bought at the cost of a fall in the glomerular filtration rate from 55 to 50 ml per min.[29] In general, the dihydropyridine (DHP) calcium antagonists such as amlodipine are less effective at reducing proteinuria than the non-DHPs such as verapamil.[37]

ROLE OF BRADYKININ

Bradykinin is the crucial vasoactive agent of the vasodilator and natriuretic kallikrein-kinin system (Fig 1–1) that opposes the vasoconstrictor effects of angiotensin II and other constrictors.[36] Bradykinin is generally thought to have a renal vasodilator effect.[55] Furthermore, bradykinin exerts a protective effect against the development of renovascular hypertension, as shown in B_2-receptor knock out mice.[36] In humans, renal blood flow was increased substantially by ACE inhibition, but unexpectedly even more by renin inhibitors or A-I receptor blockers.[26] Possibly the biphasic nature of the response of afferent arterioles to bradykinin may explain some of these results;[55] another possibility is the importance of non-ACE paths for formation of angiotensin II.

RENAL ARTERY STENOSIS AND RENOVASCULAR HYPERTENSION

Typically, renal artery stenosis is suspected in individuals with a relatively high blood pressure, especially if refractory to conventional therapy and sensitive to ACE inhibitors, and with some of the following features: smoking, intermittent claudication, abdominal bruits, and a high plasma renin.[6]

Pathophysiology. The mechanism whereby renal artery stenosis leads to renin-dependent hypertension is well established (Fig 4–4). Increased renin is manufactured in response to a decreased renal arterial pressure. When the rate of renin release is chronically elevated, then manufacture of the renin precursor, *pro-renin,* also increases.[13] In addition, all the other components of the renin-angiotensin system are present in the kidney.[46] Hence, there is an increased intrarenal production of angiotensin II with its many complex effects besides regulation of efferent arteriolar tone.

ACE inhibitor therapy in unilateral renal artery stenosis. Because angiotensin II by efferent arteriolar constriction helps to maintain intraglomerular pressure in the affected kidney in renovascular hypertension, it may be expected on first principles that ACE inhibitor therapy would almost inevitably adversely influence the already compromised renal function,[46] especially in those with pre-existing high renin states such as therapy by high diuretic dose or a very low sodium diet. Hence, ACE inhibitor therapy should be initiated without diuretics in patients on a normal sodium diet. ACE inhibitor therapy will, at the same time, remove the adverse effects of excess circulating angiotensin II on the normal contralateral kidney. Thus, the overall effects of ACE inhibitor therapy can be expected to be beneficial despite the potentially adverse effects on the ischemic kidney.

Indeed, soon after the introduction of ACE inhibitors, it was noted that they were strikingly effective in the therapy of hypertension associated with renal artery stenosis. Preci-

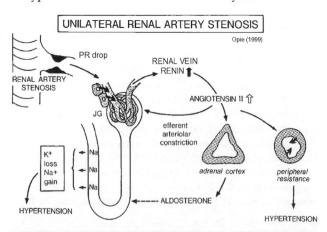

Figure 4-4. In unilateral renal artery stenosis, it is the drop in pressure (PR) that stimulates secretion of renin from the juxtaglomerular (JG) cells to form renin. Increased renin leads to increased circulating angiotensin II, which stimulates aldosterone secretion that in turn promotes hypertension, as does the effect of angiotensin II on the peripheral arterioles. Angiotensin constriction of efferent renal arterioles helps to maintain renal function on the side of the renal artery stenosis. Figure © LH Opie, 1999

pitous falls in blood pressure were also found leading to
the requirement for the more cautious introduction of ACE
inhibitors and of prior low test doses to exclude patients
with excessive hypotension. The response of the hypertension in patients with renal artery stenosis to ACE inhibitor
therapy can be correlated with the response to subsequent
corrective surgery.[50] Debate continues as to whether sustained ACE inhibitor therapy, or surgical correction, or
renal angioplasty is the optimal therapy for renal artery stenosis. Currently, the problem of restenosis following angioplasty is being tackled by stenting, a logical but not yet
well-documented procedure. An important argument is that
if renal artery stenosis is caused by localized atheroma and
is left untreated surgically or by angioplasty, complete renal
artery obstruction may occur with renal atrophy.[22]

ACE inhibitor therapy in bilateral renal artery stenosis.
In the therapy of renal artery stenosis by ACE inhibitors, it
became apparent that a subset of patients, namely those
with bilateral renal artery stenosis, were at high risk of
renal failure upon initiation of ACE inhibitor therapy
(Fig 4-5). This hazard is held to be the result of combined
preglomerular and postglomerular vasodilation. Not all patients with bilateral renal artery stenosis develop irreversible renal failure; reversible failure is also common.
Furthermore, it is possible to treat bilateral renal artery stenosis cautiously by ACE inhibitor therapy without precipitating renal failure, especially if not combined with diuretic
therapy.[53] When acute renal failure occurs upon initiation

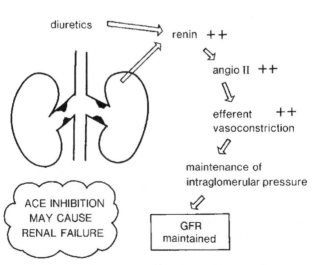

BILATERAL RENAL ARTERY STENOSIS

Opie (1999)

diuretics

renin ++

angio II ++

efferent ++
vasoconstriction

maintenance of
intraglomerular pressure

ACE INHIBITION
MAY CAUSE
RENAL FAILURE

GFR
maintained

Figure 4-5. *In bilateral renal artery stenosis, maintenance of intraglomerular pressure and glomerular-filtration rate (GFR) may be critically dependent on formation of angiotensin II. ACE inhibitor therapy, therefore,
may precipitate renal failure so that this condition is generally a contraindication to therapy by ACE inhibitors, unless cautiously applied and under careful observation. Figure © LH Opie, 1999*

of ACE inhibitor therapy, one of the conditions that must be considered is bilateral renal artery stenosis or, equally probable, renal artery stenosis affecting a solitary kidney.[48] Thus, in the presence of severe renovascular hypertension, ACE inhibitor therapy can permanently interfere with renal autoregulation, with marked initial deterioration and subsequent improvement without full recovery of normality.[2]

Other permutations of severe renovascular hypertension. *Unilateral stenosis in a single functioning kidney* provides a situation very similar to bilateral renal artery stenosis from the functional point of view (Fig 4-6). *After renal transplantation,* renal artery stenosis may also develop. Four patients with stenosis of the transplanted renal artery reacted adversely to the introduction of captopril therapy with acute loss of renal excretory function.[11]

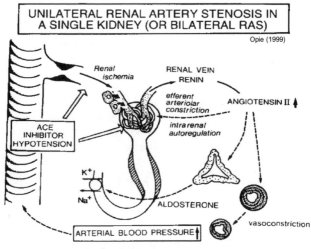

UNILATERAL RENAL ARTERY STENOSIS IN A SINGLE KIDNEY (OR BILATERAL RAS)

Opie (1999)

Figure 4-6. In unilateral renal artery stenosis in a single kidney, as in bilateral artery stenosis (RAS), there is risk of severe renal failure when the compensatory efferent arteriolar constriction is removed. In this condition, as in bilateral renal artery stenosis, intrarenal autoregulation is maintained by the efferent arteriolar constriction. Therefore, again, ACE inhibitor therapy must be started cautiously and under observation, if at all. Usually, ACE inhibitor therapy is contraindicated. Figure © LH Opie, 1999

ACE INHIBITORS IN DIAGNOSIS OF RENOVASCULAR HYPERTENSION

An extension of the above principles lies in diagnostic radiology or diagnostic nuclear renography. Because of the acute effect of ACE inhibition in decreasing renal perfusion to the affected side in renal artery stenosis, acute ACE inhibition by captopril (the quickest acting of the currently available oral agents) results in shunting of blood away from the affected kidney and thereby exaggerating the effects of renal artery stenosis. In this way, borderline isotopic perfusion abnormalities can be magnified and clarified.[39] This procedure is commonly known as the *captopril renogram.* Captopril is used only for its rapidity of action; alternatively, intravenous enalaprilat is suitable and acts even faster.[17] The captopril renogram becomes most sensitive and specific when combined with (1) measurements of plasma renin, a post-captopril increase of >5.7 ng/ml/h being significant, and (2) Doppler duplex examination of the renal arteries.[39] In black patients, however, captopril is not so effective and angiography is the preferred method of diagnosis of renal artery stenosis.[16]

ACE INHIBITORS AND RISK OF ACUTE RENAL IMPAIRMENT

The preceding studies outline the situations in which ACE inhibitor therapy can be expected to lessen renal damage or to prevent the progression of microalbuminuria. Nonetheless, it should be carefully considered that efferent arteriolar vasoconstriction, thought to be basic to the pathogenesis of the microalbuminuria, can be expected to be *beneficial* in certain conditions with activation of the renin-angiotensin system (RAS). These conditions may include excess diuresis, dehydration, severe heart failure, and renal artery stenosis especially when bilateral.[30] In heart failure, it is especially the elderly who are at risk.[54] In these clinical situations, the following sequence may predispose to acute renal failure (ARF):

> Renal ischemia or other stimulus to RAS → renin release angiotensin II formation → efferent arteriolar vasoconstriction → removed by ACE inhibition → decreased intraglomerular filtration pressure → deterioration in renal function with risk of ARF

It is not unexpected that in conditions such as severe cardiac failure in which renal blood flow is diminished, arteriolar efferent vasoconstriction can help maintain renal function. Instances of marked deterioration in renal function in patients with severe heart failure have been shown, particularly in relation to combination therapy of ACE inhibitor and diuretic[19] or in the elderly.[54] In such patients, it is the degree of diuretic-induced sodium depletion and activation of RAS, as well as the ACE inhibitor-induced hypotension that appear to play a major role. The combination of sodium depletion and poor renal perfusion should lead to a greater degree of efferent arteriolar vasoconstriction, a greater dependence on angiotensin II and, therefore, a more marked effect of ACE inhibition in causing deterioration of renal function. In addition, another factor causing potential deterioration of renal function following ACE inhibitor therapy in congestive heart failure is systemic hypotension, one of the major side-effects of this category of drugs (Fig 4-7). In reality, provided that due precautions are undertaken, ACE inhibitor use has been relatively safe in hypertensive patients with renal failure with efficacy shown by reduced progression of renal failure and fewer cardiovascular events.[30]

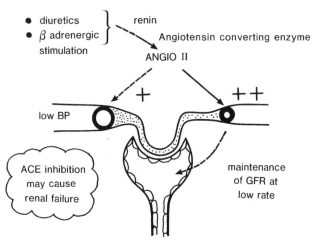

Figure 4-7. In severe congestive heart failure, there is a low renal perfusion pressure that can be further decreased by ACE inhibitor therapy. The danger is precipitation of renal failure, most marked when dealing with a severe sodium depletion state. The mechanism of the potential adverse effects of ACE inhibitors includes relief of the efferent arteriolar constriction that is helping to maintain the intraglomerular pressure. The solution is to give a small test dose of the ACE inhibitor and to avoid excess diuresis. Note preliminary evidence that perindopril may avoid first dose hypotension in heart failure. Figure © LH Opie, 1999

Renal indices and initiation of therapy. Often after the onset of ACE inhibitor therapy for heart failure, there is often a rise in serum creatinine which may cause concern. The standard advice is to avoid ACE inhibitors in patients with a raised serum creatinine. But, how high constitutes a contraindication? The limits set in the various large trials varied substantially, from 2.0 to 3.4 mg per deciliter, and from 177 to 300 μmol per liter.[9,47,49] Dehydration or excess diuresis or severe hyponatremia must all be avoided. Then therapy starts with the smallest effective dose of the ACE inhibitor,[54] and the dose is titrated upwards towards that used in clinical trials, provided that hypotension or an increase in serum creatinine did not occur. In practice small asymptomatic rises of serum creatinine, without precisely defined danger limits, are often accepted. At the other extreme is symptomatic acute renal failure (see section on renal side-effects).

HEMATOLOGICAL ASPECTS OF ACE INHIBITORS AND RENAL FAILURE

First, ACE inhibitors may depress erythrocyte and leukocyte counts. Possibly the anti-proliferative effect is at work. Originally, neutropenia was thought to be a specific complication of captopril therapy, but now a more general hematological effect of all ACE inhibitors as a class seems possible. Thus, there is the entity of anemia induced by

ACE inhibitor use (see Chapter 9), which could exaggerate the anemia that often results from chronic renal failure. Therapeutically, the capacity of ACE inhibitors to reduce hemoglobin is used to treat the erythrocytosis that may follow renal transplantation.[35]

PROGRESSIVE RENAL FAILURE, NOT DIABETIC IN ORIGIN

In progressive renal failure, from whatever cause, there is a steady rise in serum creatinine and fall in glomerular function. Another index of the severity of the disease is the degree of proteinuria. Besides dietary protein restriction, a variety of drugs have been used with apparent benefit: ACE inhibitors with or without diuretics, calcium antagonists, and combination therapy.[34] There is good evidence from a meta-analysis on 1946 patients (Fig 4-8) showing that ACE inhibitors beneficially alter the course of end-stage renal failure (ESRF), although better blood pressure reduction could also explain the results.[20] For those with urinary protein excretion more than 1 g/day, the blood pressure goal should be 125/75 mmHg.[34]

To this must be added the very impressive REIN study (*Ramipril Efficacy In Nephropathy*)[21] and its long term follow up, which makes the results of the Giatras meta-analysis even more impressive (Fig 4-8). In the initial core study,

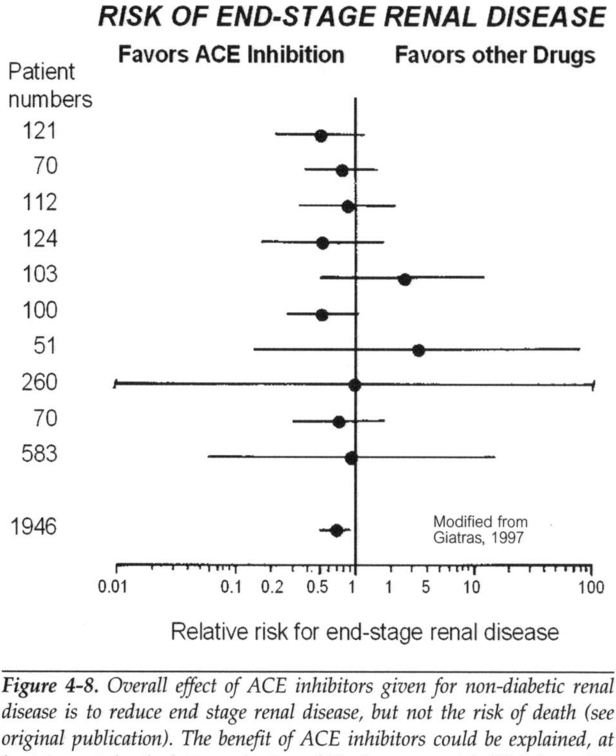

RISK OF END-STAGE RENAL DISEASE

Figure 4-8. Overall effect of ACE inhibitors given for non-diabetic renal disease is to reduce end stage renal disease, but not the risk of death (see original publication). The benefit of ACE inhibitors could be explained, at least in part, by the better reduction of blood pressure. Modified from Giatras[20] with permission of author and publishers.

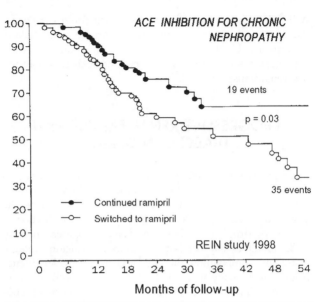

Figure 4-9. The follow up of the REIN (Ramipril Efficacy in Nephropathy) study. In the first part, extending over about 2 years, ramipril reduced the rate of decline of the glomerular filtration rate in patients with chronic nephropathy and proteinuria. For the second part of the study, those originally assigned to ramipril were continued on this drug, whereas those initially assigned to other agents were switched to ramipril. With further follow up over 30 months or more, those switched (and not on ramipril for the first part of the study) had more end stage renal failure (ESRF) than those that had had ramipril throughout (relative risk of having switched: 1.86, confidence intervals 1.07–3.26; p=0.03). Reproduced from The Lancet, 1998, 352:1252, by permission of the publishers and the authors.

patients with proteinuria of more than 3 g per 24 h were selected, and ramipril reduced the rate of GFR decline more than expected from the BP drop. In the follow up study, the incidence of ESRF at 36 months was zero in those originally allocated to ramipril, but 30% in those allocated to placebo plus conventional antihypertensive therapy. Of interest, those originally allocated to non-ramipril therapy and then switched to ramipril at the end of the initial core study, never "caught" up with those kept on ramipril from the start (Fig 4–9). This failure to improve occurred even though the BP reduction in the "switched" group was greater than in those who had continued on ramipril throughout. The following suggestions can be made, based on the results of REIN: (1) the earlier ACE inhibitor therapy is started, the better; (2) the sickest patients benefit most; and (3) the benefit is not fully explained by reduction of the BP.

RENAL SIDE-EFFECTS OF ACE INHIBITORS

Transient acute renal failure after onset of ACE inhibitor therapy. While a modest rise in serum creatinine is fairly common, renal impairment may be severe enough to cause transient oliguria or even overt anuria.[54] The true incidence of acute renal failure (ARF) during the use of ACE inhibitors is unknown, but in one French institution, 9% of all admissions to the renal intensive care unit were for ARF related to use of ACE inhibitors.[54] Major risk factors in the elderly were dehydration due to intermittent vomiting or diarrhea or the use of high doses of loop diuretics. Generally the ARF is reversible, yet occasionally protracted hypotension may cause irreversible acute tubular necrosis.[54]

Prophylaxis against renal failure. As already outlined, the risk that ACE inhibitors could impair renal function is much higher in situations where the renin-angiotensin II system (RAS) is stimulated as in severe cardiac failure, renal artery stenosis, and during excess diuretic therapy with a pre-existing negative sodium balance. Because it is impossible to predict the degree of stimulation of renin-angiotensin II in any given pathophysiologic situation in a specific patient, it is correct *always to start with a low dose* of an ACE inhibitor. Thereafter, the dose is incrementally increased before proceeding to long-term therapy, while following indices of renal function.

Doses of ACE inhibitors in renal failure. In general the doses of all ACE inhibitors should be reduced in renal failure, because most of the active diacid forms (e.g. enalaprilat) are excreted by the kidney. Taking two examples, the dose of enalapril should be reduced by half when the creatinine clearance falls below 30 ml/min (Ch 8). In the case of perindopril, the standard dose of 4 mg daily should be reduced to 2 mg or even less, depending on the severity of renal failure.[38] An exception is in the case of fosinopril which is dully excreted (liver and kidney), needing no dose adjustment in renal failure.

SUMMARY

1. *Angiotensin II is a powerful renal efferent arteriolar vasoconstrictor.* The specific sites of vasoconstriction are preglomerular, that is to say afferent renal arteriolar vasoconstriction, and, particularly, efferent vasoconstriction. Efferent vasoconstriction maintains intraglomerular filtration pressure in a variety of circumstances, such as severe heart failure, bilateral renal artery stenosis, renal artery stenosis treated vigorously with diuretics, and, theoretically, in some cases of hypertension-induced renal damage. Relief of efferent vasoconstriction can be expected to have therapeutic benefits in conditions where intraglomerular hypertension and hyperfiltration is a basic problem, such as hypertensive microalbuminuria, certain other instances of hypertension-induced renal damage, and in progressive renal disease.

2. *Angiotensin II promotes sodium reabsorption.* The mechanism includes increased secretion of aldosterone, and stimulation of the renal tubular sodium pump.

3. *Microalbuminuria.* This condition is increasingly regarded as an early harbinger of progressive renal

damage, and is an indication for tight blood pressure control. In non-hypertensives, ACE inhibitor therapy limits the progression to macroalbuminuria.

4. *Renovascular hypertension.* The marked therapeutic benefits of ACE inhibitors in renal artery stenosis can be related to the degree of increase of circulating renin, and thereby a general relief of arterial pressure elevation with an increase in preglomerular plasma flow. Nonetheless, these advantages have to be balanced against the potential disadvantage of decreased efferent vasoconstriction in response to ACE inhibitor therapy. There is the potential for severe temporary acute renal failure to occur, with permanent failure in some cases, particularly when renal artery perfusion is already impaired. Such predisposing conditions include bilateral renal artery stenosis, severe heart failure, unilateral renal artery stenosis in a solitary kidney, or renal artery stenosis in a transplant kidney, and similar situations.

5. *Acute renal failure induced by ACE inhibitors.* To prevent temporary or permanent failure, upon the use of ACE inhibitors, care should be taken to avoid significant or excess concurrent diuretic therapy, because a negative sodium balance stimulates the angiotensin-renin system. In severe heart failure with poor renal perfusion, ACE inhibitor therapy must be introduced only when excess diuresis has been avoided and after a low test dose. Conventionally, patients with significant pre-existing renal impairment, are excluded from therapy with ACE inhibitors. In all cases plasma creatinine is followed after the onset of ACE inhibitor therapy. If the rise in creatinine is excess (limits not well-defined), the ACE inhibitor is stopped.

6. *Progressive renal failure (non-diabetic).* ACE inhibitor therapy slows the progression to end-stage renal failure. In one trial on patients with proteinuria exceeding 3 g per day, ramipril given continuously over many months eliminated the development of end-stage renal failure.

REFERENCES

1. Bauer JH. Modern antihypertensive treatment and the progression of renal disease. J Hypertens 1998;16 (Suppl 5):S17–S24.

2. Bender W, La France N, Walker WG. Mechanism of deterioration in renal function in patients with renovascular hypertension treated with enalapril. Hypertension 1984;6 (Suppl 1):I-193–I-197.

3. Bianchi S, Bigazzi R, Baldari G. Microalbuminuria inpatients with essential hypertension: effects of several antihypertensive drugs. Am J Med 1992;93:108–113.

4. Bigazzi R, Bianchi S, Baldari D, et al. Microalbuminuria predicts cardiovascular events and renal insufficiency in patients with essential hypertension. J Hypertens 1998;16:1325–1333.

5. Bigazzi R, Bianchi S, Baldari D, et al. Long-term effects of a converting enzyme inhibitor and a calcium channel blocker on urinary albumin excretion in patients with essential hypertension. Am J Hypertens 1992;6:108–113.

6. Bijlstra PJ, Postma CT, de Boo T, et al. Clinical and biochemical criteria in the detection of renal artery stenosis. J Hypertens 1996;14:1033–1040.

7. Blythe WB. Captopril and renal autoregulation. N Engl J Med 1983;308:390–391.

8. Brenner BM, Schor N, Ichikawa I. Role of angiotensin II in the physiologic regulation of glomerular filtration. Am J Cardiol 1982;49:1430–1433.

9. CONSENSUS Trial Study Group. Effects of enalapril on mortality in severe heart failure: Results of the Co-operative North Scandinavian Enalapril Survival Study (CONSENSUS). N Engl J Med 1987;316:1429–1435.

10. Corman B, Vienet R. Converting enzyme inhibition prevents postprandial hyperfiltration in rats with renal mass ablation. Am J Hypertens 1991;4:253S–257S.

11. Curtis JJ, Luke RG, Whelchel JD, et al. Inhibition of angiotensin converting enzyme in renal-transplant recipients with hypertension. N Engl J Med 1983;308:377–381.

12. De Venuto G, Andreotti C, Mattarei M, et al. Long-term captopril therapy at low doses reduces albumin excretion in patients with essential hypertension and no sign of renal impairment. J Hypertens 1985;3 (Suppl 2):S143–S145.

13. Derkx FHM, Tan-thong L, Wenting GJ, et al. Asynchronous changes in prorenin and renin secretion after captopril in patients with renal artery stenosis. Hypertension 1983;5:244–256.

14. Dworkin LD, Benstein JA, Parker M, et al. Calcium antagonists and converting enzyme inhibitors reduce renal injury by different mechanisms. Kidney Int 1993;43:808–814.

15. Edwards RM. Segmental effects of norepinephrine and angiotensin-II on isolated renal microvessels. Am J Physiol 1983;244.

16. Emovon OE, Klotman PE, Dunnick NR, et al. Renovascular hypertension in blacks. Am J Hypertens 1996;9:18–23.

17. Erbsloh-Moller B, Dumas A, Roth D, et al. Furosemide-^{131}I-hippuran renography after angiotensin-converting enzyme inhibition for the diagnosis of renovascular hypertension. Am J Med 1991;90:23–29.

18. Erley CM, Haefele U, Heyne N, et al. Microalbuminuria in essential hypertension. Hypertension 1993;21:810–815.

19. Funck-Brentano C, Chatelier G, Alexandre J-M. Reversible renal failure after combined treatment with enalapril and frusemide in a patient with congestive heart failure. Br Heart J 1986;55:596–598.

20. Giatras I, Lau J, Levey AS. For the Angiotensin-Converting-Enzyme Inhibition and Progressive Renal Disease Study Group. Effect of angiotensin-converting enzyme inhibitors on the progression of nondiabetic renal disease: a meta-analysis of randomized trials. Ann Intern Med 1997;127:337–345.

21. GISEN Group. (Gruppo Italiano di Studi Epidemiologici in Nefrologia). Randomised placebo-controlled trial of effect of ramipril on decline in glomerularfiltration rate and risk of terminal renal failure in proteinuric, non-diabetic nephropathy. Lancet 1997;349:1857–1863.

22. Guzman RP, Zierler E, Isaacson JA. Renal atrophy and arterial stenosis. A prospective study with duplex ultrasound. Hypertension 1994;23:346–350.

23. Hannedouche T, Landais P, Goldfarb B, et al. Randomised controlled trial of enalapril and b blockers in non-diabetic chronic renal failure. BMJ 1994;309:833–837.

24. Himmelmann A, Hansson L, Hansson B-G, et al. Long-term renal preservation in essential hypertension. Angiotensin converting enzyme inhibition is superior to β-blockade. Am J Hypertens 1996;9:850–853.

25. Hodsman GP, Isles CG, Murray GD, et al. Factors related to the first dose hypotensive effect of captopril: prediction and treatment. Br Med J 1983;286:832–834.

26. Hollenberg NK, Fisher NDL, Price DA. Pathways for angiotensin II generation in intact human tissue. Evidence from comparative pharmacological interruption of the renin system. Hypertension 1998;32:387–392.

27. Hollenberg NK, Williams GH. Abnormal renal function, sodium, volume homeostasis, and renin system behavior in normal-renin essential hypertension. In: Laragh JH, Brenner BM, eds. Hypertension, Pathophysiology, Diagnosis and Management. New York: Raven Press, 1990.

28. Ingelfinger JR, Pratt RE, Ellison K, et al. Sodium regulation of angiotensinogen mRNA expression in rat kidney cortex and medulla. J Clin Invest 1986;78:1311–1315.

29. Janssen JJWM, Gans ROB, van der Meulen J, et al. Comparison between the effects of amlodipine and lisinopril on proteinuria in nondiabetic renal failure. Am J Hypertens 1998;11:1074–1079.

30. Keane WF, Polis A, Wolf D, et al. The long-term tolerability of enalapril in hypertensive patients with renal impairment. Nephrol Dial Transplant 1997;12 (Suppl 2):75–81.

31. Klag MJ, Whelton PK, Randall BL, et al. Blood pressure and end-stage renal disease in men. N Engl J Med 1996;334:13–18.

32. Lang. Rates and tissue sites of noninsulin- and insulin-mediated glucose uptake in diabetic rats. Proc Soc Exptl Biol Med 1992;199:81–87.

33. Lariviere R, Lebel M, Kingma I, et al. Effects of losartan and captopril on endothelin-1 production in blood vessels and glomeruli of rats with reduced renal mass. Am J Hypertens 1998;11:989–997.

34. Lazarus JM, Bourgoignie JL, Buckalew VM, et al. For the Modification of Diet in Renal Disease Study Group. Achievement and safety of a low blood pressure goal in chronic renal disease. Hypertension 1997; 29:641–650.

35. MacGregor MS, Rowe PA, Watson MA, et al. Treatment of postrenal transplant erythrocytosis. Nephron 1996;75:517–521.

36. Madeddu P, Milia AF, Salis MB, et al. Renovascular hypertension in bradykinin b_2-receptor knockout mice. Hypertension 1998;32:503–509.

37. Maki DD, Ma JZ, Lous TA, et al. Long-term effects of antihypertensive agents on proteinuria and renal function. Arch Intern Med 1995;155:1073–1080.

38. Meyrier A, Dratwa M, Sennesael J, et al. Fixed low-dose perindopril-indapamide combination in hypertensive patients with chronic renal failure. Am J Hypertens 1998;11:1087–1092.

39. Miralles M, M I Covas, Martinez Miralles E, et al. Captopril test and renal duplex scan for the primary screening of renovascular disease. Am J Hypertens 1997;10:1290–1296.

40. Miyazaki Y, Murkami H, Hirata A, et al. Effects of the angiotensin converting enzyme inhibitor temocapril on insulin sensitivity and its effects on renal sodium handling and the pressor system in essential hypertensive patients. Am J Hypertens 1998;11:962–970.

41. Navar LG, Champion WJ, Thomas CE. Effects of calcium channel blockade on renal vascular resistance responses to changes in perfusion pressure and angiotensin-converting enzyme inhibition in dogs. Circ Res 1986;58:874–881.

42. Pontremoli R, Sofia A, Ravera M, et al. Prevalence and clinical correlates of microalbuminuria in essential hypertension. The MAGIC study. Hypertension 1997;30:1135–1143.

43. Raij K, Chious X-C, Owens R, et al. Therapeutic implications of hypertension-induced glomerular injury. Comparison of enalapril and a combination of hydralazine, reserpine, and hydrochlorothiazide in an experimental model. Am J Med 1985;79 (Suppl 3C):37–41.

44. Reams GP, Bauer JH. Acute and chronic effects of angiotensin converting enzyme inhibitors on the essential hypertensive kidney. J Cardiovasc Drugs Ther 1990;7:207–219.

45. Redon J. Renal protection by antihypertensive drugs: insights from microalbuminuria studies. J Hypertens 1998;16:2091–2100.

46. Robertson JIS. Intrarenal actions of angiotensin converting enzyme inhibitors: their relevance to renal artery stenosis. ACE Report 1985;16:1–5.

47. SAVE Study. Pfeffer MA, Braunwald E, et al. Effect of captopril on mortality and morbidity in patients with left ventricular dysfunction after myocardial infarction. Results of the Survival and Ventricular Enlargement trial. N Eng J Med 1992;327:669–677.

48. Silas JH, Klenka Z, Solomon SA, et al. Captopril induced reversible renal failure: a marker of renal artery stenosis affecting a solitary kidney. Br Med J 1983;285:1702–1703.

49. SOLVD Investigators. Effect of enalapril on mortality and the development of heart failure in asymptomatic patients with reduced left ventricular ejection fractions. New Engl J Med 1992;327:685–691.

50. Staessen J, Bulpitt C, Fagard R, et al. Long-term converting-enzyme inhibition as a guide to surgical curability of hypertension associated with renovascular disease. Am J Cardiol 1983;51:1317–1322.

51. Tolins JP, Raij L. Comparison of converting enzyme inhibitor and calcium channel blocker in hypertensive glomerular injury. Hypertension 1990;16:452–461.

52. Wald G, Scgerzer O, Popovtzer MM. Na, K-ATPase in isolated nephron segments in rats with experimental heart failure. Circ Res 1991;68:1051–1058.

53. Watson ML, Bell GM, Muir AL, et al. Captopril/diuretic combinations in severe renovascular disease: a cautionary note. Lancet 1983;2:404–405.

54. Wynckel A, Ebikili B, Melin J-P, et al. Long-term follow up of acute renal failure caused by angiotensin converting enzyme inhibitors. Am J Hypertens 1998;11:1080–1086.

55. Yu H, Carretero OA, Juncos LA, et al. Biphasic effect of bradykinin on rabbit afferent arterioles. Hypertension 1998;32:287–292.

56. Zhuo J, Moeller I, Jenkins T, et al. Mapping tissue angiotensin-converting enzyme and angiotensin AT_1, AT_2 and AT_4 receptors. J Hypertens 1998;16:2027-2037.

CHAPTER 5

ACE Inhibitors, coronary artery disease, and the heart

*"ACE inhibitor use in acute myocardial infarction
has shifted from investigational to standard
therapeutics" – Pfeffer (1998)[64]*

Initially it was thought that ACE inhibitors had only an indirect effect on the heart, for example by decreasing blood pressure, thereby unloading the heart, and thereby having an indirect effect in decreasing left ventricular mass in hypertension. More recently, evidence has mounted that there are angiotensin receptors in the myocardium, that stimulation of such receptors can alter myocardial contractile function, and that, furthermore, at least some of the angiotensin involved might be manufactured in cardiac cells. This chapter will start by analyzing the effects of angiotensin receptor stimulation and ACE inhibitors on the myocardium, and then examine the possible role of ACE inhibition in the clinical manifestations of coronary artery disease including angina pectoris, acute myocardial infarction, reperfusion, and postinfarct remodeling.

MYOCARDIAL ANGIOTENSIN II RECEPTORS AND SUBTYPES

There are two myocardial angiotensin II receptor subtypes, AT_1 and AT_2. It is the AT_1 receptor that has the established role in myocardial signaling (Chapter 1), and that is upregulated by pressure overload. Although the role of the AT_2 receptor is "far from clear",[19] inhibition of this receptor might have a favorable effect on postinfarct remodeling.[45] There is ongoing controversy about the dominant receptor type in cardiac tissue. In the non-failing left ventricle, Bristow's group found that AT-1 receptor density exceeded that of AT-2 receptors by about 50%.[8] In contrast, Regitz-Zagrosek et al[70] found a dominance of AT-2 receptors in the atria and in the failing LV. To reconcile these apparently conflicting data, it may be noted that: (1) Regitz-Zagrosek et al did not report on the non-failing LV, in which AT-1 receptors are higher;[8] (2) Bristow's group did find less AT-1 than AT-2 receptor density in failing hearts from idiopathic dilated cardiomyopathy patients, the group that was dominant in the other study. Studies with mRNA support the concept that there is relative downgrading of AT-1 receptors in severe failure.[33] The downgrading of the AT-1 receptors is proportional to that of the beta-1 receptors.[8] In contrast there is unchanged expression of the AT_{-2} receptor.[8] Thus, functions of the AT_{-2} receptor, whatever they be, might be more relevant in severe heart failure. Indirect evidence suggests that AT-2 receptor blockade could be beneficial in cardiac remodeling,[54] while in ischemic-reperfusion injury, blockade of the AT-2 but not of the AT-1 receptor enhanced recovery.[28]

Significance of the resident myocardial renin-angiotensin system. That there is a myocardial renin-angiotensin system is now generally accepted (Fig 5–1). That it has pathophysiological significance is much more difficult to prove. Even more difficult to know is whether the system resides in the cardiac myocytes or in the fibroblasts or in combinations of both or even in other cells. Even cell cultures are seldom pure. Furthermore, exact enzyme that converts angiotensin I to angiotensin II may differ between the humans and the common laboratory animal, the rat. Evidence for recognition of the cardiac components of the renin-angiotensin system is summarized in Table 3-1 as are the data showing that there are myocardial angiotensin receptors. The physiological effects of such receptor stimulation could include inotropic and chronotropic changes, but it is difficult to be sure that it is the myocardial renin-angiotensin system that is involved and not circulating components, or components that are located on cardiac cells but have direct access to the extracellular space. Increasing evidence shows that the tissue system acts to stimulate growth factors (Table 3-2).

Modification of the activity of the renin-angiotensin system has obvious importance in relation to the heart (Table 3-3). However, there is no proof that it is the myocardial myocyte renin-angiotensin system that is the major target of ACE inhibitor drug action, as opposed to other systems, for

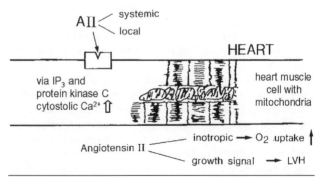

Figure 5–1. Angiotensin II and heart muscle. Proposed role of myocardial angiotensin II (AT-1) receptors in regulating cystolic calcium in heart muscle cells, with consequences for the inotropic stage and for myocardial growth. Figure © LH Opie, 1999

example those in the vascular endothelium, or the circulating renin-angiotensin system. The following challenge of Lindpainter and Ganten[49] is still not fully answered: "To date, no experiments have been reported that provide *unequivocal* evidence for direct physiological significance of intracardially synthesized angiotensin". There is, however, some evidence that the mRNA for the human AT-1 receptor can be found in both myocytes and non-myocytes.[33]

Vascular tissue and fibroblasts. Myocardial cells may participate and interact with a variety of other cells, including fibroblasts, vascular smooth muscle cells, and endothelial cells in a multiple cellular interactive manner. Thus, current evidence strongly suggests the existence of a cardiac multicellular renin-angiotensin system, probably helping to regulate cardiac growth, including fibrogenesis.[97]

Growth factors in vascular cells. Angiotensin II may induce the release of a number of growth factors from vascular smooth muscle cells. For example, the platelet-derived growth factor (PDGF) may arise not only from platelets but from smooth muscle cells and be released from them by angiotensin II. Likewise, the transforming growth factor β_1 (TGF-β_1) can thus be released. The latter growth factor may play a special role in promoting the growth of extracellular matrix, including collagen.[25]

RENIN-SODIUM PROFILE, ANGIOTENSIN AND RISK OF MYOCARDIAL INFARCTION

If angiotensin II has adverse effects on the myocardium and possibly on the coronary arteries by causing excess growth and fibrosis, then a reasonable hypothesis would be that patients with high circulating renin activities could be more prone to heart attacks than others. Laragh's group has tested their hypothesis that high-renin patients may be at increased cardiovascular risk.[7] In 1,717 patients with mild to moderate hypertension, *renin profiles* were obtained by plotting plasma renin activity against urinary excretion of sodium (Fig 5–2). Their data showed that the ratio rate for high-renin status was about five times that of the low profile group, even when allowing for other cardiovascular risk factors. Of great interest is that black men were twice as likely as white men to have a low-renin profile, which may well explain the clinical findings that (1) this ethnic group is relatively protected from myocardial infarction, and (2) there is a poor response to ACE inhibitor therapy for hypertension (see page 75). The combination of a high-renin profile with other risk factors, such as smoking, a high cholesterol level, or a high fasting blood glucose, increase the risk ratio considerably. For example, patients with the combination of a low-renin profile and a low fasting blood glucose had a risk factor for myocardial infarction of 2.1 per 1,000 patient years, whereas a high-renin profile and a high fasting blood glucose had a risk factor of

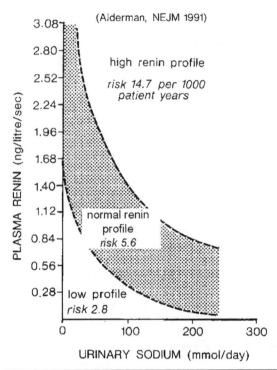

Figure 5–2. The renin profile relates plasma renin activity to simultaneously measured urinary sodium excretion. These data, taken from Alderman et al[7] with permission, are modified from Figure 1 and table 3 in the paper. The zone between the dotted lines show the normal renin profile with the renin rising in relation to the fall in urinary sodium – on a low sodium diet plasma renin is high. In the high-renin profile group, in which the patient renin values were about 2–3 times higher for the same urinary sodium excretion, the risk of acute myocardial infarction (AMI) was considerably higher. Low-renin profile patients, on the other hand, appear to be relatively protected. For further details see Alderman et al[7].

48.5 per 1,000 patient years, i.e. 23 times higher. The blood pressure itself was, however, not a direct risk factor for myocardial infarction. These data may help to explain the promising effects of ACE inhibitor therapy in lessening the incidence of myocardial reinfarction in selected patients.[65]

ACE INHIBITORS AND CORONARY ARTERY DISEASE

Coronary blood flow and relief of vasoconstriction. In general, ACE inhibitors are not vasodilators in the conventional sense, rather acting to relieve induced vasoconstriction.[26,35] Examples are as follows. First, in experimental myocardial ischemia, when there is activation of the renin-angiotensin system, there is coronary constriction that the ACE inhibitors relieve. Second, infusion of angiotensin II causes vasoconstriction, with a sustained effect large conductance vessels and a transient effect on small distal vessels.[17] Third, in patients with mild essential hypertension and no evidence of ischemic heart disease, diuretic administration (furosemide 50 mg daily for 1 week) reduced coronary blood flow, compatible with renin-angiotensin II-mediated coronary constriction.[52] Thereafter, a single dose of captopril 25 mg increased blood flow despite reducing the mean arterial pressure. Fourth, in smokers ACE inhibition by quinapril in the TREND study had a greater vasodilator effect than in non-smokers – compatible with the concept of endothelial damage and enhanced vasoconstrictor responses in smokers.[77]

Besides inhibition of coronary vasoconstriction mediated by angiotensin II[63] and involving the AT_1-receptors,[87] there are two possible additional vasodilatory mechanisms of ACE inhibitors. First, increased vasodilatory prostaglandins, such as PGI_2 formed in the wake of the increase in bradykinin, as shown in isolated hearts.[94] Second, in the case of captopril, there may be another mechanism involving SH-groups.[94] All these observations would explain why ACE inhibitors could potentially act as coronary vasodilators.

Are there antianginal effects of ACE inhibitors in humans? The decrease in myocardial oxygen consumption associated with a decreased blood pressure in the absence of any tachycardia, together with potential coronary vasodilation, should mean that ACE inhibitors have a potential antianginal effect. In some studies,[46,85] a modest antianginal effect has been found. Bartels et al[10] and Remme et al[71] paced 25 untreated normotensive patients with angina but not in heart failure. During pacing, there was neurohumoral activation. After the intravenous injection of perindoprilat (0.5 mg), the ACE inhibitor clearly reduced myocardial ischemia by preventing a catecholamine-mediated rise in total peripheral resistance.

On the other hand, in the presence of coronary stenosis, ACE inhibitors might potentially worsen myocardial ischemia because of dilation of the resistance vessels with risk of passive narrowing or even collapse of the coronary stenoses.[79] In 11 patients with coronary artery stenosis demonstrated by coronary angiography, the ACE inhibitor benazepril had no overall antianginal effect, although a benefit was noted in 6 of the patients.[90] Thus, on the whole, ACE inhibitors are not regarded as particularly efficacious antianginal agents. There might be variable results depending on the overall balance between the adverse effects of hypertension, the potential lessening of blood flow across coronary stenosis, the indirect beneficial antiadrenergic effect, and long-term vascular protection.

Hypertension and angina. As expected, in patients with this combination, ACE inhibitor monotherapy could both reduce blood pressure and anginal attacks.[6,86]

Severe heart failure and angina pectoris. It might be anticipated in patients with heart failure that the ACE inhibitors would be particularly effective as antianginal agents because of their capacity to reduce the load on the ventricle and hence to lessen left ventricular dilation. In severe heart failure and angina, however, ACE inhibitor therapy may not be successful.[16] The presumed mechanism of this adverse effect is a decreased blood pressure with impaired coronary perfusion. Concurrent therapy with nifedipine was especially harmful.

Unstable angina. In the SOLVD study,[84] patients with low ejection fractions treated by enalapril had a lower incidence of unstable angina and myocardial infarction than those treated by placebo.[100]

Nitrate tolerance during the treatment of angina pectoris. ACE inhibitors might benefit patients with angina by facilitating the effects of nitrates (Fig 5–3). Long-term nitrate treatment leads to nitrate intolerance, in part due to increased sensitivity to vasoconstrictor stimuli, particularly angiotensin II and endothelin.[34] Concomitant captopril (25 mg three times daily) prevents this supersensitivity. In another study, anginal patients not responding well to nitrates alone, appeared to respond to added captopril.[56] Are these effects specific to captopril with its SH groups? In patients,

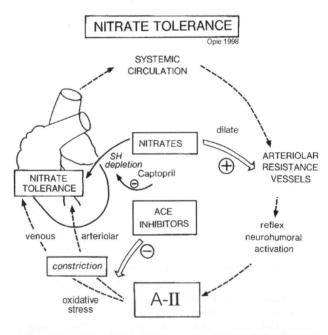

Figure 5–3. Nitrate tolerance. There are two major theories. First, there may be a deficiency of vascular SH-groups and, for this, captopril containing SH-groups, would seem logical therapy. Second, the nitrate-induced vasodilation could cause reflex neurohumoral activation with increased renin-angiotensin activity. The latter increases vascular oxidative stress. The result of either mechanism would be arteriolar and venous constriction, thereby diminishing the vascular effects of nitrates on those two systems. For the second mechanism, any type of ACE inhibitor, whether or not it contains an SH-group, should, in practice, be appropriate therapy. Clinical data suggest that different ACE inhibitors are almost equieffective for nitrate tolerance. Figure © LH Opie, 1999

maintenance of the nitrate effect and lessening of nitrate tolerance is equally achieved by enalapril (10 mg twice daily) or captopril (25 mg three times daily).[42] One proposal is that nitrate tolerance can be is prevented by any effective form of vasodilation, whether by ACE inhibition or by hydralazine.[11]

ACE INHIBITORS AND EARLY PHASE ACUTE MYOCARDIAL INFARCTION

The marked neurohumoral activation in patients with acute myocardial infarction (Fig 5-4), with angiotensin II leveis increasing up to eight times,[20] made it logical to treat left ventricular failure complicating myocardial infarction by ACE inhibitors.[14,15,53] The next and most recent step has been to use ACE inhibitors prophylactically, to avoid the onset of LV failure, especially in those with large anterior infarcts or diabetics.

Experimental reduction of infarct size. As reduction of the myocardial oxygen demand is known to be a factor decreasing ultimate infarct size, it was not surprising that continuous administration of captopril decreased estimated infarct size over 30 minutes to 6 hours of coronary occlusion in an open-chest dog model.[27] Regional myocardial

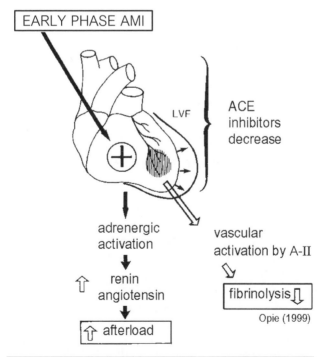

Figure 5-4. *Early phase acute myocardial infarction (AMI). Left ventricular failure (LVF) may develop with resulting adrenergic activation and an increase in afterload mediated by renin-angiotensin. Oral ACE inhibition is logical therapy, as supported by trial data (Fig 5-8). Figure © LH Opie, 1999*

blood flow improved and arterial pressure decreased, as did left atrial pressure. In rats with coronary artery ligation, perindopril improved left ventricular performance and decreased myocardial depletion of norepinephrine.[74]

Infarct reduction by ACE inhibition is mediated by bradykinin in rats, rabbits and dogs.[32,36,51,61] Bradykinin is formed during ACE inhibition because its breakdown is decreased (Fig 1-11). A reasonable argument would be that AT-1 receptor blockade failed to work because it would not mediate protection through bradykinin. Unexpectedly, perhaps, bradykinin *does* play a role in the protection against pig infarcts by the AT-1 blocker candesartan.[38] Locally unopposed AT-2 receptor activity may be responsible. Why the pig model differs from the others is not clear. However, it is not a conventional model of transmural infarction.

ACE inhibition within 24 h of onset of AMI. As will be argued, ACE inhibitors are now virtually mandatory for overt left ventricular failure or LV dysfunction after the early acute phase of myocardial infarction is over. The only possible controversy surrounds their use within 24 hours of onset of AMI (Fig 5-5). There are two major policies. The policy document issued by the American heart Association and American College of Cardiology suggests administration of ACE inhibitors to all patients within 24 hours of onset, unless there is a contraindication such as a systolic BP below 100 mmHg, then at 6 weeks determining whether or not long term ACE inhibition is needed (ACE Inhibitor Myocardial Infarction Collaborative Group).[2] The alternate policy, favored by the present author, is to give ACE inhibitors to all high risk patients: diabetics, those with anterior infarcts or tachycardia or overt LV failure. Logically, the sicker the patients, the greater the activation of the renin-

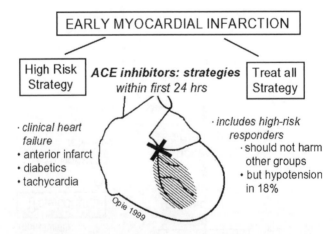

Figure 5–5. Contrasting policies for use of ACE inhibitors in early myocardial infarction. The strategy on the left selects those with heart failure or at risk of developing heart failure. ACE inhibition can start within 2 hours of streptokinase in anterior infarcts (French et al, J Am Coll Cardiol, 33;139:1999). The "treat all" strategy on the right includes the subgroup at high risk, and should not harm others except for the risk of hypotension. Fig © LH Opie, 1999

angiotensin-system, and the better the expected result with the use of an ACE inhibitor. To understand this recommendation requires a brief review of the four relevant trials: ISIS-4,[37] GISSI-3,[31] CONSENSUS II,[18] and SMILE[82] (Table 5-1).

TABLE 5–1.   TRIALS OF ACE INHIBITORS GIVEN WITHIN 24 HOURS OF ONSET OF ACUTE MYOCARDIAL INFARCTION

	CONSENSUS-II	ISIS-4	GISSI-3	SMILE
Total number treated	3,044	27,442	9,435	1,556
Drug and daily dose	Enalaprilat IV 1 mg over 2 h; then enalapril up to 20 mg 2× daily	Captopril 6.25 mg initially, increased to 50 mg 2× daily	Lisinopril 2.5-5 mg initially, increased to 10 mg 1× daily	Zofenopril 7.5 mg initially, repeated after 12 hrs then doubled to target of 30 mg 2× daily
Duration	41 to 180 days	28 days	42 days	6 weeks drug, then 48 weeks follow up
Patient population	AMI within 24 h of onset	AMI within 24 h of onset	AMI within 24 h of onset	AMI, anterior, non-thrombolysed, within 24 h of onset
Thrombolysed	56%	68%	70%	None
Age, years	66 mean	72% below 70	70 or below in 73%	64 mean
Gender male (%)	73	74	78	73
BP exclusion levels	100/60	100 systolic	100 systolic	100 systolic
Hypotension as side-effect (%)	25 (control 10)	21 (control 10)	21 (control, 10)** 8.8 (control 3.6)+	17 (control 9)
Mortality change, (absolute %)	0.8 increase	0.46 decrease*	0.88 decrease+	4.1 decrease at one year
Mortality change as risk reduction	10% increase	9% decrease* (p = 0.04)	12% decrease+ (p = 0.03)	29% decrease (p=0.011)

* 35 days; ** see Latini et al [47]; + 6 weeks.

ISIS-4: Nearly 54,000 patients were randomized to captopril or to placebo within 24 hours of the onset of symptoms.[37] The initial dose of captopril was 6.25 mg, titrated upward to 50 mg twice daily for 4 weeks. Of note, the control 5-week mortality was low, being 7.2%, so that on the average low risk patients were studied. In the first 35 days, there were 4.6 fewer deaths per 1,000 patients in the captopril-treated groups with an absolute reduction in mortality of 0.46% (2p = 0.04). Put differently, there was a 6% risk reduction in mortality. These modest benefits, to some extent offset by an increased incidence of hypotension (nearly 20% of the captopril-treated patients versus 10% in placebo patients), do not argue strongly for the routine use of oral captopril in acute infarction.

GISSI-3. In the GISSI-3 study[31] on a total of nearly 19,000 patients, lisinopril was given as an initial dose of 2.5 mg or 5 mg orally, increasing up to 10 mg once daily for 6 weeks. The mortality at 6 weeks was reduced from the already low value of 7.1% in controls to 6.3% in the lisinopril group, i.e. a reduction of 0.8% ($2p = 0.03$). Put differently, there was an 11% reduction in the relative risk of mortality. When combined with nitrates (intravenous followed by intermittent transdermal nitroglycerin), there was an impressive risk reduction of 17% in mortality. A later analysis of the subgroups showed that the mortality reduction was largely confined to the diabetic patients.[102]

CONSENSUS-II.[18] Here an intravenous ACE inhibitor, enalaprilat, did not work because of the frequent occurrence of excess hypotension which, in turn, predisposed to increased mortality.

SMILE.[82] Patients with anterior infarcts who could not be given thrombolytics, were randomly given placebo (mortality 14.1% at one year) or zofenopril, up to 30 mg twice daily (mortality 10.0%, risk reduction of 29%, $P = 0.011$). These were, by definition, high risk patients in whom the benefit was largely confined to those with anterior ST-elevation.[13]

The selective policy: use in those at higher risk. The data from ISIS-4 and GISSI-3 hasten the time frame in which ACE inhibitors can safely and beneficially be used in acute myocardial infarction. Data from GISSI-3 and SMILE show that high risk patients benefit most. The ACE inhibitor collaborative group[2] warns against the concurrent risks. Thus, persistent hypotension nearly doubled from 9 to 18%, while renal dysfunction rose from 0.6 to 1.3%. Thus these workers point out that the greatest absolute benefit of the use of ACE inhibitors in early infarct would in those at higher risk, as for example in Killip classes 2 or 3, tachycardia, anterior infarction and, one should add, diabetes.[102] The strongest recommendation (class 1) for ACE inhibitor use within 24 hrs of onset of AMI is given for high risk patients with ST-elevation in 2 or more anterior pericardial leads, or with clinical heart failure, and in the absence of hypotension or other contraindications.[1]

Hypotension. The fear of hypotension in the acute stage of myocardial infarction is real. In response to intravenous enalaprilat,[18] the incidence of first-dose hypotension increased from 12% in controls to 17% and was linked to an increased mortality. The incidence of hypotension at any time was 25% in the enalaprilat group and 10% in controls ($p < 0.001$). The cause of this increased harmful hypotension could have been the fixed high intravenous dose of enalaprilat given at the start of the study.

General policy. To other observers, the overall expected benefits in acute phase myocardial infarction although modest, are strong enough to recommend general use within the first 24 hours, provided that hypotension or other complications are absent. ACE inhibition will then give benefit to those at higher risk while not harming those at lower risk. For this use, the AHA-American College task force gives a class 2A recommendation,[1] meaning that the weight of evidence or opinion favors efficacy. To follow this policy, trial data (often ignored) suggest that the most logical therapy of choice would be an oral ACE inhibitor plus a nitrate.[31]

At present, cast-iron recommendations cannot be made, but clearly all these trials have influenced more and more cardiologists to use ACE inhibitors in early stage myocardial infarction.

ACE INHIBITORS AND REPERFUSION INJURY

Arrhythmias. Taking the broader concept of reperfusion injury which includes not only arrhythmias but also stunning as well as metabolic damage,[62] ACE inhibitors have been reported to decrease early metabolic damage such as noradrenaline overflow and creatine kinase release in a closed-chest pig model.[22] Because of their indirect antiadrenergic effect, ACE inhibitors can be expected to decrease ischemic arrhythmias. Reperfusion arrhythmias, although decreased in isolated rat heart models,[75,93] were unchanged in the closed-chest pig.[21,23] Nonetheless, our data[59] show that pretreatment of pigs by trandolapril lessens both ischemic and reperfusion arrhythmias. This accords with less sudden death in the trandolapril trial.[92] The antiarrhythmic effect, when found, is a probably a class effect (Fig 5-6).

The mechanism of the antiarrhythmic benefit may include bradykinin formation. In the isolated rat heart, arrhythmias that had been inhibited by ramiprilat were precipitated by addition of a bradykinin antagonist.[50]

Late arrhythmias, occurring days after ischemic reperfusion in closed-chest pigs, can be decreased by captopril

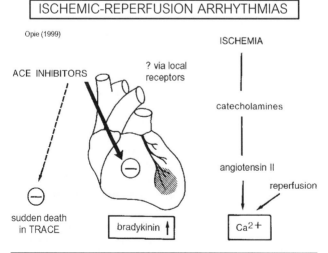

Figure 5–6. ACE inhibitors and arrhythmias. These agents may decrease adrenergic activity associated with acute myocardial infarction. In the TRACE study,[92] and in a large meta-analysis.[24] ACE inhibition decreased sudden death. Figure © LH Opie, 1999

treatment, probably by limitation of left ventricular dilation.[67]

ACE inhibitors vs AT-1 blockers in ischemic-reperfusion injury. During global ischemia followed by reperfusion, the myocardial AT-1 receptors are upgraded in rats.[99] When this change was prevented by anti-sense oligodeoxynucleotides that inhibit formation of the receptor mRNA, then reperfusion function improved. Unexpectedly, the AT-1 blocker losartan failed to give benefit. Likewise, in a similar rat model, losartan worsened post-ischemic recovery, whereas an AT-2 blocker gave improvement.[28] In coronary-ligated and reperfused rat hearts, infarct size was reduced by the ACE inhibitor ramiprilat but not by the AT-1 blocker, losartan.[51] The protection afforded by ramiprilat appeared to be mediated by bradykinin stimulation of release of nitric oxide and/or protaglandins. The uniform finding is that the AT-1 blocker did not benefit. Thus, although extrapolation of the rat data to large animals and humans must be done with considerable caution, a reasonable hypothesis (still to be tested in patients) would is that ACE inhibitors are better in this situation than AT-1 blockers.

ACE INHIBITORS, REMODELING, LV DYSFUNCTION, AND LV FAILURE

Remodeling and role of A-II. After myocardial infarction some patients undergo a progressive increase in left ventricular (LV) size manifest by a long-term increase in the end-diastolic and end-systolic volumes.[29,57] This process whereby the left ventricle progressively dilates together with an increase in mass of the surviving ventricular tissue, is called *remodeling*.[54] At a cellular level there is a greater increase in myocyte length rather than width,[30,44] explaining the increased LV volume. Sarcomere length is unchanged, so that there is no sarcomere "overstretching". Nor is there "cell slippage", according to Gerdes et al.[30] There are different intracellular signals that mediate the myocyte elongation that predominates in remodeling, and concentric hypertrophy with increased myocyte width as found in hypertension.[41] Probably the physical nature of the increased wall stress that deforms the intracellular cytoskeleton is different in progressive LV dilation, predominantly a volume load, and in hypertension, predominantly a pressure load. Such stress may be most at the border between the infarct and non-infarct tissue.[57] Increased wall stress stimulates the cardiac renin-angiotensin system.[78,98]

Fibrosis and resident renin-angiotensin system. In the areas forming fibrous tissue, local A-II generation is increased, as is the density of AT-1 receptors.[88] There is co-localization of ACE and the AT-I receptors with the expression of transforming growth factor beta (TGF-β_1) in fibroblasts. Furthermore an AT-1 receptor antagonist attenuates the formation of TGF-β_1 and the synthesis of type 1 collagen.[88] Thus it is reasonable to conclude that in the healing process following myocardial infarction, there is increased activity of the renin-angiotensin-AT-1 system in fibroblasts and that this process is associated with increased collagen formation. Note, too, the possibility that fibroblasts can generate growth factors that promote hypertrophy of cardiac myocytes (Fig 3-4).

Role of ACE inhibitor treatment. Evidence both from captopril-treated rats[68] and from patient studies[66] suggests that ventricular unloading by means of ACE inhibition can beneficially improve the remodeling process, particularly in moderate size rat infarcts (Fig 5–7). The rat heart data, showing improved postinfarct survival, has led to many clinical trials with ACE inhibitors following acute myocardial infarction, starting with Pfeffer et al.[66] As a result, ACE inhibition is now firmly ensconced in the prevention and treatment of post-infarct LV remodeling. A new but still provisional concept is that cardiac myocyte elongation can be reversed by the appropriate therapy, including ACE inhibition.[41]

ACE inhibitors in postinfarct LV dysfunction. In patients with a poor left ventricular ejection fraction (< 45%) but without clinical evidence of heart failure, captopril 25 mg three times daily compared with furosemide 40 mg daily prevents progressive left ventricular enlargement.[80] Patients in this study were started 1 week after the onset of acute myocardial infarction or later. In a second study, administration of the ACE inhibitor was started 24 to 48 hours after the onset of symptoms. One hundred patients were given either placebo or captopril 50 mg twice daily and followed

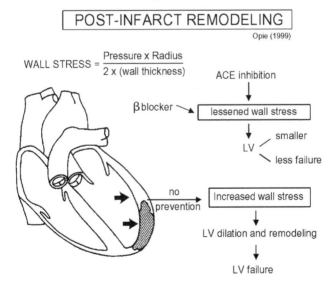

$$\text{WALL STRESS} = \frac{\text{Pressure x Radius}}{2 \times (\text{wall thickness})}$$

Figure 5–7. Postinfarction remodeling. Increased wall stress promotes adverse remodeling and left ventricular (LV) failure by the Laplace Law (see equation). The proposal, based on substantial animal data and human studies, is that ACE inhibition will attenuate postinfarct left ventricular enlargement and promote beneficial remodeling with better LV mechanical function. Figure © LH Opie, 1999

for 3 months.[81] The captopril group had a decrease in left ventricular end-systolic volume and an increase in the ejection fraction, changes not found in the placebo group. Similar data were obtained with enalapril in those with more evident heart failure.[43] These studies in relatively small numbers of patients have now been extended to show hard benefits in terms of improved morbidity and mortality in three massive studies, SAVE[76] using captopril, AIRE[4] using ramipril, and TRACE[92] using trandolapril (Tables 5-2 and 6-3). In addition, SOLVD, using enalapril, studied post infarct patients; besides improvement in clinical heart failure, there was less unstable angina.[100]

TABLE 5–2. META-ANALYSIS OF LONG-TERM ACE INHIBITOR
             TREATMENT AFTER MYOCARDIAL INFARCTION, BASED
             ON SAVE, AIRE, AND TRACE STUDIES

	ACE-inhibitor (%) N = 2995	Control N = 2971	Relative Risk (95% CI)
Deaths	23	29	0.74 (0.66–0.83)***
Hospitalization for CHF	12	16	0.73 (0.63–0.85)***
Non-fatal MI	11	13	0.80 (0.69–0.94)*
Stroke	4	4	1.10 (0.84–1.43)

(from Flather et al, Circulation, 1997; 96: 1-706)

SAVE study. In patients with recent acute myocardial infarction, captopril given to those with low ejection fractions but without symptoms improved the depressed left ventricular function better than did furosemide.[80] In the subsequent large SAVE study[76] on over 2,000 patients, captopril achieved some striking outcome benefits. It was given to patients 3 to 16 days postinfarct who had ejection fractions of below 40% but were not in overt heart failure, at an initial dose of 6.25 mg and titrated up to 50 mg three times daily. The hard benefits over an average of 42 months were several (Table 5-1). Most importantly, mortality from all causes was reduced by 19%, the development of severe heart failure was down by 37%, and (a surprise) recurrent myocardial infarction was reduced by 25%. Mortality reduction was not found until almost one year of therapy. Such studies and others in acute phase myocardial infarction (Fig 5–8) have led to the controversial recommendation that ACE inhibitors should be given for at least 6 weeks as part of the routine post-infarction treatment.[2] Strictly speaking, there should be proof that left ventricular dysfunction improves in the individual postinfarct patient given prophylactic ACE inhibition.[89]

Drug interactions. In the SAVE study,[76] captopril was beneficial even for patients given concurrent beta-blockers or thrombolytic therapy or aspirin. A retrospective analysis of SAVE showed that the protective effects of beta-blockade were additive to those of captopril.[95]

Postinfarct clinical heart failure: AIRE study with ramipril.
The AIRE (*Acute Infarction Ramipril Efficacy*)[4] trial shows

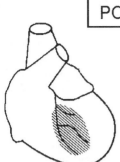

POST-INFARCT: **SAVE**

Opie (1999)

- *captopril*
- *entry point:*
  -ejection fraction < 40%
- 3-6 days post-infarct
- mean duration 42 months
- mortality ↓ 19 %

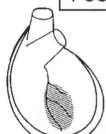

POST-INFARCT: **TRACE**

Opie (1999)

- *trandolapril*
- *entry point:*
  ejection fraction < 35%
- 3-7 days post-infarct
- treat 1-2 years
- mortality ↓ 24%
- sudden death ↓ 22%

POST-INFARCTION: **AIRE**

Opie (1999)

- *ramipril*
- *entry point:*
  -clinical heart failure
- 2-9 days post-infarct
- mean duration 15 months
- mortality ↓ 27%

Long-term use: ↓ 36%

Figure 5–8. Post-infarct ACE inhibition. Note mortality reduction by captopril, ramipril or trandolapril.

a striking benefit for ramipril given to early postinfarct patients with clinically manifest heart failure. The drug was given 3 to 10 days after the onset of acute myocardial infarction in an initial dose of 2.5 mg and titrated upwards to 5 mg twice daily. The mean follow up was 15 months, with a minimum of six months, and the mean duration of therapy was about one year.[5] All-cause mortality and a variety of softer end-points were all reduced (Table 5-2). Only a minority of these patients were also receiving digoxin, although the majority had diuretic therapy and received aspirin.

AIREX study. Long term follow-up of the AIRE patients, over 42 – 59 months, gave "robust evidence" that all cause mortality was reduced by 36% (relative risk reduction) with an absolute reduction of 11.4%.[5] These are impressive data, and very strongly argue for the compulsory use of ACE inhibitors in postinfarct patients with clinical failure.

Postinfarct LV dysfunction: TRACE study with trandolapril. The hypothesis tested by TRACE (*Tr*andolapril *C*ardiac *E*valuation)[92] was that patients having echocardiographic LV dysfunction soon after myocardial infarction, would benefit from long term ACE inhibition. Of nearly 7000 consecutive patients about one-third had left ventricular systolic dysfunction (using a wall motion abnormality score that corresponded to an ejection fraction of 35% or less). Signs of congestive heart failure were present in 74%. The initial dose of trandolapril was 1mg once daily, increased stepwise to 4 mg daily in those who could tolerate it. Trandolapril was given for one to two years. Follow up was for 2 – 4 years (maximum, 50 months). There were consistent reductions in total and cardiovascular mortality (p value for both, 0.0001), sudden death (p = 0.03), as well as decreased progression to severe heart failure (p = 0.003), the average risk reduction being by about 25% for all these events. Unexpectedly, in view of SAVE, recurrent infarction was unchanged. In all, 24 lives were saved after only 1 month of treating 2000 patients with LV dysfunction.

Postinfarct ischemic dysfunction with ST-segment changes. In postinfarct patients with a mean ejection fraction of 40%, captopril (titrated to a dose of 25 mg twice daily for 180 days) improved exercise tolerance, decreased ambulatory ST-segment changes, and lessened the heart volume.[83] Similar functional changes were found in another study wherein captopril compared favorably with digoxin;[12] ischemia was not an end-point in that study.

Mechanism of benefit of ACE inhibitors in remodeling. ACE inhibition acts both as a nonspecific load reducer and specifically. First, Jugdutt[40] compared prophylactic ACE inhibition with prophylactic nitrate administration early after acute myocardial infarction and followed the effects on left ventricular dimensions and function. Both agents had a similar prophylactic benefit on remodeling. Therefore, ACE inhibitors are nonspecific arteriolar and venous unloaders, as also shown experimentally,[69] which explains why they limit LV enlargement.[67] Second, experimental ACE inhibition limits ventricular myocyte growth and fibrosis.[60] Thus local autocrine/paracrine effects of ACE inhibition seem to be important. Third, enhanced fibrinolysis could mediate long term protection against re-infarction.[96]

Inhibition of sudden cardiac death. In a meta-analysis on 15 trials with a total of 15,104 patients, ACE inhibitors reduced the risk of death by 17%, cardiovascular death by 18%, and sudden cardiac death by 20% (confidence intervals: 0.70–0.92).[24]

Cost-effectiveness of postinfarct ACE inhibition. Postinfarct ACE inhibition, started some days after the onset of myocardial infarction, is highly cost effective especially when compared to statins in the 4s study.[55] One of three strategies for the use of ACE inhibitors were evaluated: (1) given only for high risk patients as in AIRE; (2) given also for intermediate risk SAVE-type patients; or (3) given to all patients with AMI and thereafter limiting use to AIRE or SAVE type patients. For these purposes, the TRACE type patients are probably somewhere between AIRE and SAVE. The cost of the third strategy (give to all, continue for SAVE type patients) was about $4500 per life year gained, and about $3000 for AIRE type patients. Not much was saved by an initial selective policy e.g. only AIRE type patients. Note these authors did *not* consider whether or not ACE inhibitors should be used in the first 24 hours of MI, although the different choices involved would be rather similar. Of interest, these costs were thought to be very reasonable in comparison with statins, in that the cost per life year gained in the 4S study was much more, at about $8000.

Unfortunately these calculations, favoring a "give-to-all" policy, leave out the cost of the echocardiogram and the cardiological assessment required at 6 weeks to decide whether or not the ACE inhibitor should be continued. Thus the advantage of the "initial AIRE" policy of the deliberate selection of high risk patients, is that it needs only a stethoscope and a pair of ears to define clinical heart failure and therefore to use the ACE inhibitor. Another important caveat is that the cost of the ACE inhibitor used could greatly alter the cost effectiveness. Tragically, despite clear cost-effectiveness and overwhelming data on the benefit of ACE inhibitors post infarct, the majority of high risk patients are still being discharged from American hospitals without receiving an ACE inhibitor.[9] Thus there is a major educational task in persuading physicians and cardiologists that they should not hesitate to use postinfarct ACE inhibitors whenever indicated.

LONG-TERM PROTECTION AGAINST MYOCARDIAL INFARCTION

Whether ACE inhibitors can give protection against myocardial infarction, as unexpectedly suggested by studies such as SOLVD and SAVE, needs prospective confirmation by adequately powered studies, such as HOPE with trandolapril and EUROPA with perindopril (see Ch 8). At present the results of meta-analyses are very suggestive of this benefit. As proposed mechanisms, ACE inhibitors cou' (1) enhance fibrinolysis, acting through the A-IV recer to reduce fibrinogen and plasminogen activator inhi'

(Fig 1-11); (2) exert long term protection by reversal of endothelial dysfunction, as result of increased nitric oxide formation; or (3) confer a preconditioning-like protection, acting via bradykinin BK_2-receptor activation as suggested by short term observations on human atrial tissue.[58]

ACE INHIBITORS IN OTHER CARDIAC CONDITIONS

In *chronic cor pulmonale*, captopril does not decrease pulmonary vascular resistance (hypoxic pulmonary hypertension), and any decrease in pulmonary wedge pressure reflects an effect on the left ventricle not on the pulmonary circulation.[101] Vasodilation induced by ACE inhibition may cause pulmonary vascular shunting to increase hypoxia. In *chronic aortic regurgitation*, acute administration of captopril 25 mg gave benefit by reducing the regurgitant fraction in the absence of any fall in the blood pressure.[72] The mechanism of this benefit is speculative and may include (1) effects of the ACE inhibitor on aortic compliance; and (2) reduction of the preload and thereby an improvement of myocardial wall stress. Further studies with much longer follow-up are required before ACE inhibition can be used for this indication. In *chronic mitral regurgitation* due to severe prolapse, enalapril for 6 months gave modest decreases in LV mass and end-systolic volume, with only a small increase in ejection fraction.[91]

In *murine Coxsackie myocarditis* produced experimentally, captopril whether started early or late in the disease process reduced heart weight and when given early it reduced the extent of necrosis.[73] In patients with *idiopathic dilated cardiomyopathy,* captopril is better able to reduce wall stress than is nifedipine.[3] In *anthracycline cardiomypathy,* in a small series of patients already treated by a diuretic and digoxin, addition of ACE inhibition reversed a downward trend.[39] Clearly, prospective data are required. In *pediatric cardiomyopathy,* a retrospective study suggested that captopril could improve survival.[48]

SUMMARY

1. *Role of angiotensin II.* This octapeptide helps to regulate the cardiac inotropic state and acts as a growth signal for the myocardium and blood vessels. There is increasing molecular evidence that the cardiac renin-angiotensin system participates in growth regulation during left ventricular hypertrophy and in remodeling. Nonetheless, the exact role of angiotensin-converting enzyme in the production of cardiac angiotensin II in humans is controversial. It is proposed that there is a multicellular interactive renin-angiotensin system involving cardiac myocytes, fibroblasts, vascular smooth muscle, and endothelium.

2. *Cardioprotective role of ACE inhibitors.* Theoretical grounds suggest that ACE inhibition may play a role in the control of myocardial ischemia, postreperfusion arrhythmias, and, possibly, postreperfusion stunning. At least some of the benefit of these drugs may be mediated by increased local formation of bradykinin. Nonetheless, firm data supporting the use of ACE inhibitors to lessen the severity of clinical myocardial ischemia or to decrease reperfusion stunning in patients, are still lacking. Protection from myocardial infarction, found in some studies, may be explained by enhanced fibrinolysis. Alternatively, or in addition, ACE inhibitors protect from endothelial dysfunction. A new meta-analysis shows consistent protection from death, including cardiovascular death and sudden cardiac death.[24]

3. *Nitrate tolerance.* This common condition is associated with increased sensitivity to vasoconstrictors, which can be lessened by ACE inhibitors or by hydralazine.

4. *Postinfarct left ventricular dysfunction.* Both experimental and clinical data are concordant in supporting the use of ACE inhibition even without additional diuretic therapy and, in fact, in preference to diuretic therapy.

5. *Postinfarct trials.* The results of several large-scale trials (SAVE; AIRE; AIREX; TRACE) on patients with impaired left ventricular function or failure show beyond reasonable doubt that ACE inhibition saves lives. The AIRE study[4] and its long term follow up, AIREX,[5] show that it is *compulsory* (unless there are clear contraindications) to treat postinfarct patients with clinical heart failure by ACE inhibition.

6. *Alternate policies in acute stage myocardial infarction.* One current trend is to treat all patients with AMI prophylactically within 24 hours of admission, and then to re-evaluate the need for ACE inhibitors at 6 weeks. Alternatively, high risk patients may be selected: anterior infarcts, patients with tachycardia or diabetes or clinical heart failure. The selective policy is probably more cost-effective.

REFERENCES

1. ACC/AHA Guidelines. Ryan TK, Anderson JL, Antman EM, et al. ACC/AHA guidelines for the management of patients with acute myocardial infarction: Executive summary. Circulation 1996;94:2341–2350.

2. ACE Inhibitor Myocardial Infarction Collaborative Group. Indications for ACE inhibitors in the early treatment of acute myocardial infarction. Circulation 1998;97:2202–2212.

3. Agostoni PG, De Cesare N, Doria E, et al. Afterload reduction: a comparison of captopril and nifedipine in dilated cardiomyopathy. Br Heart J 1986;55:391–399.

4. AIRE Study. The effect of ramipril on mortality and morbidity of survivors of acute myocardial infarction with clinical evidence of heart failure. Lancet 1993;342:821–828.

5. AIREX Study. Hall AS, Murray GD, Ball SG. On behalf of the AIREX Study Investigators. Follow-up study of patients randomly allocated ramipril or placebo for heart failure after acute myocardial infarction: AIRE Extension (AIREX) Study. Lancet 1997;349:1493–1497.

6. Akhras F, Jackson G. The role of captopril as single therapy in hypertension and angina pectoris. Int J Cardiol 1991;33:259–266.

7. Alderman MH, Madhavan S, Ooi WL, et al. Association of the renin sodium profile with the risk of myocardial infarction in patients with hypertension. N Engl J Med 1991;324:1098–1104.

8. Asano K, Dutcher D, Port J, et al. Selective downregulation of the angiotensin II AT_1 receptor subtype in failing human ventricular myocardium. Circulation 1997;95:1193–1200.

9. Barron HV, Michaels AD, Maynard C, et al. Use of angiotensin-converting enzyme inhibitors at discharge in patients with acute myocardial infarction in the United States: Data from the National Registry of Myocardial Infarction 2. J Am Coll Cardiol 1998;32:360–367.

10. Bartels L, Remme WJ, van der Ent M, et al. ACE inhibitors reduce myocardial ischemia through modulation of ischemia-induced catecholamine activation, experience with perindoprilat. J Am Coll Cardiol 1993;21:19A.

11. Bauer JA, Fung H-L. Concurrent hydralazine administration prevents nitroglycerin-induced hemodynamic tolerance in experimental heart failure. Circulation 1991;84:35–39.

12. Bonaduce D, Petretta M, Arrichielo P, et al. Effects of captopril treatment on left ventricular remodeling and function after anterior myocardial infarction: comparison with digitalis. J Am Coll Cardiol 1992;19:858–863.

13. Borghi C, Ambrosioni E. Clinical aspects of ACE inhibition in patients with acute myocardial infarction. Cardiovasc Drugs Ther 1996;10:519–525.

14. Bounhoure JP, Kayanakis JG, Fauvel M, et al. Beneficial effects of captopril in left ventricular failure in patients with myocardial infarction. Br J Clin Pharmacol 1982;14:187S–191S.

15. Brivet F, Delfraissy J-F, Guidicelli J-F, et al. Immediate effects of captopril in acute left ventricular failure secondary to myocardial infarction. Eur J Clin Invest 1981;11:369–373.

16. Cleland JGF, Henderson E, McLenachan J, et al. Effect of captopril, an angiotensin-converting enzyme inhibitor, in patients with angina pectoris and heart failure. J Am Coll Cardiol 1991;17:733–739.

17. Cohen MV, Kirk ES. Differential response of large and small coronary arteries to nitroglycerin and angiotensin. Autoregulation and tachyphylaxis. Circ Res 1973;33:445–453.

18. CONSENSUS II. Swedberg K, Held P, Kjekshus J, Rasmussen K. Effects of the early administration of enalapril on mortality in patients with acute myocardial infarction. Results of the Co-operative Scandinavian Enalapril Survival Study II (CONSENSUS II). N Engl J Med 1992;327:678–684.

19. Csikos T, Chung O, Unger T. Receptors and their classification: focus on angiotensin II and the AT_2 receptor. J Human Hypertens 1998;12:133–318.

20. Dargie HJ, McAlpine M, Morton JJ. Neuroendocrine activation in acute myocardial infarction. J Cardiovasc Pharmacol 1987;9 (Suppl 2):S21–S24.

21. de Graeff, van Gilst WK, Bel K, et al. Conentration-dependent protection by captopril against myocardial damage during ischemia and reperfusion in a closed chest pig mdel. J Cardiovasc Pharmacol 1987;9 (Suppl 2):S37–S42.

22. de Graeff PA, de Langen CDJ, van Gilst WH, et al. Protective effects of captopril against ischemia/reperfusion-induced ventricular arrhythmias in vitro and in vivo. Am J Med 1988;84 (Suppl 3A):67–74.

23. de Langen C, de Graeff P, van Wilst WH, et al. Effects of angiotensin II and captopril on inducible sustained ventricular tachycardia two weeks after myocardial infarction in the pig. J Cardiovasc Pharmacol 1989;13:186–191.

24. Domanski MJ, Exner DV, Bordowf CB, et al. Effect of angiotensin converting enzyme inhibition on sudden cardiac death in patients following acute myocardial infarction. A meta-analysis of randomized clinical trials. J Am Coll Cardiol 1999;33:598–604.

25. Dostal DE, Baker KM. Evidence for a role of an intracardiac renin-angiotensin system in normal and failing hearts. Trends Cardiovasc Med 1993;3:67–74.

26. Ertl G. Coronary vasoconstriction in experimental myocardial ischemia. J Cardiovasc Pharmacol 1987;9 (Suppl 2):S9–S17.

27. Ertl G, Kloner RA, Alexander W, et al. Limitation of experimental infarct size by an angiotensin-converting enzyme inhibitor. Circulation 1982;65:40–48.

28. Ford WR, Clanachan AS, Jugdutt BI. Opposite effects of angiotensin AT_1 and AT_2 receptor antagonists on recovery of mechanical function after ischemia-reperfusion in isolated working rat hearts. Circulation 1996;94:3087–3089.

29. Gadsboll N, Hoilund-Carlson P-F, Badsberg JS, et al. Late ventricular dilatation in survivors of acute myocardial infarction. Am J Cardiol 1989;64:961–966.

30. Gerdes AM, Kellerman SE, Moore JA, et al. Structural remodeling of cardiac myocytes in patients with ischemic cardiomyopathy. Circulation 1992;86:426–430.

31. GISSI-3 Study Group. GISSI-3: effects of lisinopril and transdermal glyceryl trinitrate singly and together on 6-week mortality and ventricular function after acute myocardial infarction. Lancet 1994;343:1115–1122.

32. Hartman JC, Wall TM, Hullinger TG, et al. Reduction of myocardial infarct size in rabbits by ramiprilat: reversal by the bradykinin antagonist HOE 140. J Cardiovasc Pharmacol 1993;21:996–1003.

33. Haywood GA, Gullestad L, Katsuya T, et al. AT_1 and AT_2 angiotensin receptor gene expression in human heart failure. Circulation 1997;95:1201–1206.

34. Heitzer T, Just H, Brockhoff C, et al. Long-term nitroglycerin treatment is associated with supersensitivity to vasoconstrictors in men with stable coronary artery disease: prevention by concomitant treatment with captopril. J Am Coll Cardiol 1998;31:83–88.

35. Holtz J, Busse R, Sommer O, et al. Dilation of epicardial arteries in consious dogs induced by angiotensin-converting enzyme inhibition with enalaprilat. J Cardiovasc Pharmacol 1987;9:348–355.

36. Hu K, Gaudron P, Anders H-J, et al. Chronic effects of early started angiotensin converting enzyme inhibition and angiotensin AT_1-receptor subtype blockade in rats with myocardial infarction: role of bradykinin. Cardiovasc Res 1998;39:401–412.

37. ISIS-4 Study. ISIS-4 Collaborative Group. A randomised factorial trial assessing early oral captopril, oral mononitrate, and intravenous magnesium in 58,050 patients with a suspected acute myocardial infarction. Lancet 1995;345:669–685.

38. Jalowy A, Schulz R, Dorge H, et al. Infarct size reduction by AT_1-receptor blockade through a signal cascade of AT_2-receptor activation, bradykinin and prostaglandins in pigs. J Am Coll Cardiol 1998;32:1787–1796.

39. Jensen BV, Nielsen SL, Skovsgaard T. Treatment with angiotensin-converting-enzyme inhibitor for epirubicin-induced dilated cardiomyopathy. Lancet 1996;347:297–299.

40. Jugdutt BI. Nitrates in myocardial infarction. Cardiovasc Drugs Ther 1994;8:635–646.

41. Katz AM. Regression of left ventricular hypertrophy. New hope for dying hearts (Editorial). Circulation 1998;98:623–624.

42. Katz RJ, Levy WS, Buff L, et al. Prevention of nitrate tolerance with angiotensin converting enzyme inhibitors. Circulation 1991;83:1271–1277.

43. Konstam MA, Rousseau MF, Kronenberg MW, et al. Effects of the angiotensin-converting enzyme inhibitor enalapril on the long-term progression of left ventricular dysfunction in patients with heart failure. Circulation 1992;86:431–438.

44. Kramer CM, Rogers WJ, Park CS, et al. Regional myocyte hypertrophy parallels regional myocardial dysfunction during post-infarct remodeling. J Moll Cell Cardiol 1998;30:1773–1778.

45. Kurabayashi M, Yazaki Y. Downregulation of angiotensin II receptor type 1 in heart failure. Circulation 1997;95:1104–1107.

46. Lai C, Onnis E, Orani E, et al. Antiischaemic activity of ACE inhibitor enalapril in normotensive patients with stable effort angina (Abstract). J Am Coll Cardiol 1987;9:192A.

47. Latini R, Avanzini F, Nicolao AD. GISSI-3 Investigators. Effects of lisinopril and nitroglycerin on blood pressure early after myocardial infarction: the GISSI-3 pilot study. Clin Pharmacol and Therapeutics 1994;56:680–692.

48. Lewis AB, Chabot M. The effect of treatment with angiotensin-converting enzyme inhibitors on survival of pediatric patients with dilated cardiomyopathy. Pediatr Cardiol 1993;14:9–12.

49. Lindpainter K, Ganten D. The cardiac renin-angiotensin system. An appraisal of present experimental and clinical evidence. Circ Res 1991;68:905–921.

50. Linz W, Martorana PA, Grotsch H, et al. Antagonizing bradykinin (BK) obliterates the cardioprotective effects of bradykinin and angiotensin-converting enzyme (ACE) inhibitors in ischemic hearts. Drug Development Res 1990;19:393–408.

51. Liu Y-H, Yang X-P, Sharov VG, et al. Paracrine systems in the cardioprotective effect of angiotensin-converting enzyme inhibitors on myocardial ischemia/reperfusion injury in rats. Hypertension 1996;27:7–13.

52. Magrini F, Shimizu M, Roberts N, et al. Converting enzyme inhibition and coronary blood flow. Circulation 1987;75 (Suppl I):I-168-I-174.

53. McAlpine HM, Morton JJ, Leckie B, et al. Haemodynamic effects of captopril in acute left ventricular failure complicating myocardial infarction. J Cardiovasc Pharmacol 1987;9 (Suppl 2):S25–S30.

54. McDonald K, Garr M, Carlyle P, et al. Relative effects of α-adrenoceptor blockade, converting enzyme inhibitor therapy, and angiotensin II sub-

type 1 receptor blockade on ventricular remodeling in the dog. Circulation 1994;90:3034–3046.

55. McMurray JJV, McGuire A, Davie AP, et al. Cost-effectiveness of different ACE inhibitor treatment scenarios post-myocardial infarction. Eur Heart J 1997;18:1411–1415.

56. Metelitsa WI, Marsevich SY, Kozyreva MP, et al. Enhancement of the efficacy of isosorbide dinitrate by captopril in stable angina pectoris. Am J Cardiol 1992;69:291–296.

57. Mitchell GF, Lamas GA, Vaughan DE, et al. Left ventricular remodeling in the year after first anterior myocardial infarction: a quantitative analysis of contractile segment lengths and ventricular shape. J Am Coll Cardiol 1992;19:1136–1144.

58. Morris SD, Yellon DM. Angiotensin-converting enzyme inhibitors potentiate preconditioning through bradykinin B_2 receptor activation in human heart. J Am Coll Cardiol 1997;29:1599–1606.

59. Muller CA, Opie LH, Peisach M, et al. Chronic oral pretreatment with the angiotensin converting enzyme inhibitor, trandolapril decreases ventricular fibrillation in acute ischaemia and reperfusion. Eur Heart J 1994;15:988–996.

60. Nguyen T, Salibi EE, Rouleau JL. Postinfarction survival and inducibility of ventricular arrhythmias in the spontaneousy hypertensive rat. Effects of ramipril and hydralazine. Circulation 1998;98:2074–2080.

61. Noda K, Sasaguri M, Ideishi M. Role of locally formed angiotensin-II and bradykinin in the reduction of myocardial infarct size in dogs. Cardiovasc Res 1993;27:334–340.

62. Opie LH. Reperfusion injury and its pharmacologic modification. Circulation 1989;80:1049–1062.

63. Perondi R, Saino A, Tio RA, et al. ACE inhibition attenuates sympathetic coronary vasoconstriction in patients with coronary artery disease. Circulation 1992;85:2004–2013.

64. Pfeffer MA. ACE inhibitors in acute myocardial infarction: patient selection and timing. Circulation 1998;97:2192–2194.

65. Pfeffer MA, Braunwald E, Moye LA, et al. Effect of captopril on mortality and morbidity in patients with left ventricular dysfunction after myocardial infarction. Results of the Survival and Ventricular Enlargement Trial. N Engl J Med 1992;327:669–677.

66. Pfeffer MA, Lamas GA, Vaughan DE, et al. Effect of captopril on progressive ventricular dilatation after anterior myocardial infarction. N Engl J Med 1988;319:80–86.

67. Pfeffer MA, Pfeffer JM. Ventricular enlargement and reduced survival after myocardial infarction. Circulation 1987;75 (Suppl IV):IV-93–IV-97.

68. Pfeffer MA, Pfeffer JM, Steinberg C, et al. Survival after an experimental myocardial infarction: beneficial effects of long-term therapy with captopril. Circulation 1985;72:406–412.

69. Raya TE, Gay RG, Aguirre M, et al. Importance of venodilation in prevention of left ventricular dilatation after chronic large myocardial infarction in rats: A comparison of captopril and hydralazine. Circ Res 1989;64:330–337.

70. Regitz-Zagrosek V, Friedel N, Heymann A, et al. Regulation, chamber localization, and subtype distribution of angiotensin II receptors in human hearts. Circulation 1995;91:1461–1471.

71. Remme WJ, Kruyssen DA, Look MP, et al. Systemic and cardiac neuroendocrine activation and severity of myocardial ischemia in humans. J Am Coll Cardiol 1994;23:82–91.

72. Reske SN, Heck I, Kropp J, et al. Captopril mediated decrease of aortic regurgitation. Br Heart J 1985;54:415–419.

73. Rezhalla S, Kloner RA, Khatib G, et al. Beneficial effects of captopril in acute Coxsackie virus B_3 murine myocarditis. Circulation 1990;81:1039–1046.

74. Ribout C, Mossiat C, Devissaguet M, et al. Beneficial effect of perindopril, an angiotensin-concerting enzme inhibitor, on left ventricular performance and noradrenaline myocardial content during cardiac failure development in the rat. Can J Physiol Pharmacol 1990;68:1548–1551.

75. Rochette L, Ribuot C, Belichard P, et al. Profective effect of angiotensin converting enzyme inhibitors (CEI): captopril and perindopril on vulnerability to ventricular fibrillation during myocardial ischemia and reperfusion in rat. Clin Exp Theory Pract 1987;A9:365–368.

76. SAVE Study. Pfeffer MA, Braunwald E, Moye LA. Effect of captopril on mortality and morbidity in patients with left ventricular dysfunction after myocardial infarction. Results of the Survival and Ventricular Enlargement trial. N Eng J Med 1992;327:669–677.

77. Schlaifer JD, Mancini J, O'Neill BJ, et al. Influence of smoking status on angiotensin-converting enzyme inhibition-related improvement on coronary endothelial function. Cardiovasc Drugs Therap 1999;In press.

78. Schunkert H, Sadoshima J-I, Cornelius T, et al. Angiotensin II-induced growth responses in isolated adult rat hearts. Circ Res 1995;76:489–497.

79. Schwartz JS, Bache RJ. Pharmacologic vasodilators in the coronary circulation. Circulation 1987;75 (Suppl 1):I-162–I-167.

80. Sharpe N, Murphy J, Smith H, et al. Treatment of patients with symptomless left ventricular dysfunction after myocardial infarction. Lancet 1988;1:255–259.

81. Sharpe N, Smith H, Murphy J, et al. Early prevention of left ventricular dysfunction after myocardial infarction with angiotensin-converting enzyme inhibition. Lancet 1991;337:872–876.

82. SMILE Study. Ambrosioni E, Borghi C, Magnani B. For the Survival of Myocardial Infarction Long-Term Evaluation Study Investigators. The effect of the angiotensin-converting-enzyme inhibitor zofenopril on mortality and morbidity after anterior myocardial infarction. N Engl J Med 1995;332:80–85.

83. Sogaard P, Gotzsche CO, Ravkilde J, et al. Effects of captopril on ischemia and dysfunction of the left ventricle after myocardial infarction. Circulation 1993;87:1093–1099.

84. SOLVD Investigators. Effect of enalapril on mortality and the development of heart failure in asymptomatic patients with reduced left ventricular ejection fractions. New Engl J Med 1992;327:685–691.

85. Strozzi C, Cocco G, Portaluppi F, et al. Effects of captopril on the physical work capacity of normotensie patients with stable effort angina pectoris. Cardiology 1987;74:226–228.

86. Stumpe KO, Overlack A on behalf of the Perindopril Therapeutic Safety Study Groups (PLUTS). A new trial of the efficacy, tolerability and safety of angiotensin-converting enzyme inhibition in mild systemic hypertension with concomitant diseases and therapies. Am J Cardiol 1993;71:32E–37E.

87. Sudhir K, MacGregor JS, Gupta M, et al. Effect of selective angiotensin II receptor antagonism and angiotensin-converting enzyme inhibition on the coronary vasculature in vivo. Intravascular two-dimensional and Doppler ultrasound studies. Circulation 1993;87:931–938.

88. Sun Y, Zhang JQ, Zhang J, et al. Angiotensin II, transforming growth factor-ß$_1$ and repair in the infarcted heart. J Moll Cell Cardiol 1998;30:1559–1569.

89. Sutton M, Pfeffer MA, Plappert T, et al. Quantitative two-dimensional echocardiographic measurements are major predictors of adverse cardiovascular events after acute myocardial infarction. The protective effects of captopril. Circulation 1994;89:68–75.

90. Thurmann P, Odenthal HJ, Rietbrock N. Converting enzyme inhibition in coronary artery disease: a randomized, placebo-controlled trial with benazepril. J Cardiovasc Pharmacol 1991;17:718–723.

91. Tischler MD, Rowan M, Winter MML. Effect of enalapril therapy on left ventricular mass and volumes in asymptomatic chronic, severe mitral regurgitation secondary to mitral valve prolapse. Am J Cardiol 1998;82:242–245.

92. TRACE Study. Kover L, Torp-Pedersen C, Carsen JE, et al. A clinical trial of the angiotensin-converting-enzyme inhibitor trandolapril in patients with left ventricular dysfunction after myocardial infarction. N Engl J Med 1995;333:1670–1676.

93. van Gilst WH, de Graeff PA, Wesseling H, et al. Reduction of reperfusion arrhythmias in the ischemic isolated rat heart by angiotensin converting enzyme inhibitors: a comparison of captopril, enalapril and HOE 498. J Cardiovasc Pharmacol 1986;8:722–728.

94. van Gilst WH, Wijngaarden J, Scholtens E, et al. Captopril induced increase in coronary flow: An SH-dependent effect on arachidonic acid metabolism. J Cardiovasc Pharmacol 1987;9 (Suppl 2):S31–S36.

95. Vantrimpont P, Rouleau JL, Wun C-C, et al. Additive beneficial effects of ß-blockers to angiotensin converting enzyme inhibitors in the survival and ventricular enlargement (SAVE) study. JACC 1997;29:229–236.

96. Vaughan DE. Fibrinolytic balance, the renin-angiotensin system and atherosclerotic disease. Eur Heart J 1998;19 (Suppl G):G9–G12.

97. Weber KT, Sun Y, Tyagi SC, et al. Collagen network of the myocardium: function, structural remodeling and regulatory mechanisms. J Mol Cell Cardiol 1994;26:279–292.

98. Yamagishi H, Kim S, Nishikimi T, et al. Contribution of cardiac renin-angiotensin system to ventricular remodelling in myocardial-infarcted rats. J Mol Cell Cardiol 1993;25:1369–1380.

99. Yang BC, Phillips MI, Zhang YC, et al. Critical Role of AT$_1$ receptor expression after ischemia/reperfusion in isolated rat hearts. Beneficial effect of antisense oligodeoxynucleotides directed at AT$_1$ receptor mRNA. Circ Res 1998;83:552–559.

100. Yusuf S, Pepine CJ, Garces C, et al. Effect of enalapril on myocardial infarction and unstable angina in patients with low ejection fractions. Lancet 1992;340:1173–1178.

101. Zielinski J, Hawrylkiewicz I, Gorecka D, et al. Captopril effects on pulmonary and systemic hemodynamics in chronic cor pulmonale. Chest 1986;90:562–565.
102. Zuanetti G, Latini R, Maggioni AP, et al. Effect of ACE inhibitor lisinopril on mortality in diabetic patients with acute myocardial infarction. Circulation 1997;96:4239–4245.

CHAPTER 6

ACE Inhibitors
for congestive heart failure

"ACE inhibitors are now part of established therapeutic practice for congestive heart failure" (Braunwald, 1991).[5]

"ACE inhibitors should be used routinely and early in patients with congestive heart failure, especially those with low ejection fractions" (Garg and Yusuf, 1995)[21]

There is a tendency to use ACE inhibitors earlier and earlier including now even for the milder degrees of heart failure. Extensive hemodynamic studies have shown acute and chronic benefit with these agents, generally without the development of tolerance. Three major outcome studies in congestive heart failure, in patients mostly already treated by diuretics and digoxin, have shown improved mortality.[9,67,75] Two major outcome trials in patients with left ventricular systolic dysfunction but without advanced heart failure attest to the preventative benefits of these agents.[64,67] A large and still unpublished meta-analysis, involving about 12,000 patients, attests to the safety and efficacy of ACE inhibitors.[19] Specifically, there is a consistent effect in reduction of mortality especially from progressive heart failure.[21]

Despite these persuasive data, which justify the widespread and increasing use of ACE inhibitors, many aspects of their role in the therapy of congestive heart failure remain unanswered, particularly because the typical patient enrolled in these trials has been white, male, about 60, and with a previous myocardial infarction. Data on females, blacks, and valvular heart disease are strikingly absent. This chapter will first briefly review the presumed stages of development of heart failure. The possible use of ACE inhibitors at each stage will be considered, with particular reference to the information made available by each of the therapeutic trials. Emphasis will be laid on factors that govern the success of addition of ACE inhibitors to existing therapy, as well as factors that may predict their likely failure.

RATIONALE FOR ACE INHIBITORS AT EACH STAGE OF DEVELOPMENT OF MYOCARDIAL FAILURE

Meerson[35] has proposed that excess mechanical loading of the left ventricle leads to myocardial failure through three phases (Fig 6-1): (1) an acute adaptation to the hemodynamic load, which leads to (2) compensatory ventricular hypertrophy, and eventually to (3) myocardial failure. In the phase of left ventricular failure, the well known neurohumoral adaptation is thought to be a reaction to systemic hypotension, according to the proposals of Harris:[24]

> "In these ways the syndrome of congestive heart failure may be regarded as one which arises when the heart becomes chronically unable to maintain an appropriate arterial pressure without support".

This basic role of hypotension in the vicious circle that exists in severe congestive heart failure is shown in Fig 6-2. Compensatory vasoconstrictive and volume-retaining mechanisms having their origin in baroreceptor control overwhelm opposing vasodilatory mechanisms mediated through atrial natriuretic peptide and having their origin in atrial distension,[25] as shown in Fig 6-3.

In the early stages of the Meerson progression, ACE inhibitors should act both on the early first loading stage of myocardial hypertrophy as well as during the phase of left ventricular hypertrophy. ACE inhibitors reduce the load on the myocardium (Table 6-1) by acting both as arteriolar and venous dilators, by reducing the blood pressure and decreasing ventricular dimensions. By similar logic, ACE inhibitors decrease left ventricular hypertrophy, which in itself is the cause of diastolic dysfunction and predisposes to the third phase of the failing left ventricle. Whereas the second phase is characterized by normal indices of systolic

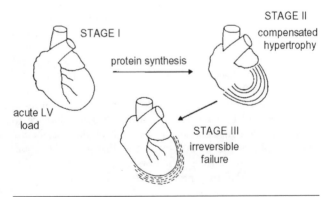

CARDIAC HYPERTROPHY AND FAILURE

Meerson's 3 stages modified

Figure 6-1. Meerson's three stages, as modified for clinical application. The acute hemodynamic load (Stage I) calls forth protein synthesis and compensated hypertrophy (Stage II) before failure develops (Stage III). Figure © LH Opie, 1999

function but abnormal diastolic function, the third phase is characterized by abnormalities both of systolic and diastolic function and is symptomatically divided by the severity of dyspnea according to the New York Heart Association (NYHA) classification.

TABLE 6-1: STAGES OF DEVELOPMENT OF CONGESTIVE HEART FAILURE WITH POSSIBLE ROLE OF ACE INHIBITORS

Meerson stage	Clinical modification of Meerson classification	Rationale for ACE Inhibition
Acute load	Initial loading stage, normal left ventricle (early post-AMI, early valve disease, early hypertension).	Load reduction prevents left ventricular hypertrophy (hypothetical).
Compensatory hypertrophy	Left ventricular hypertrophy often with diastolic failure.	Load reduction improves left ventricular hypertrophy and diastolic function.
Failure	Left ventricular hypertrophy and dilation with systolic and diastolic failure. Neurohumoral adaptation.	Load reduction lessens dilation. Decrease of angiotensin-II and plasma norepinephrine. Sometimes aldosterone levels fall.

AMI : acute myocardial infarction

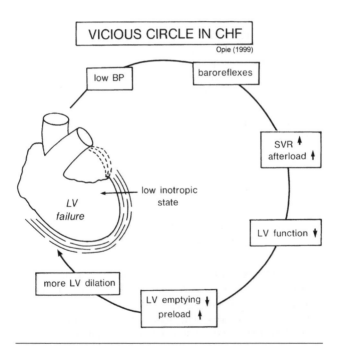

Figure 6-2: *Potential vicious circle in congestive heart failure (CHF) in which a low inotropic state of the left ventricle (LV) causes a low arterial blood pressure (BP), which activates the baroreflexes to increase the systemic vascular resistance (SVR) and the afterload. Consequently, the failing left ventricle must work against a greater resistance so that left ventricular function falls, left ventricular emptying is depressed, left ventricular preload is increased, and there is more left ventricle dilation. Figure © LH Opie, 1999*

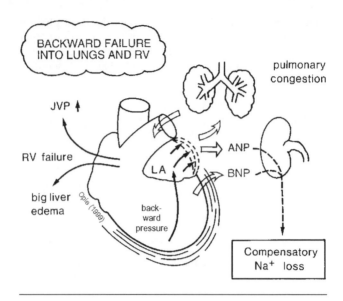

Figure 6-3: *Backward failure. Note association with pulmonary congestion and abnormalities of left atrial emptying or LV relaxation. RV, right ventricle; LA, left atrium; JVP, jugular venous pressure; ANP, atrial natriuretic peptide; BNP, brain natriuretic peptide. Figure © LH Opie, 1999*

EARLY RENAL SODIUM ABNORMALITIES

In early asymptomatic heart failure there is an impairment of sodium reabsorption in the proximal nephron, so that sodium is retained in response to an increased sodium intake.[76] This defect occurs even in those with normal plasma renin and aldosterone levels, and is reversed by enalapril. The latter which acts independently of changes in renal or systemic hemodynamics, showing a specific intrarenal effect. Also in such patients, an infusion of amino acids failed to elicit an increase in glomerular filtration rate or in renal plasma flow, as found in normals.[34] Both the ACE inhibitor, enalapril, and the AT-1 receptor blocker, losartan, reversed these abnormalities, suggesting a major causative role for A-II.

ESTABLISHED HEART FAILURE

Effects on neurohumoral activation. ACE inhibitors are commonly used in advanced failure, in which a neurohumoral syndrome is elicited that includes enhanced renin secretion by the kidney (Fig 6-4). It may be supposed that circulating renin and angiotensin-II levels should therefore be elevated in all patients with congestive heart failure and that the degree of elevation should bear relation to the severity of the congestive heart failure. However, in untreated early congestive heart failure, in patients with NYHA Disability Class I or Class II, plasma renin activity is not raised, although atrial natriuretic peptide values and plasma adrenaline are increased.[60] Likewise, in untreated patients with slightly more severe congestive heart failure

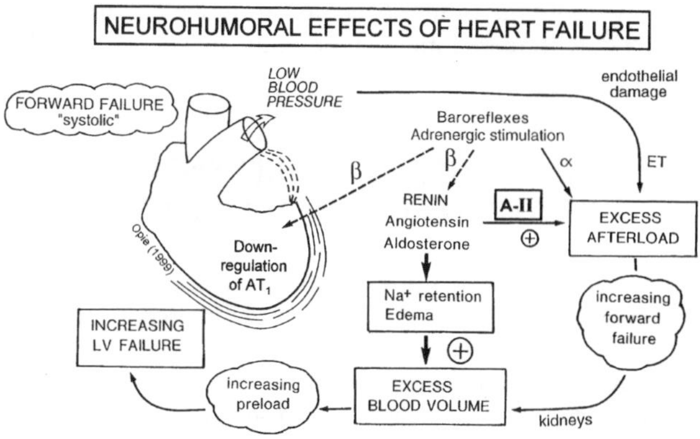

Figure 6-4: Forward failure. Note association of forward failure with hypotension and neurohumoral activation with consequent afterload increase to which increased angiotensin II (AII) and endothelin (ET) contribute. α = alpha-adrenergic; ß = beta-adrenergic. Figure © LH Opie, 1999.

(NYHA Classes II and III), plasma renin and aldosterone levels were normal, although plasma norepinephrine levels were high.[4]

In untreated patients with severe congestive heart failure, almost all in NYHA Class III or IV, the major consistent finding was water and sodium retention as well as an increased plasma norepinephrine.[2] Plasma renin activity was increased in only some patients. On the other hand, in diuretic-treated patients, plasma renin activity is consistently elevated.[4] An elevation in plasma renin activity may only follow an increase in plasma catecholamines.[60] Thus, logically, ACE inhibitors should be especially effective in patients with heart failure treated by diuretics (which increase renin activity). Because ACE inhibitors can prophylactically avoid the development of heart failure, there must be factors other than plasma renin that are involved, such as the cardiac renin-angiotensin system.

Cardiac renin-angiotensin. Cardiac A-II may be an important site of ACE inhibition.[63] Of interest, cardiac AT-1 receptors become relatively down-regulated in heart failure, when compared with AT-2 receptors.[27]

Additional mechanisms of benefit. In early pre-symptomatic heart failure, as already discussed, even when renin values are normal, there are defects of response to acute salt, water and amino-acid loading that are improved by ACE inhibition.[34,76,77] Cardiac parasympathetic activity may be increased by ACE inhibition, which may also benefit heart failure.[18]

Bradykinin. In experimental heart failure, endothelium-derived vasodilation is reduced.[69] The response is restored by bradykinin, whether infused or locally generated. In human heart failure, there is also impaired endothelial function, which is better restored by quinaprilat than by enalaprilat, hypothetically the result of the greater tissue affinity of the former,[28] with more formation of bradykinin.[79]

ACE INHIBITORS AS PREVENTATIVE THERAPY IN POSTINFARCT FAILURE

Preventative role in the postinfarct phase: SAVE study.
In patients with recent acute myocardial infarction, ACE inhibitor therapy given to those with low ejection fractions but without symptoms improved the depressed left ventricular function better than did furosemide.[66] In the large SAVE study[54] on over 2,000 patients, captopril achieved some striking benefits. Most importantly, mortality from all causes was reduced by 19%, the development of severe heart failure was down by 37%, and (a surprise) recurrent myocardial infarction was reduced by 25%. ACE inhibitors do not appear to act beneficially in postinfarct remodeling by only arteriolar dilation – it seems as if the added venous dilation is crucial, both shown by Jugdutt et al[30] and by the failure of hydralazine to improve postinfarct remodeling in rats.[59] The knowledge that there is a tissue renin-angiotensin system, which is a potential site at which ACE inhibitors could work, provides a satisfactory explanation for the prophylactic benefit.

Other etiologies for early myocardial failure. Does the benefit extend to other clinical conditions that predispose to eventual left ventricular failure? Two such conditions would be *early valvular heart disease* and early hypertension. Logically, patients with aortic stenosis or mitral stenosis should be excluded from such therapy with ACE inhibitors. Equally logically, ACE inhibition that improves the hemodynamics of mitral and aortic regurgitation could be given at an early stage as part of prophylactic therapy to prevent eventual left ventricular hypertrophy and dilation. This particular use is, as yet, largely unexplored although there is provisional evidence for the benefit of ACE inhibition in mitral vale prolapse with a normal ejection fraction.[72] Likewise, in early *hypertension*, before the development of left ventricular hypertrophy, prophylactic use of ACE inhibitors would also be logical. Nonetheless, there are no outcome trials nor data to support this proposed use. In none of these situations can it be expected that plasma renin activity would be elevated, so that the logical basis for the use of ACE inhibitors postinfarct would be the mechanical unloading effect or an effect on LV growth.

Early symptomatic left ventricular hypertrophy with diastolic dysfunction. The symptoms, chiefly exertional dyspnea, are thought to result from diastolic dysfunction, which is a consequence of left ventricular hypertrophy. Because ACE inhibition can lessen left ventricular hypertrophy, such therapy is likely to improve symptoms. Nonetheless, this seemingly logical sequence of events has not yet been established.

POSSIBLE USE OF ACE INHIBITORS AS FIRST-LINE THERAPY IN HEART FAILURE

Strictly speaking, there have been only three studies on the possible use of ACE inhibitors as *sole therapy* (i.e. no diuretics, no digoxin) in clinical heart failure. First, Richardson et al[61] studied 14 patients who were previously stable on diuretic therapy. Patients were randomly assigned to either captopril 25 mg three times daily or a loop diuretic once daily (furosemide 40 mg, amiloride 5 mg). After 8 weeks patients were crossed over without washout to the other therapy. Captopril by itself was as effective as prior diuretic therapy in 10 of 14 patients in that this group remained stable, whereas in the other 4 patients who had had a history of pulmonary edema, captopril was not sufficient as monotherapy.

Second, Riegger[62] studied the effects of quinapril given as monotherapy to 26 patients with heart failure (NYHA Class II and III). The increase of exercise time in patients receiving quinapril monotherapy was greater than in those receiving placebo. However, the data are not given in detail, so this report must be regarded as provisional. Third, in 5 patients with untreated but severe heart failure, Anand et al[3] gave an acute dose of enalapril and found surprisingly few hemodynamic changes; systemic vascular resistance fell and cardiac index rose, but pulmonary wedge and pulmonary artery pressures did not fall. Thereafter, 3 of the 5 patients responded to 1 month of enalapril therapy by weight loss. The authors felt unable to recommend a longer formal trial for ACE inhibition as monotherapy in patients with severe congestive heart failure.

SOLVD preventative study. In the huge SOLVD study[67] on over 4,000 patients, most postinfarct, only 17% were taking diuretics and 66% were in NYHA Class I (Table 6-2) – so that the question was whether enalapril could prevent the development of overt heart failure. Not surprisingly, the most striking benefits were found in patients with the lowest initial ejection fractions, below 28%, with only borderline results in those with values of 33% to 35%. Enalapril in a mean daily dose of 17 mg was associated with less hospitalization and less development of symptomatic heart failure. It is the data from this arm of SOLVD that influences a still unpublished meta-analysis to show that the mortality benefit of ACE inhibitors can be found even in the absence of initial diuretic therapy.[19] Thus, both the European and American Guidelines recommend ACE inhibitors as first line treatment for mild LV dysfunction without symptoms of volume overload.[44,70]

ACE INHIBITORS AS SECOND-LINE THERAPY WITH DIURETICS FOR CONGESTIVE HEART FAILURE

Diuretic therapy is still universally accepted as first-step and first-line therapy in clinically evident left ventricular

TABLE 6-2 : THREE TREATMENT TRIALS WITH ACE INHIBITORS IN
PATIENTS WITH OVERT CHRONIC HEART FAILURE,
THE MAJORITY RECEIVING DIURETIC THERAPY;
COMPARISON WITH ONE PREVENTION TRIAL

	CONSENSUS-I (treatment)	SOLVD-I (treatment)	V-Heft-II (treatment)	SOLVD-II (prevention)
Total number treated	127	1,285	403	2,111
Drug & dose (daily)	Enalapril[+] 18.4 mg	Enalapril[+] 16.6 mg	Enalapril 5–20 mg	Enalapril mean dose 16.7 mg
Mean duration (months)	6	41	24	37
Patient population	Severe heart failure	Chronic heart failure	Chronic heart failure	"Asymptomatic"; EF 35% or less; no antifailure drugs
Age (years) mean	71	61	61	60
Gender, male (%)	70	81	100	89
Race, white (%)	100	79	70	86
NYHA (%) I	0	11	6	66
II	0	57	52	33
III	0	30	42	0
IV	100	2	0.5	0
Post-infarct (%)	47	66	46	81
Hypertension (%)	24	43	50	37
Diuretics (%)	100	86	100	16
Digitalis (%)	92	66	100	12
Ejection fraction (%), mean	?	25	29	28
Mortality reduction (%)	40	16	28	8
(NS) Worsening of or development of new heart failure (%) (reduction in risk)	13*	26	None	37
Sudden death (reduction)	None	NS	38**	Not stated

NS, not significant; EF, LV ejection fraction
+ mean daily dose
* improvement in mean NYHA classification, calculated from Table 4 of the study
** calculated from Table 2 of the study

failure and in congestive heart failure. This is because of
symptomatic benefit. There is no trial evidence that life is
prolonged, although it would be intuitively clear that an
intravenous loop diuretic could be life saving when given
to a patient with severe LV failure and pulmonary edema.

***ACE inhibition versus digoxin versus the combination in
early left ventricular failure.*** An important study by Kromer et al[31] on only 19 patients, clearly shows that relatively
short-term therapy with an ACE inhibitor is preferable to
digoxin in early heart failure already treated by diuretics.
Digoxin exerted no benefit of note. While these data cannot
be extrapolated to longer periods and need further follow-

up and supportive studies, nonetheless the data support a widespread clinical impression that ACE inhibitor therapy combined with a mild diuretic is highly effective in early heart failure.

When should an ACE inhibitor be added to the diuretic? Cowley et al[11] clearly showed that, from the short-term symptomatic point of view, an increase of diuretic dose may achieve at least as much as ACE inhibition in selected patients. Their study did not go on to show that there are long-term benefits of the increase of diuretic dose and, on first principles, it could be supposed that there would be many adverse effects including activation of the renin-angiotensin axis. Of interest is the finding that in postinfarct patients with modestly depressed left ventricular function, the ACE inhibitor captopril was better able to maintain left ventricular function and size than the diuretic furosemide.[66] Clearly, longer term observations are required to settle the comparable symptomatic benefits of addition of ACE inhibition and increased diuretic therapy in early heart failure. The general protective effects of ACE inhibition in early heart failure, as shown by the SOLVD preventative study, mean that these drugs are now used earlier and earlier.

Dose of ACE inhibitor added to furosemide. In a fascinating report,[39] the addition of a minute dose of captopril (1 mg) was able to facilitate a diuresis when added to furosemide (median dose 80 mg/day). In contrast, 25 mg captopril decreased blood pressure and glomerular filtration and slightly decreased the diuretic response to furosemide in the same study. Possibly the higher dose of captopril had a negative pharmacokinetic interaction with furosemide (see Chapter 10).

Captopril-Digoxin Multicenter study in mild to moderate heart failure. Three hundred patients with mild to moderate heart failure and an average functional classification (NYHA) of 2.3 were allocated randomly in a double-blind manner to captopril, digoxin, or placebo.[6] Most were maintained on furosemide. Captopril was better than digoxin in increasing the effort tolerance and the functional classification as well as decreasing ventricular premature beats. However, only digoxin increased the ejection fraction. The improvement in the effort tolerance with captopril and in mechanical performance with digoxin correspond well to the data of Kromer.[31]

ACE INHIBITORS AS THIRD COMPONENT THERAPY IN COMBINATION WITH DIURETICS AND DIGOXIN

The fundamental logic for triple therapy (diuretic-ACE inhibitor-digoxin) lies in the mortality benefit of ACE-inhibitors and the symptomatic benefit of digoxin.[14] From the hemodynamic point of view, the combination ACE inhibitor-digoxin gives better results than either therapy alone both in mild heart failure[31] and in severe heart failure.[22] Withdrawal of digoxin from triple therapy results in deterioration.[57]

Can ACE inhibition reduce diuretic requirements in congestive heart failure? In patients with severe congestive heart failure (NYHA Class IV), captopril did not do so.[42] In patients with NYHA Class III heart failure, about half of a small series required a lower diuretic dose.[42] Likewise, the addition of enalapril to patients already treated by digoxin and a diuretic required reduction of diuretic dose in about half but eventually the diuretic dose was increased in the other half.[65]

Neurohumoral effects of ACE inhibitors added to digoxin and diuretics. Administration of ACE inhibitors has, as shown in Table 5-4 of the previous edition, a consistent effect in increasing plasma renin, decreasing angiotensin-II and aldosterone, and a fall in norepinephrine and vasopressin. Parasympathetic activity, reduced in heart failure, is improved by ACE inhibition. Although there are some exceptions to the patterns noted, most of the results are reasonably consistent. From these data it can be concluded that chronic ACE inhibition ameliorates the neurohumoral changes found in congestive heart failure. Generally, such changes are thought to be adverse because of increased vasoconstriction following enhanced levels of angiotensin-II and norepinephrine, because of fluid and sodium retention associated with increased aldosterone levels, and the dilutional hyponatremia associated with increased vasopressin levels.

ENTER THE NEW ERA OF ß-BLOCKERS

As ACE inhibitors are so effective in suppressing the neurohumoral response, it is no surprise that β-blockers, that also inhibit renin and the effects of norepinephrine, also benefit heart failure. The consistently positive results of the CIBIS II study with bisoprolol,[7] and the MERIT study with metoprolol,[37] were such that both trials were stopped early because of mortality reduction. Taken together with the previous positive data from the carvedilol studies, β-blockers are now increasingly viewed as an integral part of the standard therapy of heart failure (Fig 6-6). The chosen drug should be introduced carefully at a very low dose which is then worked up over several months. The β-blocker should be introduced when the patient is stable, not when there is hemodynamic deterioration.

Can the β-blocker therapy be combined with an ACE inhibitor? The answer is certainly yes, as almost all the patients in these trials were already receiving an ACE inhibitor. Furthermore, in the Yusuf meta-analysis, mortality reduction with the combination of an ACE inhibitor and a β-blocker was better than with an ACE inhibitor alone, the data being a relative risk of 0.68 for the combination, versus 0.83 for the ACE inhibitor alone.[19] Of concern, however, is that very few patients with class IV heart failure have been

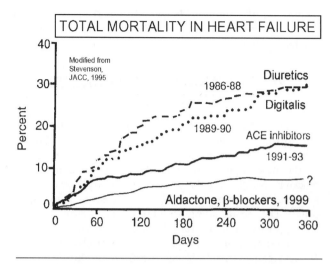

Figure 6-5. *Hypothetical total mortality in heart failure and the influence of various types of therapy. Although ACE inhibitors have made a substantial difference, it can be speculated that the further addition of Aldactone (spironolactone) or of beta-blockade could reduce mortally much further. This figure represents composite data and projections derived from the literature.*

studied. Carvedilol, for example, is only licensed for class II and III heart failure. In all these trials, a fair number of patients were not receiving digoxin.

A new triple therapy? There is no good formal evidence for the new triple therapy of diuretics, ACE inhibitors, with β-blockers (but without digoxin), as recommended by the American Consensus statement.[44] Nonetheless, the arguments for this triple therapy are strong,[44] especially because of the marginal benefits of digoxin in heart failure.[14]

"RALES": A THERAPEUTIC SURPRISE

Because the production of aldosterone in heart failure may "escape" during ACE inhibitor therapy, and because there is a correlation between aldosterone production and mortality in heart failure, the effect of addition of the aldosterone antagonist spironolactone, has been studied.[55] In RALES, **R**andomized **A**ldactone **E**valuation **S**tudy, a low dose of *spironolactone,* often only 25 mg daily, was added to prior therapy in NYHA class III-IV by an ACE inhibitor, a loop diuretic and sometimes digoxin, with very positive results.[58] There was only a small rise in serum potassium, but it should be stressed that these patients did not have renal impairment, a risk factor for serious hyperkalemia. Cardiac mortality was reduced by 27%, due to decreases in both progressive heart failure and sudden death. As many of the patients were not receiving prior digoxin, this trial is an indirect argument for another type of triple therapy (ACE inhibitor, loop diuretic and spironolactone). The surprise is that the standard advice to doctors prescribing ACE inhibitors, is to avoid the addition of potassium retainers because of the implicit danger of hyperkalemia. Yet in RALES the rise in serum potassium was limited and the results positive.

ROLE OF ADDED CONVENTIONAL VASODILATORS

Logically, there should be scope for added vasodilator therapy to the previous standard triple therapy in congestive heart failure, consisting of diuretics-ACE inhibition-digoxin, or the new triple therapy of diuretics-ACE inhibition-β-blockers. *Nitrates* are better able to decrease pulmonary arteriolar resistance and right atrial pressure than captopril.[52] The acute administration of isosorbide dinitrate 40 mg every 6 hours for 24 hours relieved pulmonary hypertension and improved left ventricular filling in 10 of 14 patients with chronic heart failure already treated with captopril.[36] In the CONSENSUS study[9] 47% of patients were already receiving nitrates, while in the treatment arm of SOLVD[67] 40% were on nitrates. In the Hy-C trial,[20] 84% of the patients were on nitrate therapy. Thus, in nitrate-treated patients, ACE inhibition can produce further clinical benefit. Conversely, however, there is little evidence that the chronic addition of nitrates to diuretics and ACE inhibitors gives long term benefit in heart failure.[45]

Hydralazine. In these trials, very few patients were receiving hydralazine. There is a specific disadvantage of hydralazine in that active arteriolar dilation increases reflex sympathetic output. Furthermore, when either captopril or hydralazine was added to the therapy of patients mostly already receiving digitalis, furosemide, and nitrates, mortality was worse in the hydralazine group.[20]

DIASTOLIC DYSFUNCTION

The preceding discussion has concentrated on the role of ACE inhibition in systolic heart failure and the indices of improvement in systolic function. Currently, however, the emphasis is shifting to diastolic heart failure, thought to be an early event particularly in left ventricular hypertrophy. There are relatively few studies with ACE inhibitor therapy in diastolic heart failure, and results depend on the technique used to assess diastolic dysfunction (see Chapter 5). Results are controversial. More data are required on the effects of ACE inhibitors on diastolic dysfunction.

SKELETAL MUSCLE METABOLISM IN HEART FAILURE

Poor blood flow to working skeletal muscle may be one cause of fatigue and exercise intolerance in congestive heart failure and, furthermore, there may be chronic metabolic abnormalities in such muscle.[78] It is, therefore, logical to ask whether ACE inhibitor therapy can improve blood flow and metabolism in the leg muscle of patients with congestive heart failure. Chronic but not acute ACE inhibitor therapy improved the oxygen uptake of exercising leg muscle,[15] probably because of increased formation of locally acting vasodilatory prostaglandins as shown during chronic therapy with perindopril.[29]

ACE INHIBITOR THERAPY FOR CONGESTIVE HEART FAILURE: SUCCESS AND FAILURE

Variable individual responses. Why do some patients appear not to respond to ACE inhibitor therapy? An analogy could be made with hypertension in which mean values of blood pressure in a group of patients are consistently reduced by, for example, thiazide therapy, but when the individual patient response is considered, there may be only about a 60% response. Thus, in considering the individual patients, there may be failures with ACE inhibitor therapy. The question of the estimated one-third to one-quarter of patients who do not respond well to ACE inhibitor therapy[40] merits much more intense study. In the USA, Africa the UK and elsewhere, it is well accepted that black patients respond less well in hypertension, but the situation in heart failure is not clear. In this group, standard vasodilators might work better or the doses of ACE inhibitors should be higher. In some, severe hepatic dysfunction might reduce the rate of conversion of enalapril-like compounds to the active enalaprilat-like form.[41]

The response to ACE inhibitor therapy in congestive heart failure, depending on how measured, varies from a high positive response, to a very high failure rate of 100%.[71] When large numbers of patients are studied as in SAVE, SOLVD, and CONSENSUS, and especially TRACE, then the overall mortality benefits are obvious (Table 6-3). For the individual patient, ACE inhibitor therapy may achieve more or less than expected. There are no crucial differences between the available ACE inhibitors, according to the 1999 American Consensus committee.[44] Therefore if one ACE inhibitor does not work, there is little point in switching to another in the treatment of congestive heart failure.

Exercise response. Besides mortality reduction, the most obvious symptom that requires improvement is exercise intolerance. Increases in exercise time were found in 12 of the 13 trials summarized in the previous edition of this book (Table 5-3). In a review of 35 trials involving 3411 patients in total, improved exercise duration was prolonged in 23 studies, while symptoms improved in 25 of 33 studies.[40] The drugs included (in alphabetical order): benazepril, captopril, cilazapril, enalapril, fosinopril, lisinopril, perindopril, and quinapril. Yet strangely, a large well designed study on trandolapril showed improved exercise in both placebo and drug groups, with no specific benefit for the active agent over 16 weeks.[23] It should be recalled that the mortality

TABLE 6-3: Treatment Trials with ACE Inhibitors in Early
Postinfarct Patients with Left Ventricular
Dysfunction or Overt Heart Failure.

	SAVE	AIRE	TRACE
Total number drug-treated	1,115	1,014	876
Drug and dose (daily)	Captopril 50 mg 3× in 79%	Ramipril 2.5–5 mg 2×	Trandolapril 1–4 mg 1×
Mean duration (months)	42	15	12-24 drug 24–50 follow up
Days since onset of infarct	3–16 days post-infarct	2–9 days post-infarct	3–7 days post-infarct
Entry criteria	Ejection fraction 40% or less	Clinical heart failure	Ejection fraction 35% or less
Age (years) mean	59	65	68
Gender, male (%)	83	74	72
Clinical classification	60% Killip Class I	Severe heart failure excluded (all received ACE inhibitors)	74% signs of CHF
Hypertension (%)	43	28	23
Diuretics (%)	32 at end	60	64
Digitalis (%)	?	12	26
Ejection fraction (%), mean	31	?	?
Mortality reduction (%)	19	27	12
Worsening heart failure % (reduction in risk)	37	29	29
Sudden death (reduction)	? none	Reduced	24%↓

CHF = Congestive Heart Failure

benefit of ACE inhibition only became evident after 1 year
in the SAVE study (Fig 6-6), and that altered skeletal muscle metabolism in heart failure is a complex ill-understood
event that may take long to improve. The overall evidence
is that exercise does improve and symptoms do become
less, but that improvements may be slow.

**Chronic hemodynamic and echocardiographic studies
with ACE inhibitors.** The nearly consistent effects of captopril or enalapril include: reduction of the preload and afterload, decreased echocardiographic size, increased indices of
function such as fractional shortening, as well as an increased ejection fraction measured by radionuclide techniques (Table 5-3 of the second edition of this book).

Predictors of response to ACE inhibitor therapy. Because
activation of the renin-angiotensin-aldosterone axis has adverse effects in congestive heart failure, it might be supposed that the higher the initial renin value, the better the
response to ACE inhibitor therapy. That expectation has not
been met in at least four studies.[13,38,50,53] The reason could
be that tissue renin-angiotensin activation and local tissue
concentrations of angiotensin II are of greater importance,
or that there are variable degrees of endothelial dysfunction

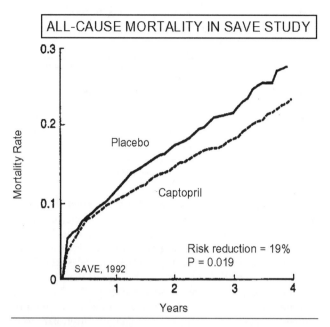

Figure 6-6. All-cause mortality in SAVE study. Overall risk reduction of 19% over 4 years, but note that the curves only clearly separate after one year. Reproduced with permission of authors and publishers, New England Journal of Medicine.[64]

and bradykinin response.[79] Thus according to these concepts, the myocardial and peripheral vasodilatory effects of ACE inhibitors cannot be predicted. The group of *non-responders* includes those in whom the initial serum creatinine exceeds 1.5 mg/dl.[46] In most large trials, exclusion criteria have included serum creatinine values exceeding certain arbitrary elevations such as 2.0 – 3.4 mg per deciliter (177-300 μmol per liter).[9,64,67]

The *sodium status* may be an important factor determining the response to ACE inhibitor therapy. In many studies in congestive heart failure, the exact sodium intake is not stipulated. Variations in the sodium status could help determine the response to ACE inhibitor therapy. Thus, dietary sodium depletion appears highly desirable.

Atrial natriuretic peptide (ANP) is released in response to angiotensin-II stimulation and therefore would act as a natural vasodilator to counter vasoconstriction induced by angiotensin-II.[17,25] One reason why a patient might not respond to ACE inhibitor therapy is that with a decrease in circulating angiotensin-II there could be a tendency to decreased ANP.

ACE INHIBITORS FOR CONGESTIVE HEART FAILURE: CONTRAINDICATIONS AND CAUTIONS

Renal function in congestive heart failure. Whereas hemodynamic and hormonal effects of ACE inhibition are uniformly favorable, some of the renal effects can be construed

TABLE 6-4: META-ANALYSIS OF EFFECTS OF ACE INHIBITOR
THERAPY ON MORTALITY IN CONGESTIVE HEART
FAILURE [21]

	ACE inhibitors	Controls	Relative risks, CI
Mortality	611/3870	709/3235	0.77 (0.67–0.88)
Mortality or hospitalization	854/3810	1036/3178	0.65 (0.57–0.74)
Mortality and EF >25%	209/1335	208/1138	0.98 (0.78–1.23)
Mortality, EF 25% or less	287/1129	351/1039	0.69 (0.57–0.85)

CI = 95% confidence intervals, EF = ejection fraction

as being unfavorable. Packer et al[47] have argued that renin-angiotensin activation serves to preserve glomerular function in heart failure, in keeping with the known hemodynamic effects of angiotensin-II on efferent renal arteriolar tone. Thus, it is not surprising that there may be a tendency for urea and creatinine to rise, with a fall in the glomerular filtration rate and creatinine clearance (Fig 4-7). These occur despite an increase in the effective plasma flow and presumably reflect a decrease in efferent arteriolar tone, thereby decreasing intraglomerular filtration pressure (see Chapter 4). Among the benefits of chronic ACE inhibition is a sodium diuresis and improved handling of a water load.

Practical policies: hypotension and renal function in heart failure. *Temporary renal failure* is most likely to develop in patients with excess diuretic therapy and volume depletion, in whom there is a greater hypotensive response to ACE inhibitor therapy.[48] Thus it is logical to start ACE inhibitors with low initial doses, such as captopril 6.25 mg or enalapril 2.5 mg. A low initial dose of perindopril (2 mg) is less likely to cause initial hypotension (for details see chapter 9) than a low first dose of either enalapril (2.5 mg) or captopril (6.25 mg).[33] A preliminary report[68] shows that a second dose of enalapril (2.5 mg) is again more likely to reduce the blood pressure than a second dose of perindopril (2 mg) despite equivalent degrees of inhibition of plasma ACE. In *diabetics*, renal failure is a particular hazard[49] doubtlessly because diabetes predisposes to renal disease.

Hyponatremia, if present, indicates that the neurohumoral response is sufficiently severe to call forth a vasopressin response, as can result from intense diuretic therapy. Patients with *severe hyponatremia* (sodium <130 mmol/liter) are 30 times more likely to develop hypotension in response to ACE inhibitor therapy and require special care.[51] Yet in the SOLVD study,[67] hyponatremia (sodium <140 mmol/liter) was not associated with any special adverse effect during the use of enalapril at a mean dose of 17 mg daily. To prevent hyponatremia in patients who are not volume-depleted, restriction of water intake is important to avoid the delayed water diuresis of severe congestive heart failure that contributes to water retention and hyponatremia.

Risk of hyperkalemia in pre-existing renal failure. In such patients, a potassium-retaining diuretic should not routinely be used nor should potassium supplements be added because of the risk of hyperkalemia. In other patients with severe heart failure already stabilized on captopril, furosemide, and digitalis, the addition of spironolactone to low-dose captopril can improve the clinical status without excess hyperkalemia.[12] As shown by the RALES study, spironolactone can improve outcome.[58]

Nonsteroidal anti-inflammatory drugs (NSAIDs). Also contributing to the risk of hyperkalemia is associated therapy by NSAIDs, because NSAIDs inhibit the formation of vasodilatory prostaglandins that help to maintain renal blood flow in severe heart failure.[43] NSAIDs in their own right sometimes precipitate renal failure and are known to cause sodium retention. For these reasons, they should not be prescribed in patients with congestive heart failure.

Which ACE inhibitor? Are the data obtained from the large-scale studies only applicable to the actual ACE inhibitor used? This possibility seems highly unlikely for several reasons. First, both captopril and enalapril have been used, and these two agents belong to two different pharmacokinetic categories of ACE inhibitors (see Chapter 8). There are clear structural differences between them, with captopril possessing an SH-group and enalapril not. Second, in the Hy-C trial, captopril was able to reduce mortality in advanced heart failure, when compared with hydralazine.[20] Third, enalapril is representative of a large group of ACE inhibitors that become activated by liver metabolism (see Chapter 8). Ramipril, another representative of this group, is likely to have similar effects on mortality, morbidity and functional capacity as other ACE inhibitors.[32] Fourth, the benefits found are likely to be those of the specific inhibition of the renin-angiotensin axis, not just the consequences of nonspecific vasodilation, as shown by the V-HeFT-II study.[75] All ACE inhibitors are by definition able to interrupt a sequence leading from renin to angiotensin-II. It is this pathway that is activated in the myocardium by either post-infarct remodeling or in heart failure.

Which doses of ACE inhibitors? Whereas an extremely low dose (1 mg) of captopril can enhance the diuretic effect of furosemide,[39] when the aim is suppression of neurohumoral activation and long-term survival, then the ideal dose of captopril is "high", 75 mg or more per day, rather than low.[57] A similar conclusion was based on the retrospective analysis of data on severe heart failure.[56] High dose ACE inhibition is better able to improve exercise capacity than is low dose.[74] The still unpublished ATLAS study (Assessment of Treatment with Lisinopril and Survival), presented at the American College of Cardiology Meeting in 1998, was an outcome mortality study that compared low and high dose lisinopril, using 2.5 mg and 35 mg as "low" and "high" doses. The differences were slight, for example hospitalization was less in the high dose group, and there was a trend to decreased mortality (8% reduction, P = 0.128). Thus ATLAS[8] does not provide convincing evidence for high-dose therapy. Rather, first principles would say that it is desirable to use the doses of ACE inhibitors already shown to reduce mortality in placebo-controlled trials.

Hypotension may, unfortunately, often be a limiting factor. In that case, the addition of spironolactone may suppress urinary aldosterone excretion and achieve clinical benefit even in the presence of low-dose captopril.[12] The strategy of adding spironolactone receives indirect support from the RALES trial.[58] In studies on patients with heart failure, both captopril and enalapril caused more first-dose hypotension than did another ACE inhibitor, perindopril,[33] raising the possibility that not all ACE inhibitors are equal when it comes to this side-effect.

Cost-effectiveness of ACE inhibitors in treatment of heart failure. While all calculations of cost-effectiveness must be based on extrapolations, Hart and McMurray[26] worked out that the cost per life year gained varied from $300 to $1,000 according to the dose and according to whether the treatment was initiated in hospital or outside hospital by a general practitioner. These calculations were based on the SOLVD treatment arm study. Furthermore, some calculations from SOLVD show that enalapril was actually cost-saving.[10] Other calculations from the AIRE study, in which there was overt heart failure, show that it cost about $2,000 to $4,000 per life year gained.[16] Calculations made from SAVE with captopril, suggest that it is much more expensive to gain a life year in a younger than an older patient.[73] In an 80-year old it would cost $3,600 to achieve the gain of one quality-adjusted life year, whereas in a 50-year old patient, it would cost over $60,000. All these costs compare very well with other accepted preventative therapies, such as the use of β-blockers postinfarct.[73]

It is therefore apparent that the use of ACE inhibitors in the treatment of heart failure, whether caused by those diseases covered by the SOLVD study or whether caused by acute infarction,[1] is highly cost-effective. At a time when governments are examining their policy in relation to drugs that might often be considered relatively expensive, such as the ACE inhibitors, their cost-effectiveness needs to be considered as a further argument in favor of the use of these agents.

HOW TO START ACE INHIBITOR THERAPY IN GENERAL PRACTICE

First, *confirm the clinical diagnosis of heart failure, a condition in which effort intolerance is due to a cardiac cause.* Current opinion is that an ACE inhibitor should be started sooner rather than later. Next, check for contraindications: hypotension, impaired renal function, hyponatremia, and pregnancy. Consider the remote possibility of bilateral renal artery stenosis. Assess concomitant therapy — NSAIDs reduce the efficacy of ACE inhibitors. Decrease the aspirin dose. Avoid overdiuresis, and cut back for a few days on the diuretic doses. To avoid hypotension, start with a test dose of captopril (6.25 mg) or perindopril (2 mg). Then gradually increase the dose of the ACE inhibitor you know best to the dose required by trial data, or in the case of mild or early heart failure to an average dose. Repeat renal investigations about 1–2 weeks after starting the ACE inhibitor, and if the rise of creatinine is too much, reduce the dose. Follow the patient up long term to assess clinical improvement. These procedures are no more difficult than the use of digoxin, without the need to check on blood levels of the drug, and without numerous contraindications and side-effects. Furthermore, the benefit of ACE inhibitors in reducing mortality is established, whereas digoxin leaves mortality unchanged.

SUMMARY

1. *The benefits of ACE inhibitor therapy* have now become abundantly clear in the modern therapeutic approach to congestive heart failure. In early studies the benefits were proven as add-on therapy after digitalis and diuretics. More recent studies have shown that as second-line therapy ACE inhibition may be preferable to digoxin. The current trend to the early use of ACE inhibitors is reinforced by the large number of patient studies that show an overall reduction in mortality.

2. *The data base is very solid.* Seven major trials on nearly 14,000 treated patients, and about an equal number of controls, have established the beneficial effects and safety of ACE inhibition in heart failure, both in its treatment and its prevention. In the SOLVD prevention trial, ACE inhibitor monotherapy by enalapril helped to prevent the development of heart failure. Similar data were obtained in the SAVE study. The postinfarct trials (SAVE, SOLVD preventative arm, AIRE and TRACE) showed that ACE inhibition could help prevent or treat congestive heart failure and also reduce all-cause mortality.

3. *Diastolic dysfunction.* When there is diastolic dysfunction on the basis of left ventricular hypertrophy, then the arguments favoring early ACE inhibitor therapy are strong, because both high-dose diuretics and digitalis are theoretically contraindicated.

4. *The hemodynamic benefits* of ACE inhibitor therapy are shown by reduction of preload and afterload, and increased left ventricular performance, as monitored both by classic invasive hemodynamic techniques and by echocardiography, the latter showing decreased left ventricular dimensions. Ejection fractions have increased.

5. *The neurohumoral changes* associated with chronic ACE inhibitor therapy include increased plasma renin, decreased angiotensin-II, decreased aldosterone, decreased plasma norepinephrine, a tendency to

decreased epinephrine, and decreased vasopressin. These changes are thought to be beneficial in the therapy of congestive heart failure. Many workers now believe that these neurohumoral changes are essential in explaining the benefits of ACE inhibitor therapy and explain the benefits of ACE inhibitor therapy over conventional vasodilators. In addition, *increased bradykinin* may promote formation of nitric oxide with its vasodilatory and endothelial protective qualities.

6. *Contraindications or cautions* when ACE inhibitors are used for heart failure include the following: pre-existing hypotension, a high serum creatinine, high-renin states such as bilateral renal artery stenosis with hypertensive heart failure, aortic stenosis combined with congestive heart failure, and of course pregnancy. Overdiuresis and a low serum sodium both predispose to hypotension.

7. *Renal function in heart failure.* ACE inhibitor therapy may have deleterious effects for example by decreasing the glomerular filtration rate. In general, it is likely that serum urea and creatinine will rise slightly and the glomerular filtration rate fall slightly during ACE inhibitor therapy.

8. *Initiation of therapy* by an ACE inhibitor is relatively simple, with the chief dangers being hypotension and increasing renal failure. Practical guidelines allow the use of ACE inhibitors by general practitioners, provided that the clinical diagnosis of heart failure is securely based on the definition of effort intolerance due to a cardiac cause.

9. *New therapies.* Several recent positive trials show that beta-blockade added to ACE inhibitor therapy with a diuretic, reduces mortality in heart failure. One recent trial shows that the addition of low dose spironolactone, also to ACE inhibitor and diuretic therapy, was safe and reduced mortality, even in class III and class IV patients. Such combinations of ACE inhibitors with other agents are likely to be used increasingly, and correspondingly the use of digoxin is likely to fall.

REFERENCES

1. AIRE Study. The effect of ramipril on mortality and morbidity of survivors of acute myocardial infarction with clinical evidence of heart failure. Lancet 1993;342:821–828.

2. Anand IS, Ferrari R, Kalra GS, et al. Edema of cardiac origin. Studies of body water and sodium, renal function, hemodynamic indexes, and plasma hormones in untreated congestive cardiac failure. Circulation 1989;80:299–305.

3. Anand IS, Kalra GS, Ferrari R, et al. Enalapril as initial and sole treatment in severe chronic heart failure with sodium retention. Int J Cardiol 1990;28:341–346.

4. Bayliss J, Norrell M, Canepa-Anson R, et al. Untreated heart failure: clinical and neuroendocrine effects of introducing diuretics. Br Heart J 1987;57:17–22.

5. Braunwald E. Stunning of the myocardium: an update. Cardiovasc Drugs Ther 1991;5:849–851.

6. Captopril-Digoxin Multicenter Research Group. Comparative effects of therapy with captopril and digoxin in patients with mild to moderate heart failure. JAMA 1988;259:539–544.

7. CIBIS II Study. The Cardiac Insufficiency Bisoprolol Study II (CIBIS-II): a randomised trial. Lancet 1999;353:9–13.

8. Cohn JN. The ATLAS Trial (Editorial). International Newsletter. Valsartan Heart Failure Trial 1998;3:1.

9. CONSENSUS Trial Study Group. Effects of enalapril on mortality in severe heart failure: Results of the Co-operative North Scandinavian Enalapril Survival Study (CONSENSUS). N Engl J Med 1987;316:1429–1435.

10. Cook JR, Glick HA, Gerth W, et al. The cost and cardioprotective effects of enalapril in hypertensive patients with left ventricular dysfunction. Am J Hypertens 1998;11:1433–1441.

11. Cowley A, Stainer K, Wynne R, et al. Symptomatic assessment of patients with heart failure: double-blind comparison of increasing doses of diuretics and captopril in moderate heart failure. Lancet 1986;2:770–772.

12. Dahlstrom U, Karlsson E. Captopril and spironolactone therapy for refractory congestive heart failure. Am J Cardiol 1993;71:29A–33A.

13. Davis R, Ribner H, Keung E, et al. Treatment of chronic congestive heart failure with captopril, an oral inhibitor of angiotensin-converting enzyme. N Engl J Med 1979;301:117–121.

14. DIGITALIS Investigation Group. The effect of digoxin on mortality and morbidity in patients with heart failure. New Engl J Med 1997;336:525–533.

15. Drexler H, Banhardt U, Meinertz T, et al. Contrasting peripheral short-term and long-term effects of converting enzyme inhibition in patients with congestive heart failure. Circulation 1989;79:491–502.

16. Erhardt L, Ball S, Andersson F, et al. Cost effectiveness in the treatment of heart failure with ramipril. A Swedish substudy of the AIRE Study. Pharmacoeconomics 1997;12:256–266.

17. Ferrari R, Anand I. Neurohumoral changes in untreated heart failure. Cardiovasc Drugs Ther 1989;3:979–986.

18. Flapan AD, Nolan J, Neilson JMM, et al. Effect of captopril on cardiac parasympathetic activity in chronic cardiac failure secondary to coronary artery disease. Am J Cardiol 1992;19:842–850.

19. Flather MD, Yusuf S, Kober L, et al. Systematic overview of individual patient data fromt he large randomized trials of long term ACE inhibition or therapy in patients with heart failure or left ventricular dysfunction following myocardial infarction. Submitted for publication 1999.

20. Fonarow G, Chelimsky-Fallick C, Stevenson L, et al. Effect of direct vasodilation with hydralazine versus angiotensin-converting enzyme inhibition with captopril on mortality in advanced heart failure: The Hy-C Trial. J Am Coll Cardiol 1992;19:842–850.

21. Garg R, Yusuf S. For the Collaborative Group on ACE Inhibitor Trials. Overview of randomized trials of angiotensin-converting enzyme inhibitors on mortality and morbidity in patients with heart failure. JAMA 1995;273:1450–1456.

22. Gheorghiade M, Hall V, Lakier J, et al. Comparative hemodynamic and neurohumoral effects of intravenous captopril and digoxin and their combinations in patients with severe heart failure. J Am Coll Cardiol 1989;13:134–142.

23. Hampton JR, Cowley AJ, Wnuk-Wojnar AM. For the Trandolapril study group. Failure of ACE inhibitor to improve exercise tolerance. Eur Heart J 1998;19:1823–1828.

24. Harris P. Congestive cardiac failure: central role of the arterial blood pressure. Br Heart J 1987;59:190–203.

25. Harris P. Congestive cardiac failure: the syndrome of volume expansion. Cardiovasc Drugs Ther 1989;3:941–945.

26. Hart W, McMurray J. The cost-effectiveness of enalapril in the treatment of heart failure (Abstract). Eur Heart J 1993;14 (Suppl):14.

27. Haywood GA, Gullestad L, Katsuya T, et al. AT_1 and AT_2 angiotensin receptor gene expression in human heart failure. Circulation 1997;95:1201–1206.

28. Hornig B, Arakawa N, Haussmann D, et al. Differential effects of quinalaprilat and enalaprilat on endothelial function of conduit arteries in patients with chronic heart failure. Circulation 1998;98:2842–2848.

29. Jeserich M, Pape L, Just H, et al. Effect of long-term angiotensin-converting enzyme inhibition on vascular function inpatients with chronic congestive heart failure. Am J Cardiol 1995;76:1079–1082.

30. Jugdutt B, Tymchak W, Humen D, et al. Prolonged nitroglycerin versus captopril therapy on remodeling after transmural myocardial infarction (abstract). Circulation 1990;82 (Suppl III):III–442.

31. Kromer E, Elsner D, Riegger G. Digoxin, converting-enzyme inhibition (quinapril), and the combination in patients with congestive heart failure function class II and sinus rythm. Cardiovasc Pharmacol 1990;16:9–14.

32. Lubsen J, Chadha DR, Yotof YT, et al. Meta-analysis of morbidity and mortality in five exercise capacity trials evaluating ramipril in chronic congestive heart failure. Am J Cardiol 1996;77:1191–1196.

33. MacFadyen RJ, Lees KR, Reid JL. Tissue and plasma angiotensin converting enzyme and the response to ACE inhibitor drugs. Br J Clin Pharmacol 1991;31:1–13.

34. Magri P, Rao MAE, Cangianiello S, et al. Early impairment of renal hemodynamic reserve in patients with asymptomatic heart failure is restored by angiotensin II antagonism. Circulation 1998;1998:2849–2854.

35. Meerson FZ. The myocardium in hyperfunction, hypertrophy and heart failure. Circ Res 1969;25 (suppl 2):1–163.

36. Mehra A, Ostrzega E, Shotan A, et al. Persistent hemodynamic improvement with short-term nitrate therapy in patients with chronic congestive heart failure already treated with captopril. Am J Cardiol 1992;70:1310–1314.

37. MERIT Trial. Metroprolol has MERIT in HF. Inpharma 1998;1168:12.

38. Mettauer B, Rouleau J-L, Bichet D, et al. Differential long-term intrarenal and neurohormonal effects of captopril and prazosin in patients with chronic congestive heart failure: Importance of initial plasma renin activity. Circulation 1986;73:492–502.

39. Motwani J, Fenwick M, Morton J, et al. Furosemide-induced natriuresis is augmented by ultra-low dose captopril but not by standard doses of captopril in chronic heart failure. Circulation 1992;86:439–445.

40. Narang R, Swedberg K, Cleland GF. What is the ideal study design for evaluation of treatment for heart failure. Eur Heart J 1996;17:120–134.

41. Oberg K, Just V, Bauman J, et al. Reduced bioavailability of enalapril in patients with severe heart failure (Abstr). J Am Coll Cardiol 1994;23:381A.

42. Odemuyiwa O, Gilmartin J, Kenny D, et al. Capropril and the diuretic requirements in moderate and severe chronic heart failure. Eur Heart J 1989;10:586–590.

43. Orme LEM. Non-steroidal anti-inflammatory drugs and the kidney. Br Med J 1986;292:1621–1622.

44. Packer M, Cohn JN. Consensus recommendations for the management of chronic heart failure. Am J Cardiol, 1999;82(2A):1A–38A

45. Packer M, Gheorghiade M, Young J, et al. On behalf of the RADIANCE study. Randomized, double-blind, placebo-controlled, withdrawal study of digoxin in patients with chronic heart failure treated with converting-enzyme inhibitors (abstr). J Am Coll Cardiol 1992;19:260A.

46. Packer M, Lee W, Yushak M, et al. Comparison of captopril and analapril in patients with severe chronic heart failure. N Engl J Med 1986a;315:847–853.

47. Packer M, Lee WH, Kessler PD. Preservation of glomerular filtration rate in human heart failure by activation of the renin-angiotensin system. Circulation 1986b;74:666–774.

48. Packer M, Lee WH, Medina N, et al. Functional renal insufficiency during long-term therapy with captopril and enalapril in severe chronic heart failure. An Intern Med 1987a;106:346–354.

49. Packer M, Lee WH, Medina N, et al. Influence of diabetes mellitus on changes in left ventriular performance and renal function produced by converting enzyme inhibition in patients with severe chronic heart failure. Am J Med 1987b;82:1119–1126.

50. Packer M, Medina N, Yushak M. Efficacy of captopril in low-renin congestive heart failure: importance of sustained reactive hyperreninemia in distinguishing responders from non-responders. Am J Cardiol 1984a;54:771–777.

51. Packer M, Medina N, Yushak M. Relation between serum sodium concentration and the hemodynamic and clinical responses to converting enzyme inhibition with captopril in severe heart failure. J Am Coll Cardiol 1984b;3:1035–1043.

52. Packer M, Medina N, Yushak M, et al. Comparative effects of captopril and isosorbide dinitrate on pulmonary arteriolar resistance and right ventricular function in patients with severe left ventricular failure: results of a randomized crossover study. Am Heart J 1985a;109:1293–1299.

53. Packer M, Medina N, Yushak M, et al. Usefulness of plasma renin activity in predicting hemodynamic and clinical responses and survival during long-term converting enzyme inhibition in severe chronic heart failure. Experience in 100 consecutive patients. Br Heart J 1985b;54:298–304.

54. Pfeffer MA, Braunwald E, Moye LA, et al. Effect of captopril on mortality and morbidity in patients with left ventricular dysfunction after myocardial infarction. Results of the Survival and Ventricular Enlargement Trial. N Engl J Med 1992;327:669–677.

55. Pitt B. "Escape" of aldosterone production in patiens with left ventricular dysfunction treated with an angiotensin converting enzyme inhibitor: implications for therapy. Cardiovasc Drugs Ther 1995;9:145–149.

56. Pouleur H, Rosseau MF, Oakley C, et al. For the Xamoterol in Severe Heart Failure Study Group. Difference in mortality between patients treated with captopril or enalapril in the Xamoterol in Severe Heart Failure Study. Am J Cardiol 1991;68:71–74.

57. RADIANCE Study. Packer M, Gheorghiodes M, Young JB. Withdrawal of digoxin from patients with chronic heart failure treated with angiotensin converting enzyme inhibitors. N Engl J Med 1993;329:1-7.

58. RALES Study. Spironolactone for heart failure? Inpharma 1998;1168:12.

59. Raya TE, Gay RG, Aguirre M, et al. Importance of venodilation in prevention of left ventricular dilatation after chronic large myocardial infarction in rats: A comparison of captopril and hydralazine. Circ Res 1989;64:330–337.

60. Remes J, Tikkanen I, Fyhrquist F, et al. Neuroendocrine activity in untreated heart failure. Br Heart J 1991;65:249–255.

61. Richardson A, Bayliss J, Scriven A, et al. Double-blind comparison of captopril alone against frusemide plus amiloride in mild heart failure. Lancet 1987;2:709–711.

62. Riegger G. Effects of quinapril on exercise tolerance in patients with mild to moderate heart failure. Eur Heart J 1991:705–711.

63. Ruzicka M, Leenen FHH. Relevance of blockade of cardiac and circulatory angiotensin-converting enzyme for the prevention of volume overload-induced cardiac hypertrophy. Circulation 1995;91:16–19.

64. SAVE Study, Pfeffer MA, Braunwald E, Moye LA. Effect of captopril on mortality and morbidity in patients with left ventricular dysfunction after myocardial infarction. Results of the Survival and Ventricular Enlargement trial. N Eng J Med 1992;327:669–677.

65. Sharpe N, Murphy J, Coxon R, et al. Enalapril in patients with chronic heart failure: a placebo-controlled, randomized, double-blind study. Circulation 1984;70:271–278.

66. Sharpe N, Murphy J, Smith H, et al. Treatment of patients with symptomless left ventricular dysfunction after myocardial infarction. Lancet 1988;1:255–259.

67. SOLVD Investigators. Effect of enalapril on mortality and the development of heart failure in asymptomatic patients with reduced left ventricular ejection fractions. New Engl J Med 1992;327:685–691.

68. Squire IB, MacFayden RJ, Lees KR, et al. Different blood pressure and renin angiotensin system responses to ACE inhibition in heart failure (abstract). Am Coll Cardiol 1994;23:376A.

69. Su JB, Barbe F, Houel R, et al. Preserved vasodilator effect of bradykinin in dogs with heart failure. Circulation 1998;98:2911–2918.

70. The Task Force of the Working Group on Heart Failure of the European Society of Cardiology. The treatment of heart failure. Eur Heart j 1997;18:736–753.

71. Timmis A, Bojanowski L, Najm Y, et al. Captopril versus placebo in congestive heart failure: effects on oxygen delivery to exercising skeletal muscle. Eur Heart J 1987;8:1295–1304.

72. Tischler MD, Rowan M, Winter MML. Effect of enalapril therapy on left ventricular mass and volumes in asymptomatic chronic, severe mitral regurgitation secondary to mitral valve prolapse. Am J Cardiol 1998;82:242–245.

73. Tsevat J, Duke D, Goldman L, et al. Cost-effectiveness of captopril therapy after myocardial infarction. J Am Coll Cardiol 1995;26:914–919.

74. van Veldhuisen DJ, Genth-Zotz S, Brouwer J, et al. High- versus low-dose ACE inhibition in chronic heart failure. A double-blind, placebo-controlled study of imidapril. J Am Coll Cardiol 1998;32:1811–1818.

75. V-HeFT II Study. Cohn JN, Johnson G, Ziesche S. A comparison of enalapril with hydralzine – isosorbide dinitrate in the treatment of chronic congestive cardiac failure. N Engl J Med 1991;325:303–310.

76. Volpe M, Magri P, Rao MAE, et al. Intrarenal determinants of sodium retention in mild heart failure. Effects of angiotensin-converting enzyme inhibition. Hypertension 1997;30:168–176.

77. Volpe M, Tritto C, De Luca N, et al. Angiotensin-converting enzyme inhibition restores cardiac and hormonal responses to volume overload in patients with dilated cardiomyopathy and mild heart failure. Circulation 1992;86:1800–1809.

78. Wilson JR, Mancini D, Chance B. Skeletal muscle metabolism in congestive heart failure. Cardiovasc Drugs Ther 1989;3:995–1000.

79. Zisman LS. Inhibiting tissue angiotensin-converting enzyme. A pound of flesh without the blood? Circulation 1998;98:2788–2790.

CHAPTER 7

ACE Inhibitors and the Central Nervous System

"Behavioral studies have provided clear evidence that the ACE inhibitors have potential to improve cognitive performance" (Barnes et al, 1989)[5]

Angiotensinogen is locally made in the brain.[12] ACE in the brain is found in the endothelium of the blood vessels, cells of the choroid plexus and astrocytes.[54] ACE, angiotensin II, and angiotensin II (AT-1) receptors all co-localize in dopamine synthesizing neurones in the nuclei of the vagal nerve. There are also angiotensin IV receptors.[54] ACE inhibitors are likely to interact with brain tissue and cerebrovascular ACE, and also indirectly at several other levels of the central and autonomic nervous systems. First, ACE inhibitors could modify the release of neurotransmitters such as dopamine and norepinephrine; second, there may be effects on baroreceptors; third, cerebral blood flow regulation could be altered; and fourth, there could be direct effects on mood and other higher functions.

CENTRAL ANGIOTENSIN RECEPTORS

Autoradiography shows that ACE and AT-1 receptors co-localize in the dopamine synthesizing neurons found in the neurones of the basal ganglia, as found in the caudate nucleus, putamen, and subtantia nigra.[54] Thus A-II may modulate dopamine synthesis through the AT-1 receptor. A-II (AT-1) receptors also localize to the principal cardio-vascular control centres, and the brain renin-angiotensin system has been implicated in several types of experimental and genetic hypertension.[15] AT-1 receptors are also found in the anterior pituitary and related sites outside the blood brain barrier, where blood A-II may modulate drinking, salt balance, and pituitary hormone release. Secondly, the density of the AT-2 receptors varies with the species, being widely distributed in the rat but in humans limited to one layer of the cerebellum. AT-4 receptors (see Chapter 1) are strikingly distributed with cholinergic nuclei. Their function is not known. They may respond not only to angiotensin IV, which is very low in the brain, but to a decapeptide, unrelated to angiotensin, that occurs as an internal component of human globulin.

Dopamine and Parkinson's disease (Paralysis Agitans).
AT-1 receptors are found especially in the basal ganglia of the human brain and localize with dopamine synthesizing neurones.[54] Depressed levels of dopamine are found in the corresponding cells of patients with Parkinson's disease, a movement disorder also called paralysis agitans. Dopamine depletion may explain the over-activity of the acetylcholine cholinergic system that promotes the movement disorder. In Parkinson's disease, the AT-1 receptors are completely absent in the dopamine synthesizing neurones. When rats are chronically fed with perindopril, then the extracellular and the total brain dopamine content rises (Fig 7-1). ACE inhibitors are currently undergoing evaluation as possible therapeutic agents in Parkinson's disease.

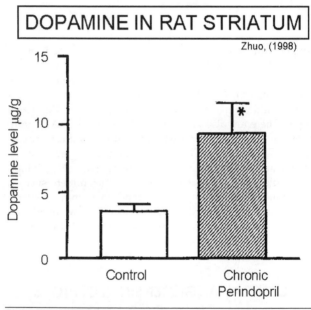

Figure 7-1. *ACE inhibitors given experimentally can increase levels of dopamine in the rat striatum. Data from Zhuo et al[54] with permission of the publisher, Journal of Hypertension.*

AUTONOMIC NERVOUS SYSTEM

Modulation of sympathetic activity. Angiotensin II is thought to have a "permissive" role in the release of norepinephrine from the terminal adrenergic neurons, both by enhancing the release of norepinephrine and by inhibiting the re-uptake of norepinephrine into the terminal neurons. Furthermore, angiotensin II facilitates ganglionic transmission and also has a role in central adrenergic activation (Fig 1-8). Normally, exercise induces a rise in plasma catecholamine levels. During ACE inhibition therapy, this rise is attenuated probably because less norepinephrine is released from terminal neurons.[32] This indirect antiadrenergic effect of ACE inhibition may be important not only in blood pressure reduction[28] but also in helping to explain the mechanism of benefit in congestive heart failure, as well as the antiarrhythmic effects in myocardial ischemia.

Enhanced parasympathetic activity. ACE inhibitor therapy reduces the blood pressure without any reflex tachycardia. Logically, this could result from resetting of baroreflexes[38,51] or enhanced activity of the parasympathetic nervous system. A relative increase of the activity of the parasympathetic nervous system compared with that of the sympathetic nervous system has been found after captopril,[11] lisinopril[1], perindopril,[2] enalapril,[8] and benazepril.[53] By enhancing parasympathetic outflow, baroreceptor activity can be reset without any change in the actual sensitivity of the receptors.[53] In diabetics with mild vagal impairment, a single dose of 25 mg captopril enhanced the reflex bradycardic response to apneic face immersion in water.[31]

EFFECTS ON CEREBRAL PERFUSION

Cerebral autoregulation. Cerebral autoregulation is the process whereby the cerebral vascular bed maintains a constant blood flow in the face of variations in the perfusion pressure,[42] the latter for practical purposes corresponding to the blood pressure. Regulation of cerebral blood flow is of dual importance in relation to hypertensive patients, particularly in the elderly in whom autoregulation may be impaired by several possible concurrent disease processes, such as stroke, diabetes, and dementia.[36,46] First, limits of autoregulation are altered by the hypertensive process and, second, various drugs may have different influences on the patterns of autoregulation. Thus, the lowest tolerated mean blood pressure in normotensives is about 43 mmHg.[45] In treated hypertensive patients, this lower limit is about 53 mmHg and, in ineffectively treated severe hypertension, the limit is about 65 mmHg.[45]

Effect of angiotensin II on cerebral circulation. In general, there is a lack of response of cerebral blood flow to intraluminal angiotensin II.[10] Degradation products of angiotensin II, such as angiotensin III, and the combination of angiotensin II-(3-8) with L-arginine may produce vasodilatory rather than vasoconstrictory responses in cerebral arterioles.[21] Local generation of angiotensin II by the renin-angiotensin system in the vascular wall does, however, occur[41] and may have different effects. As in the case of other tissues, it is unclear to what extent the circulating renin-angiotensin system and locally synthesized components interact. Nonetheless, it is the luminal ACE activity of large cerebral arteries that probably plays the most important role in determining the effects of ACE inhibitors on cerebral blood flow. Thus, whether or not ACE inhibitors penetrate to deeper sites in the central nervous system is not crucial to the control of the cerebral circulation by these agents.[43]

ACE inhibitors and autoregulation. ACE inhibitor therapy alters autoregulation of cerebral blood flow, bringing down the upper and lower limits in hypertensive rats.[6,9,33] In humans, ACE inhibitors also reset cerebral autoregulation at lower blood pressures.[42] Such resetting seems protective against sudden decreases of blood pressure, especially during the treatment of congestive heart failure, so that low arterial blood pressure values during ACE inhibitor therapy are not associated with symptoms of cerebral ischemia.[35] Conversely, Brown and Brown[10] propose that the decrease in the upper limit of autoregulation by ACE inhibitor therapy, for example from 200 to 140 mmHg,[6] could be harmful because it would not protect against any sudden upward surges of the blood pressure.

ACE INHIBITORS AND STROKE

Angiotensin II and circulation in cerebral ischemia. Currently, there are two opposing hypotheses on the possible effects of angiotensin II in cerebral ischemia. These hypotheses are particularly important in the evaluation of cerebral vascular disease. First, it is proposed that the activity of angiotensin II, by potentially increasing collateral flow to ischemic brain tissue, could protect the brain.[18] In keeping with this hypothesis, Brown and Brown[10] proposed that angiotensin II normally plays a protective role in the cerebral circulation, acting by (1) maintenance of the blood pressure during hypotensive episodes, by maintenance of the upper limit of cerebral autoregulation, and by (2) vasodilation of smaller cerebral vessels by release of prostacyclin or other vasodilator prostaglandins.[49]

Conversely, angiotensin II by virtue of its vasoconstrictive effect can be expected to exaggerate the cerebral vascular spasm associated with stroke and, hence, to make stroke worse. Furthermore, by generally elevating blood pressure, angiotensin is likely to predispose to stroke, and when stroke does occur, to make it worse. Evidence supporting the potential harmful effects of angiotensin II is summarized by Werner et al.[52]

Existing data on therapy of hypertension and stroke. A large prospective study has defined the risks for stroke in middle-aged men: a high systolic blood pressure, smoking, heavy alcohol consumption, and ischemic heart disease with left ventricular hypertrophy.[40] Another equally large retrospective survey found that an elevated diastolic blood pressure was an even greater risk.[34] In general, a fall of diastolic blood pressure of 5 to 10 mmHg should reduce the incidence of stroke by 34% to 56%.[29] The blood pressure reduction should be effective however achieved. Currently, this proposal would appear to be the most logical is supported by animal data showing that an ACE inhibitor, perindopril, reduces stroke mortality in renovascular hypertension.[4] In patients with recent ischemic cerebral stroke, the perindopril reduces blood pressure without im-

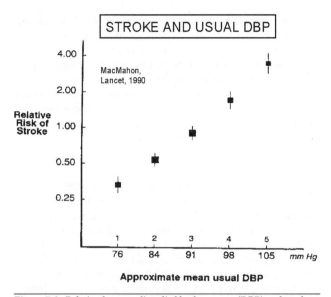

Figure 7-2. Relation between diastolic blood pressure (DBP) and stroke, estimated from the combined results of seven major prospective trials with a mean follow-up period of several years. Reproduced by permission of the authors[29] and publishers of The Lancet.

pairing overall cerebral blood flow.[17] Therefore ACE inhibitor therapy by reducing the blood pressure should be beneficial in patients with previous stroke. Clinically, this proposal is under test in PROGRESS (last section of this chapter).

Does ACE inhibitor therapy protect against the development of the initial stroke? There are as yet no good outcome data on the effect of ACE inhibitors on the occurrence of stroke in hypertensive patients. One comparative study has been completed.[13] Captopril was marginally less effective in preventing stroke than conventional therapy by a beta-blocker and/or a diuretic. Captopril is however a short acting agent, licensed for example in the USA for use three times daily. In CAPP, captopril was given once or twice daily, so that sustained 24 hour blood pressure reduction can not be assured.

Could there be a special protective effect of ACE inhibitors? Laragh and his group in New York have proposed that there could basically be two different forms of hypertension with different consequences for stroke, the first being sodium-dependent and related to abnormal membrane function, while the second is renin-dependent and related to vasoconstriction. Simply put, the former is "wet" hypertension and the latter "dry" hypertension. The proposed hypothetical difference between these two types is that vascular sequelae, such as stroke and heart attack, are more likely to occur in the high-renin "dry" type.[26] Although Laragh's concept has been much criticized, support for the proposed relationship has been forthcoming in the case of heart attacks but not stroke.[3]

Possible vascular protective role of ACE inhibitors.
Nonetheless, the vascular hypothesis lives on. Angiotensin
II is an important regulator of vascular growth (Figs 2-5, 3-4)
and, hence, of vascular hypertrophy. Vascular disease may
predispose to stroke or cognitive impairment even in the
absence of hypertension.[43] Hypothetically, ACE inhibitors
could be protective against stroke even in the absence of
any antihypertensive effect, by correction of cerebral vascular remodeling, as shown in an animal model with perindopril.[13A]

Stroke-prone spontaneously hypertensive rats. There is
a specific strain of spontaneously hypertensive rat, namely
the stroke-prone animal.[25] As the rats mature, there are
higher adrenal levels of angiotensin I and angiotensin II. In
addition, the circulating levels of plasma renin, angiotensin
I, and angiotensin II, as well as aldosterone, are all high in
the adult animal, even after bilateral nephrectomy. Therefore, there must have been a non-renal source for the renin.
Both ACE inhibitors and AT-1 blockers can prevent stroke
and increase survival.[20] Even a low non-antihypertensive
dose of dose ramipril prolongs life of these animals, though
not as effectively as anti-hypertensive high doses.[27]

Comment: Angiotensin II and stroke. Clearly, there are
three different situations to consider in relation to the possible harm of angiotensin II in relation to stroke. First, in relation to the general mechanism of stroke development,
increased circulating angiotensin II activity has a hypertensive effect, in part central, that must promote the risk of
stroke. Second, angiotensin II as a growth factor may promote cerebral vascular disease and predispose to stroke
even in the absence of hypertension. Third, in at least some
special situations, angiotensin II may be able to maintain
collateral circulation to the ischemic zone of the brain and,
thereby, exert a paradoxical protective effect against cerebral ischemia. In humans, it is likely that cerebral vaso-
spasm contributes to the overall symptomatology of
cerebrovascular accidents, as shown by the benefits of ni-
modipine in subarachnoid hemorrhage. Therefore, it may
be anticipated that, in general, the therapy of hypertension
by ACE inhibitors should be beneficial in the prevention of
cerebral vascular disease. However, a firm answer to this
important question could only be given when the outcome
data on the incidence of stroke from large and reliable clinical trials such as PROGRESS (see last section of this chapter) become available.

EFFECTS OF ACE INHIBITORS ON MOOD
AND OTHER HIGHER FUNCTIONS

In contrast to several other antihypertensive agents acting
centrally or having central effects such as methyldopa and
propranolol, ACE inhibitors are thought to improve
mood.[14] In addition, it has been proposed that ACE inhibi-

tors have unique behavioral and cognitive actions unlike those of other antihypertensive agents.[5,19]

Memory and behavior. When angiotensin is given intra-peritoneally to animals or into a brain ventricle, there is fa-cilitation of certain types of motivated behavior[19] or reversal of the helpless behavior induced by repetitive elec-trical shocks.[30] There is some evidence that angiotensin II may promote memory. In humans, there is less definitive evidence for such central effects (see review by Jern).[24] When an ACE inhibitor was given to 23 normal volunteers in an antihypertensive dose, it had no effect on memory performance nor on sleep patterns.[16] Isolated case reports have suggested that the ACE inhibitor, captopril, has a mood elevating effect in depressed patients,[55] but these patients were suffering from heart failure or from diastolic hypertension. Thus, it is not certain that the benefits in mood were achieved as a direct result of the ACE inhibitor therapy or indirectly by improving the symptomatology of heart failure or hypertension.

Hypertensive patients with psychological depression. Depression may be an organic syndrome caused by de-creased formation of certain biogenic amines. Especially re-serpine and methyldopa are therapies for hypertension that may actually cause depression.[7] Also, patients receiving propranolol are five times more likely to be given concur-rent antidepressants, and in the users of beta-blockers aged 20 to 39 years, the relative risk of antidepressant therapy use was 17 times higher.[48] This risk of depression is much less in the case of other beta-blockers.[48] Hence, in patients subject to depression, beta-blockade especially by proprano-lol should be avoided, and the agents of choice include ACE inhibitors. Although ratings of "well being" improved during ACE inhibitor therapy in hypertensive patients,[14] it is not clear that the effect is specific.[23] In a randomized, double-blind parallel group study on 360 hypertensive men, captopril but not enalapril improved the depressed mood when compared with propranolol or atenolol.[44] An-other tantalizing result was found in 379 hypertensive men: captopril preserved a high quality of life, which worsened with enalapril.[47] In neither study was there a concurrent placebo group.

CENTRAL ANTIHYPERTENSIVE MECHANISMS OF ACE INHIBITORS

Unger et al[50] review evidence for a central mechanism, at least in part, for the antihypertensive effects of ACE inhibi-tors. Such effects of ACE inhibitors, exerted chiefly at the level of the brain stem, might be more important in blood pressure reduction than the peripheral vasodilation.[43] A number of peptides besides angiotensin, such as kinins, substance P, and opioid peptides such as beta-endorphin,[22] all thought to participate in central blood pressure regulation, are substrates for converting enzyme activity or closely related enzymes that are also inhibited by ACE inhibitor therapy. Angiotensin II acts in part through release of vasopressin which is a major component of the central blood pressure controlling system.[43] Of great interest is that atrial natriuretic peptide (ANP) in general opposes the effects of angiotensin II on the brain.[43] Thus, the proposal is that ACE inhibitors have central effects that may make a major contribution to the antihypertensive action, at least in part by suppression of central peptidergic blood pressure regulation and/or of brain ACE activity.[39] Because the centers involved in blood pressure control lie outside the blood brain barrier, there is no particular difference between those ACE inhibitors, such as zofenopril, that penetrate this barrier and those, such as enalapril, that do not.

THE PROGRESS STUDY

The hypothesis under test is in PROGRESS (**P**erindopril **pRO**tection a**G**ainst **RE**current **S**troke **S**tudy) is that in those with a history of stroke, whether hypertensive or not, BP lowering by an ACE inhibitor should be protective against secondary stroke.[37] The ACE inhibitor chosen was perindopril, given first as 2mg daily and then 4 mg and then in combination with the diuretic indapamide 2 or 2.5 mg daily. Six thousand patients have been included, and will be followed for a minimum of 4 years after randomization. After six months of follow-up, the average BP reductions were 10.2/4.5mmHg. Judging from previous data, the risk of stroke should be reduced by almost 33%.[29] Results are expected in mid-2001.

SUMMARY

1. *Central receptors.* Besides cerebrovascular A-II receptors, there are also cerebral tissue AT-1 receptors that co-localize with ACE activity in the dopamine synthesizing cells of the brain. Hypothetically, ACE inhibitors could help promote the formation of dopamine in Parkinson's disease with possible clinical benefit. AT-2 receptors are scarce in the human brain. AT-4 receptors, also found in the brain, are of unknown function.

2. *Autonomic nervous system.* ACE inhibitors affect the autonomic nervous system by indirectly diminishing adrenergic activity and by relatively increasing parasympathetic activity. Thereby baroreceptor control may be altered without changing the sensitivity of the receptors.

3. *Cerebral autoregulation.* ACE inhibitors decrease the limits of cerebral autoregulation, clearly beneficial in patients with congestive heart failure and low blood pressure levels. The effects of ACE inhibitors on stroke in hypertensive patients is not yet established. First principles would suggest that a reduction of blood

pressure by any means should induce a corresponding fall in the stroke rate. Nonetheless, there are some conflicting experimental data that need to be considered.

4. *Quality of life and mood.* ACE inhibitors maintain the quality of life at normal levels. Some claim that ACE inhibitors positively improve the quality of life and that there may be differences between captopril and enalapril.

5. *PROGRESS study.* Six thousand patients with prior stroke are under study, with the aim of reducing recurrent stroke by the BP lowering effect of an ACE inhibitor, perindopril, and a diuretic, indapamide. A reasonable guess is that the results, to be declared only in mid-2001, will be positive, and that stroke reduction by about one third may be anticipated.

REFERENCES

1. Ajayi AA, Campbell BC, Howie CA, et al. Acute and chronic effects of the converting enzyme inhibitors enalapril and lisinopril on reflex control of heart rate in normotensive man. J Hypertens 1985;3:47–53.

2. Ajayi AA, Lees KR, Reid JL. Effects of angiotensin-converting enzume inhibitor, perindopril, on autonomic reflexes. Eur J Clin Pharmacol 1986;30:177–182.

3. Alderman MH, Madhavan S, Ooi WL, et al. Association of the renin sodium profile with the risk of myocardial infarction in patients with hypertension. N Engl J Med 1991;324:1098–1104.

4. Atkinson J, Bentahila S, Scalbert E, et al. Perindopril and cerebral ischaemia in renovascular hypertension (Abstract). Eur J Pharmacol 1990; 183:2066–2067.

5. Barnes JM, Barnes NM, Costall B, et al. ACE inhibition and cognition. In: MacGregor GA, Sever P, eds. Current Advances in ACE Inhibition. Churchill Livingstone, Edinburgh, 1989.

6. Barry DI, Paulson OB, Jarden JO, et al. Effects of captopril on cerebral blood flow in normotensive and hypertensive rats. Am J Med 1984; 76:79–85.

7. Beers MH, Passman LJ. Antihypertensive medications and depression. Drugs 1990;40:792–799.

8. Boni E, Alicandri C, Fariello R, et al. Effect of enalapril on parasympathetic activity. Cardiovasc Drugs Ther 1990;4:265–268.

9. Bray L, Lartaud I, Muller F, et al. Effects of the angiotensin I converting enzyme inhibitor perindopril on cerebral blood flow in awake hypertensive rats. Am J Hypertens 1991;4:246S–252S.

10. Brown MJ, Brown J. Does angiotensin II protect against strokes? Lancet 1986;2:427–429.

11. Campbell BC, Sturani A, Reid JL. Evidence of parasympathetic activity of the angiotensin converting enzyme inhibitor, captopril, in normotensive man. Clin Sci 1985;68:49–56.

12. Campbell DJ, Bouhnik J, Mernard J, et al. Identity of angiotensinogen precursors of rat brain and liver. Nature 1984;308:206–208.

13. CAPP Study Group, Hansson L, Lindholm LH, Niskanen L. Effect of angiotensin-converting-enzyme inhibition compared with conventional therapy on cardiovascular morbidity and mortality in hypertension: the Captopril Prevention Project (CAPPP) randomised trial. Lancet 1999; 353:611–616.

13A. Chillon C-M, Baumbach GL. Effects of an angiotensin-converting enzyme inhibitor and a β-blocker on cerebral arterioles in rats. Hypertension 1999;33:856–861.

14. Croog S, Levine S, Testa M, et al. The effect of antihypertensive therapy on the quality of life. N Eng J Med 1986;314:1657–1664.

15. Davisson RL, Yang G, Beltz TG, et al. The brain renin-angiotensin system contributes to the hypertension in mice containing both the human renin and human angiotensinogen transgenes. Circ Res 1998;83:1047–1058.

16. Dietrich B, Hermann WM. Influence of cilazapril on memory functions and sleep behaviour in comparison with metroprolol and placebo in healthy subjects. Br J Clin Pharmacol 1989;27:249S–261S.

17. Dyker AG, Grosser DG, Lees K. Perindopril reduces blood pressure but not cerebral blood flow in patients with recent cerebral ischemic stroke. Stroke 1997;28:580–583.

18. Fernandez LA, Spencer DD, Kaczmar T. Angiotensin-II decreases mortality rate in gerbils with unilateral carotid ligation. Stroke 1986;17:82–85.

19. Ferrario CM, Block CH, Zelenski SG. Behavioural and cognitive effects of ACE inhibitors. ACE Report 1990;70:7.

20. Gohlke P, Linz W, Scholkens A, et al. Cardiac and vascular effects of long-term losartan treatment in stroke-prone spontaneously hypertensive rats. Hypertension 1996;28:397–402.

21. Haberl RL, Decker PJ, Einhaupl KM. Angiotensin degradation products mediate endothelium-dependent dilation of rabbit brain arterioles. Circ Res 1991;68:1621–1627.

22. Handa K, Sasaki J, Tanaka H, et al. Effects of captopril on opioid peptides during exercise and quality of life in normal subjects. Am Heart J 1991;122:1389–1446.

23. Hjemdahl P, Wiklund IK. Quality of life on antihypertensive drug therapy: scientific end-point or marketing exercise? J Hypertens 1992; 10:1437–1446.

24. Jern S. Evaluation of mood and the effect of angiotensin-converting enzyme inhibitors. Drugs 1988;35 (Suppl 5):86–88.

25. Kim S, Hosoi M, Shimamoto K, et al. Increased production of angiotensin-II in the adrenal gland of stroke-prone spontaneously hypertensive rats with malignant hypertension. Biochem Biophys Res Comm 1991;178:151–157.

26. Laragh JH. Two forms of vasoconstriction in systemic hypertension. Am J Cardiol 1987;60:82G–93G.

27. Linz W, Jessen T, Becker RHA, et al. Long-term ACE inhibition doubles lifespan of hypertensive rats. Circulation 1997;96:3164–3172.

28. Lyons D, Roy S, O'Byrne S, et al. ACE Inhibition. Postsynaptic adrenergic sympatholytic action in men. Circulation 1997;96:911–915.

29. MacMahon S, Peto R, Cutler J, et al. Blood pressure, stroke, and coronary artery disease. Lancet 1990;335:765–774.

30. Martin P, Massol J, Scalbert E, et al. Involvement of angiotensin-converting enzyme inhibition in reversal of helpless behaviour evoked by perindopril in rats. Eur J Pharmacol 1990;187:165–170.

31. Moore MV, Jeffcoate WJ, MacDonald IA. Apparent improvement in diabetic autonomic neuropathy induced by captopril. J Human Hypertens 1987;1:161–165.

32. Morioka S, Simon G, Cohn JN. Cardiac and hormonal effects of enalapril in hypertension. Clin Pharmacol Ther 1983;34:583–589.

33. Muller F, Lartaud I, Bray L, et al. Chronic treatment with the angiotensin-I converting enzyme inhibitor, perindopril, restores the lower limit of autoregulation of cerebral blood flow in the awake renovascular hypertensive rat. J Hypertens 1990;8:1037–1042.

34. Palmer AJ, Bullpitt CJ, Fletcher AE, et al. Relation between blood pressure and stroke mortality. Hypertension 1992;20:601–605.

35. Paulson OB, Jarden JO, Vorstrup A, et al. Effect of captopril on the cerebral circulation in chronic heart failure. Eur J Clin Invest 1986;16:124–132.

36. Paulson OB, Strandgaard S. The brain. In: Messerli FH, ed. The ABCs of Antihypertensive Therapy. New York: Authors' Publishing House, 1994, pp 59–68.

37. PROGRESS Management Committee. PROGRESS: Perindopril Protection Against Recurrent Stroke Study: status in March 1997. J Human Hypertens 1998;12:627–629.

38. Raman GV, Waller DG, Warren DJ. The effect of captopril on autonomic reflexes in human hypertension. J Hypertens 1985;3 (Suppl 2):S111–S115.

39. Sakaguchi K, Chai S-Y, Jackson B, et al. Differential angiotensin-converting enzyme inhibition in brain after oral administration of perindopril demonstrated by quantitative in vitro autoradiography. Neuroendocrinology 1988;48:223–228.

40. Shaper AG, Phillips AN, Pocock SJ, et al. Risk factors for stroke in middle-aged British men. Br Med J 1991;302:1111–1115.

41. Speth RC, Harik SI. Angiotensin-II receptor binding sites in brain microvessels. Proc Natl Acad Sci 1985;82:6340–6343.

42. Squire IB. Actions of angiotensin II on cerebral blood flow autoregulation in health and disease. J Hypertens 1994;12:1203–1208.

43. Starr JM, Whalley LJ. ACE inhibitors: Central Actions. New York: Raven Press, 1994, pp 1–254.

44. Steiner SS, Friedhoff AJ, Wilson BL, et al. Antihypertensive therapy and quality of life: a comparison of atenolol, captopril, enalapril and propranolol. J Human Hypertens 1990;4:217–225.

45. Strandgaard S. Autoregulation of cerebral blood flow in hypertensive patients. The modifying influence of prolonged antihypertensive treatment

on the tolerance to acute, drug-induced hypotension. Circulation 1976;53:720–727.

46. Strandgaard S. Cerebral blood flow in the elderly: impact of hypertension and antihypertensive treatment. Cardiovasc Drugs Ther 1990; 4:1217–1222.

47. Testa MA, Anderson RB, Nackley JF, et al. The Quality of Life Hypetension Study Group. Quality of life and antihypertensive therapy in men. A comparison of captopril with enalapril. New Engl J Med 1993;328:907–913.

48. Thiessen BQ, QWallace SM, Blackburn JL, et al. Increased prescribing of antidepressants subsequent to beta-blocker therapy. Arch Intern Med 1990;150:2286–2290.

49. Toda N, Miyazaki M. Angiotensin-induced relaxation in isolated dog renal and cerebral arteries. Am J Physiol 1981;240. H247–H254.

50. Unger T, Rockhold RW, Kaufmann-Buhler I, et al. Effects of angiotensin converting enzyme inhibitors on the brain. In: Horovitz ZP, ed. Angiotensin Converting Enzyme Inhibitors. Baltimore: Urban and Schwarzenberg, 1981.

51. Vidt DG, Bravo EL, Fonad FM. Captopril. N Engl J Med 1982;306:214–219.

52. Werner C, Hoffman WE, Kochs E, et al. Captopril improves neurologic outcome from incomplete cerebral ischemia in rats. Stroke 1991;22:910–914.

53. West JNW, Champion de Crespigny PC, et al. Effects of the angiotensin converting enzyme inhibitor, benazepril, on the sino-aortic baroreceptor heart rate reflex. Cardiovasc Drugs Ther 1991;5:747–752.

54. Zhuo J, Moeller I, Jenkins T, et al. Mapping tissue angiotensin-converting enzyme and angiotensin AT_1, AT_2 and AT_4 receptors. J Hypertens 1998;16:2027–2037.

55. Zubenko GS, Nixon RA. Mood-elevating effect of captopril in depressed patients. Am J Psychiatry 1984;141:110–111.

CHAPTER 8

ACE Inhibitors. Specific agents: pharmacokinetics

"Trust all but verify everything"
(Russian proverb, quoted by Ronald Reagan
to Mikhail Gorbachev)

CLASSIFICATION

Chemical classification. The best known classification is that based on the nature of the ligand to the zinc ion of the enzyme (Table 8-1). The three major groups are the sulfhydryl-containing inhibitors, such as captopril, the carboxyl-containing inhibitors, such as enalapril, and the phosphoryl-containing inhibitors, such as fosinopril. Nonetheless, in current clinical practice, there seems to be little direct relevance in groupings based on these chemical properties. It would seem more natural to separate the drugs on their marked pharmacokinetic differences.

Pharmacokinetic classification. There are three types of ACE inhibitors from the pharmacokinetic point of view. The first class of compound is captopril-like (Fig 8-1), already in the active form, yet undergoing further metabolism. Such metabolic conversion produces disulfides with pharmacological activity. Both the parent compound and the disulfides are eliminated by the kidney. The second class of compounds are prodrugs (Fig 8-2). For example, enalapril becomes active only on conversion to enalaprilat, which occurs chiefly in the liver. This diacid form can then either be eliminated in the kidneys or may be taken up into the tissues where it is thought inhibition of tissue ACE activity may occur. Examples of such prodrugs include benazepril, cilazapril, perindopril, quinapril and ramipril. In the case of very highly lipophilic compounds such as fosinopril, there is also biliary excretion following hepatic cellular uptake of the diacid. The third class of compound is water-soluble and does not undergo metabolism (Fig 8-3). Lisinopril is the prototype. Such compounds do not need any further metabolic conversion to be activated. They circulate unbound to plasma protein and undergo renal elimination in the unchanged form. The only determinants of the plasma levels are therefore the oral dose, the rate of absorption,

TABLE 8-1:   CHEMICAL CLASSIFICATION OF ACE INHIBITORS.
COMPARATIVE DATA ON ACE ACTIVITY, LIPID
SOLUBILITY, AND EXCRETORY PATTERNS OF ACTIVE
FORMS

Agent	ACE activity IC_{50} nM Rabbit lung	ACE activity IC_{50} nM Human plasma	MW of parent Compound	Lipid Solubility	Excretion
Sulfhydryl-Containing					
Captopril	23	22	217	+	K
Zofenoprilat	8	ND	325	+++	K,B
Non-sulfhydryl-Containing					
Benazeprilat	2	1	424	+	K(B)
Cilazaprilat	2	1	389	?	ND
Delaprilat(OH)	40	ND	424	++	K(B)
Enalaprilat	1-5	3	348	+	K
Lisinopril	1	5	405	0	K
Perindoprilat	2	2	340	++	K
Quinaprilat	3	6*	396	++	K(B)
Ramiprilat	4	2	388	++	K(B)
Spiraprilat	1		521	?	B(K)
Trandolaprilat	(2)**	2**	430	+++	B(K)
Phosphoryl-Containing					
Fosinoprilat	11	ND	453	+++	K,B

* Kaplan et al. Angiology 1989; 40: 335. ** Roussel Investigators Brochure;
rat not rabbit lung
Lung ACE and other data from Thind.[152] Human ACE data from Mac-
Fadyen et al.[91]
IC_{50} = active ACE inhibitor concentration required for 50% inhibition of rabbit lung or human plasma ACE.
Lipid solubility based on log P = logarithm of the octanol:water partition
coefficient where + = values between 0.5 and 1.0; ++ = 1.1 to 2.0; and +++ =
2.1 or more.
For original data, see Thind[152] and Duc and Brunner.[39]
It is proposed that the higher the lipid solubility and molecular weight, the
greater the biliary excretion. K, kidney; B, biliary; ND, no data; MW, molecular weight, Delaprilat = both delaprilat and hydroxy (OH) form.

and the rate of renal excretion. It is this pharmacokinetic
classification that will be followed in this chapter.

Trough-Peak ratios: not a simple issue. According to the
provisional guidelines of the American FDA (Food and
Drug Administration) for the registration of antihypertensive agents, not only should such an agent decrease the
blood pressure, but it should do so smoothly and for a prolonged period. In technical terms, the trough and peak effect should be close to each other, the ratio of the trough
effect being no less than one half to two thirds of the peak
effect. By trough is meant the net change in blood pressure
at the end of the dosing interval, and by peak is meant the
maximum net fall in blood pressure at the time of peak
blood pressure lowering effect.[104] There are some major
problems and inconsistencies with this concept:
1.   The guidelines of the FDA were only given in draft
     and never officially implemented.[110]

2. The methods used to measure and to calculate peak and trough effects vary considerably. Placebo effects (in the same patient) and diurnal variations must be considered.[100] How are non-responders dealt with? Is the trough time that of blood pressure reduction, or of trough blood levels?

3. The T:P ratio can vary by as much as two-fold according to the dose of enalapril,[96] lisinopril,[42] and probably several other agents. Thus the T:P ratio can be incorrectly elevated by measurements after a dose higher than normal, with greater risk of side-effects.

4. There are major differences between the published T:P ratios even by the same author,[174, 175] which may also differ from the FDA-approved value.

5. The T:P ratio of a drug may be of less importance in reducing end organ damage than the 24 BP mean values.[110]

Therefore, T/P ratios give useful but not crucial information. Of greater importance are the actual dosing frequencies, as approved by the FDA, and given where available in this Chapter. Of interest, none of the ACE inhibitor drugs is given unequivocal once a day dosing approval by the FDA, although perindopril comes close. In addition, some information is now becoming available on antihypertensive effects after drug withdrawal; here trandolapril seems particularly well studied. For example there is a clear advantage for trandolapril over enalapril after a missed dose (Fig 8-4).

Lipophilicity. Some ACE inhibitors are more lipid soluble (lipophilic) than others. Examples of highly lipophilic agents are ramiprilat and quinaprilat, whereas enalaprilat is hydrophilic. It might be supposed that these differences become more important when considering the central nervous system, yet a clinical comparison of ramipril and enalapril showed no differences.[172] It should also be considered that lisinopril, which is hydrophilic, is licensed for three indications in the USA, whereas lipophilic ramipril is licensed for two. It is not clear whether ACE inhibitors can reach the site of the tissue enzyme by penetrating the extracellular fluid, accessible to hydrophilic agents, or whether actual tissue penetration is required with an advantage for lipophilic inhibitors. When considering endothelial function in patients with heart failure, quinaprilat improved flow-dependent dilation, mediated by nitric oxide, whereas enalaprilat did not.[63] Again, it is not clear that this difference is definitely due to better tissue penetration of the lipophilic quinaprilat.

Genotypes and response to ACE inhibitors. ACE gene polymorphism is often considered as a possible genetic factor that could predispose to cardiovascular disease, although the evidence remains incomplete. A different issue is whether the ACE genotype could regulate the response, for example, to infused angiotensin I in normotensive subjects, and whether the response to ACE inhibitors could likewise be sensitive to the genotype. In a small series of normotensives, the ACE DD genotype was associated with a greater elevation of blood pressure by intravenous angiotensin I than the ACE II genotype, and with a greater response to intravenous enalaprilat.[161] DD is also associated with the highest level of cardiac ACE activity in the human heart.[30] Thus variable clinical responses in different individuals to the same dose of an ACE inhibitor could potentially be explained on a genetic base.

ALACEPRIL

Although alacepril is strictly a prodrug, it has a unique feature in that its active metabolite is captopril. Thus, it is in effect a long-acting captopril preparation.

Pharmacokinetics. *Absorption and metabolism.* There is relatively rapid absorption and metabolism so that the peak value of free captopril is reached in 2.5 hours and of total captopril in 3 hours. Total captopril includes mixed disulfides. *Plasma levels.* The maximum concentration of free captopril is about 30 ng/ml after a single dose and about 40 ng/ml after consecutive doses. Corresponding values for total captopril are 150 and 190 ng/ml. *Plasma protein binding.* This is similar to captopril (30%). *Elimination, distribution and clearance.* The area under the curve is about 200 to 400 ng.h/ml for free captopril and about 1700 to 1800 ng.h/ml for total captopril. Elimination half-life for total captopril is about 8 hours. Most of the free captopril is eliminated in the urine within 8 to 10 hours, while the elimination of total captopril first has a fast phase up to about 8 to 10 hours and then a slow phase up to 24 hours when about 40% of the dose has been eliminated in that form.[138]

Pharmacodynamics. *In hypertensive patients,* a single dose of 12.5 mg reduces blood pressure maximally for 2 to 8 hours and then less for the remaining 24 hour period when the dose is given 2× daily.[138] Plasma ACE inhibition is significantly reduced at 4 to 8 hours after dosage.

Dose and concurrent disease. *In hypertension,* the dose varies from 6.25 mg to 25 mg 2× daily with an average dose of 12.5 mg 2× daily.[138] In the *elderly,* in those with *renal failure,* and in those with *hepatic failure,* similar precautions should be taken as for captopril.

BENAZEPRIL

Benazepril, a prodrug, is converted to benazeprilat chiefly by hepatic metabolism and gives a high degree of inhibition of tissue ACE activity.[67]

Pharmacokinetics. After oral administration the active metabolite benazeprilat starts to appear in the blood within 30 minutes and reaches peak values after 1 hour. The plasma half-life is approximately 11 hours with a terminal half-life of 21 to 22 hours. Conversion of benazepril to benazeprilat occurs in the liver. Both compounds are then excreted by the kidneys. Plasma protein binding is 95 to 97%.

Pharmacodynamics. Plasma converting enzyme activity is very substantially inhibited within 1 hour of administration of benazepril 2 to 20 mg or more. Nearly complete and prolonged (up to 24 hours) inhibition is obtained with all doses above 5 mg.[129] Tissue ACE inhibition may be an important pharmacodynamic site of action of ACE inhibitors. According to Johnston et al,[67] benazeprilat is about as effective in the inhibition of plasma ACE activity as most other prodrugs, and there is also a substantial degree of inhibition of renal ACE activity (over 60%). Benazeprilat is claimed to prevent left ventricular dilation following coronary artery occlusion in the rat.[147] *Trough-peak ratios.* Trough values represent reductions of about 50% of that seen at the peak (FDA-approved package insert).

Dose and concurrent disease. *In hypertension,* the only indication approved in the USA, the dose can vary from an initial response at 5 mg to maximal response at 80 mg given once daily. In the majority of studies 20 mg was chosen,[170] with a usual range of 20–40 mg according to the USA package insert. In a double-blind crossover study, benazepril given as 10 mg 2× daily had a better antihypertensive effect than 20 mg once daily, plasma renin increased more, while plasma ACE activity decreased more.[57] According to the FDA-approved package insert, in studies comparing the same daily dose given as a single morning dose or as a twice daily dose, blood pressure reductions at the time of morning trough blood levels were greater with the divided regime. *In heart failure,* a mean dose of 12 mg daily improved exercise tolerance and decreased mortality over 12 weeks.[25] *In elderly subjects,*[89] the area under the curve increased by 38% compared with young subjects, the dose being 10 mg daily. There were no significant differences between young and elderly for peak concentrations. Only a slight dose reduction appears appropriate in the elderly. *In black patients,* benazepril 10 mg 2× daily reduced blood pressure adequately in 44%, which rose to 72% when combined with nifedipine 20 mg 2× daily.[84] *In renal disease,* the glomerular filtration rate has to drop below 30 ml/min before the dose of benazepril needs reduction.[68] Even in very severe renal disease there is some non-renal mechanism of clearance,[68] probably by increased biliary excretion. *In hepatic cirrhosis,* no dose alteration is required.[68]

Combination therapy and drug interactions. When combined with furosemide the plasma concentrations of benazepril and benazeprilat are unchanged, but that of furosemide falls by about one-third.[36] When combined with the calcium antagonist nicardipine, the concomitant tachycardia induced by nicardipine is reduced,[13] suggesting that benazepril was able to minimize reflex sympathetic stimulation induced by the calcium antagonists.

CAPTOPRIL

Captopril, the first of the ACE inhibitors and still the "gold standard", was originally thought to be a drug with a high incidence of adverse side-effects and particularly feared were serious complications, such as neutropenia and renal impairment. Today, paradoxically, the drug is being promoted for absence of side-effects and for a good "quality of life". This major difference has come about because it is now known that many adverse side-effects were related to excess captopril doses in the initial studies. However, in addition, the presence of the SH-group was originally thought to be harmful and specifically to cause side-effects such as skin rashes, neutropenia, and loss of taste (ageusia). Now with lower doses currently used, these side-effects seem rare. Furthermore, consideration is being given to the possibility that the SH-groups of captopril may act to scavenge free radicals, the formation of which is thought to be an adverse side-effect of post-ischemic reperfusion. Furthermore, the SH-group may specifically account for the benefit of captopril therapy in rheumatoid arthritis. Nonetheless, for practical purposes there is little or no clinical proof that captopril has a greater therapeutic range than other drugs not containing SH-groups.

Pharmacokinetics. *Absorption.* Absolute absorption for captopril is about 70% and absolute bioavailability is about 60%.[40] Absorption is rapid and blood levels are detected within 15 minutes.[72] Despite the delay in absorption when captopril is taken together with food, from the practical point of view food does not influence the kinetics or pharmacodynamics.[127] *Sublingual captopril* has been used in patients with severe hypertension (page 72). However, the availability of the sublingual form is only marginally better than the oral form when judged by the peak effects on blood pressure and peripheral hemodynamics.[83] *Metabolism.* Captopril is partially metabolized, apparently in liver and in blood, to the disulfide and to polar metabolites. *Plasma levels.* In plasma, captopril is partially free, partially bound covalently to plasma proteins, and partially in the form of mixed disulfides with endogenous thiols, such as cysteine and glutathione.[108] One proposal is that the bound forms of captopril form a reservoir to replenish free captopril as it distributes to tissues. Total captopril levels are higher and stay elevated for much longer than those of free captopril. Hence kinetic parameters depend on the form of captopril measured (Table 8-2). Noteworthy is the much longer half-life of total captopril than of free captopril. There is also evidence that during chronic administration captopril blood levels are higher and the area under the curve greater.[65] *Plasma protein binding.* This is about 30%.[74] *Elimination, distribution and clearance.* About two-thirds of an oral single 100 mg dose is excreted within 4 hours in the urine either unchanged or converted to polar metabolites.[72] Within 24 hours 95% of the oral dose is excreted either unchanged or as metabolites. In volunteers, the elimination half-life of

TABLE 8-2: SOME PHARMACOKINETIC PROPERTIES OF CAPTOPRIL

Author	Captopril	Subjects	Conc max ng/ml	Tmax h	Elim T1/2 h	AUC ng.h/ml
Kripalani[72]	100 mg	Normal	Free 1580 Total	1.0 No data	1.7 4	1150 7160
Creasey[27]	100 mg	Healthy elderly	Free 803 Total 3350	1.0 1.4	1.4 –	1390 17320
Ohman[108]	25 mg	Essential hypt., diuretic treated	Total 400-650	1-2	6.2(t) 3.4*(t)	–
Shionoiri[142]	25 mg	Essential hypt.	Free 120	1.5	1.2	275
Richer[124]	1 mg/kg orally	Hypertension	Free 1310	1.0	0.7	–
Cody[24]	25 mg	Severe CHF	Free 122–142 Total 510–840	0.9–1.4 1.2–1.7	1-1.4 > 4	250 2350– 4000
Onoyama[111]	50 mg	Chronic renal failure	Free 430	0.9	Prolonged from 0.4 to 0.7	793

Conc, concentration; Tmax, time for maximal concentration; Elim T1/2, elimination (terminal) half-life; AUC, area under the curve; Hypt, hypertension; CHF, congestive heart failure.
* Non-protein bound. t = terminal

the terminal phase is less than 2 hours.[40] The volume of distribution in volunteers is 0.7 L/kg for the steady state.[40]

Pharmacodynamics. Captopril is already in the active form and does not require metabolic conversion (Fig 8-1). The onset of the blood pressure lowering effect is within 15 minutes with a peak effect at 1 to 2 hours and a total duration of effect of 6 to 10 hours. Serum ACE activity falls to about 40% of control values for 1 to 3 hours after a single dose of 12.5 mg captopril and large doses will have a more significant effect.[142] *Trough-peak ratios.* Captopril was registered before the advent of these ratios. When given twice daily, the T:P ratio is between 0.66 and 0.73.[94]

Indications and doses. In the USA, it is approved for use in hypertension, heart failure, LV dysfunction after myocardial infarction and diabetic nephropathy. *In hypertension,* the USA package insert recommends 25 mg bid or tid, and once 50 mg tid has been reached, the addition of a diuretic. Doses of 100 or 150 bid or tid are also approved, with a maximum of 450 mg daily. These doses would now be regarded as generally too high, with risk of serious side-effects. Today, a standard dose would be 25 mg 2× daily, as confirmed by ambulatory intra-arterial blood pressure measurements in patients with essential hypertension.[136] Sodium restriction is helpful (Fig 3-11). *In heart failure,* captopril kinetics are virtually unchanged.[24] Concentrations of free captopril rise and fall rapidly as in normals, but plasma renin activity stays elevated much longer. In the SAVE

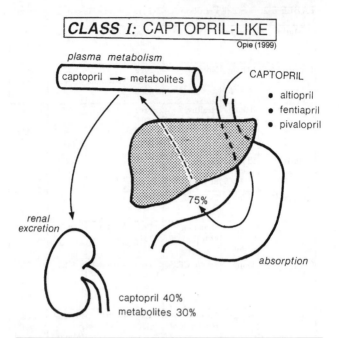

Figure 8-1. *Class I. Pharmacokinetic pattern of captopril-like drugs of which only captopril is generally available. Note conversion of captopril to metabolites and renal excretion. Figure © LH Opie, 1999*

study, in patients with asymptomatic postinfarct LV dysfunction, a test dose of 6.25 mg was given, followed by 12.5 mg, with a target of 25 mg tid, which was then gradually increased to 50 mg tid. Doses lower than 75 mg daily (25 mg 3× daily) may be associated with inadequate control of heart failure and a greater than expected mortality.[117] *In post-infarct left ventricular dysfunction,* starting as early as 3 days postinfarct, the same dosage is followed as in the SAVE study. *In diabetic nephropathy,* the standard dose is 25 mg tid. In the UK, the licence is for diabetic microalbuminuria greater than 30 mg per day.

Concomitant diseases and special situations. In *renal failure,* the captopril dose may need reduction by half or more.[143] not only because of the decreased urinary excretion of the compound and its metabolites,[111] but also because of the inherently greater risk of neutropenia in patients with collagen vascular disease. During dialysis, captopril is still eliminated.[143] *In hepatic failure,* no change in dose is required. *In elderly patients,* no change in dose is required unless there is decreased renal function. The *pediatric dose* is 0.3 to 1.3 mg/kg every 8 hours.[81] *In black subjects,* captopril is not recommended as monotherapy for hypertension, but works well in combination with a diuretic.[167] *In diabetic patients,* there is no adverse effect on glucose metabolism.[162]

Specific side-effects. It is not clear whether anaphylactoid reactions or agranulocytosis in collagen vascular diseases, as well as other side effects such as ageusia, are specific to captopril or not. High doses seem to predispose to serious side-effects.

Combination therapy and drug interactions. As in the case of all ACE inhibitors, there is an additive therapeutic effect with diuretics and low-dose initial treatment is required in such circumstances. Potassium-retaining diuretics or potassium supplements should be used with caution, particularly in the presence of renal failure. NSAIDs, such as indomethacin, may reduce the antihypertensive effect of captopril especially in cases of low-renin hypertension. Even aspirin may have this effect. Increased serum lithium levels and even lithium toxicity have been reported in patients receiving lithium and ACE inhibitor therapy together. Concomitant beta-blockade, although thought not to have a full additive antihypertensive effect according to the package insert, is often used without proof of full efficacy.

Large outcome trials. In the massive ISIS-IV study in *early phase acute myocardial infarction*, not a licensed indication in the USA, oral captopril added to fibrinolysis by streptokinase and antiplatelet therapy decreased mortality by only 0.46% (absolute reduction) at the cost of increased hypotension (Table 5-1). In *post-infarct LV dysfunction*, in those with ejection fractions of 40% or less, the risk reduction was 21% for cardiovascular death, and 37% for the development of severe heart failure (Table 6-3).[128] In *type 2 diabetics*, a careful trial over 9 years showed that captopril reduced fatal and nonfatal cardiovascular events.[162] The dose was 25–50 mg twice daily. In *hypertension* the CAPP study used incorrect dosing of captopril (page 65).

CILAZAPRIL

Cilazapril is a prodrug, being converted to its active form cilazaprilat which has a long terminal half-life with a longer duration of action than enalapril.[34, 105]

Pharmacokinetics. *Absorption.* The drug is rapidly absorbed with peak plasma levels of cilazapril reached within 1 to 2 hours.[133] *Metabolism.* Cilazapril is rapidly metabolised by deesterification to its active form, cilazaprilat, mainly in the liver and blood. *Plasma levels.* The peak plasma concentration of cilazapril is about 120 ng/ml after a single dose and about 145 ng/ml after consecutive doses; the respective values for cilazaprilat are about 25 and 30 ng/ml.[133] *Plasma protein binding.* Not known.[34] *Elimination, distribution and clearance.* Both cilazapril and cilazaprilat are found in the urine following dosage of the compound to patients. Cilazaprilat is eliminated almost entirely by the kidneys, possibly in part by active tubular secretion.[34] Almost all the cilazapril has been excreted by 6 to 8 hours, whereas there is progressive excretion of cilazaprilat in two phases, first an early phase and then a later phase of approximately 8 to 24 hours with much slower excretion.[85] The calculated terminal half-lives vary greatly.[47, 133] The manufacturers give an effective half-life of 9 hrs. Much depends on the exact elimination phases under consideration and the techniques used. Despite the prolonged terminal phase, there is no accumulation of cilazaprilat with repeated administration.[107]

Pharmacodynamics. Following a single dose of cilazapril peak inhibition of serum ACE activity is reached at 2 hours (90% or more), levels stayed down for 8 hours, then 24 hours after the initial dose there was only about 30% inhibition.[45] The percentage inhibition and drop of blood pressure is very closely related to the plasma levels of cilazaprilat.[85, 133] When the blood pressure of volunteers was increased by an intravenous infusion of Angiotensin I, then the effects of cilazapril declined with an elimination half-life of about 4 hours, very similar to enalapril.[169] *Trough-peak ratios.* No FDA-approved data are available. T:P ratios of 59–65% were found by Guntzel et al with single doses of 2.5 and 5 mg.[56]

Indications and doses. In the UK, it is approved for hypertension and heart failure. *In hypertension*, the registered dose is 1-1.25 mg daily, going up to 2.5-5 mg daily. A dose of 2.5 mg/day is the antihypertensive equivalent of propranolol 120 mg/day.[70] Doses above 5 mg achieved no greater benefit.[77] In *congestive heart failure*, the initial dose is 0.5 mg,[34] then increased to 1 mg daily, with a usual maintenance dose of 12–2.5 mg daily.

Concurrent diseases and special situations. *Renal failure.* As the renal function and creatinine clearance falls, the area under the curve (AUC) for cilazaprilat increases[133] especially with repeated doses (Table 8-3). If the average dose for hypertension is 2.5 mg, then in patients with severe renal failure only half that dose, i.e. 1.25 mg, inhibits serum ACE activity by nearly 70% 24 hours after the initial dose.[133] During *dialysis*, elimination of cilazapril and cilazaprilat is very low, so that a dose of 0.5 mg cilazapril after alternate hemodialysis sessions is recommended.[34] *Hepatic failure.* Plasma clearance of cilazapril and cilazaprilat is reduced in hepatic cirrhosis, so that the dose may need reduction.[34] *Elderly patients.* The initial dose for hypertension is 1.25 mg daily.

TABLE 8-3: SOME PHARMACOKINETIC PROPERTIES OF CILAZAPRILAT

Author	Cilazapril dose	Subjects	Conc max ng/ml	Tmax h	AUC* ng.h/ml
Francis[47]	2.5 mg	Volunteers	36	2.1	170
	10 mg		165	–	550
Shionoiri[133]	1.25 mg	Hypertension	25	3.2	227
	1.25 mg repeated	Hypertension	31	3.2	305
	1.25 mg repeated	Hypertension with CRF	117	4.3	1541
Louis[85]	2.5 mg	Hypertension	–	3.0	–

For abbreviations, see Table 8-2. CRF, chronic renal failure. *0–24 hours

Combination therapy and drug interactions. As for other ACE inhibitors, there should be caution when combining with potassium-retaining diuretics or potassium supplements (risk of hyperkalemia especially in renal failure). The dose should be reduced during concurrent diuretic therapy. Indomethacin impairs the antihypertensive effect.[34] There are no other known adverse drug interactions.

Outcome study. In 149 hypertensives studied over 3 years, the glomerular filtration rate was better preserved with cilazapril 2.5–5 mg daily, than with atenolol 50–100 mg daily.[60]

DELAPRIL

Delapril is a prodrug with two active metabolites, the first being the diacid derivative, which can then form the 5-hydroxy delapril diacid.

Pharmacokinetics. *Absorption and metabolism.* After oral administration of delapril, peak concentrations of delapril and delaprilat are reached within 1 hour, and of the metabolite 5-hydroxy delaprilat within 2 hours.[140] Delapril is an ester-type prodrug with an indane ring instead of the proline ring in enalapril. The conversion to metabolites presumably occurs in liver and blood. After a single dose of 15 mg of delapril, peak plasma concentrations (ng/ml) are about 120 for delapril, 375 to 390 for delaprilat, and 170 to 190 for 5-hydroxy delaprilat, and these concentrations are reached at about 1 to 2 hours.[102] *Plasma protein binding.* Not known. *Lipophilicty.* This is higher than with most ACE inhibitors.[121] *Elimination, distribution and clearance.* The elimination half-lives following single doses are 0.3 hours for delapril, 1.2 hours for delaprilat, and 1.4 hours for 5-hydroxy delaprilat[140] with, however, the latter value rising to 6.2 hours during consecutive dosing.[102] Elimination is largely renal because the area under the curve increases in renal failure.[102]

Pharmacodynamics (Table 8-4). After a single dose the blood pressure falls significantly in hypertensive patients for 12 hours.[140, 141] Plasma ACE activity is reduced for 24 hours, while plasma renin activity rises for 24 hours with the peak occurring between 1 and 8 hours.[140] *Trough-peak ratio.* No FDA-approved data are available, nor are there indications that are approved in the USA. Delapril is, however, used in Japan and some European countries.

Dose and concurrent disease. *In hypertension,* a single dose of 15 mg lowers the blood pressure for 1 to 8 hours and, just significantly, up to 24 hours.[141] Similar patterns are found during prolonged dosing with 15 mg 2× daily. *In heart failure,* the doses are 7.5 to 30 mg twice daily.[22] *In renal failure,* the excretion of delapril and its metabolites is impaired and the drop is proportional to the fall in creatinine clearance.[102] The peak values of metabolites and their area under the curve (AUC) values are higher.[140] A dose of

TABLE 8-4: DELAPRIL. SOME PHARMACOKINETIC PROPERTIES OF DELAPRILAT (DT) AND 5-HYDROXY-DELAPRILAT (5-HOD)

Author	Delapril dose	Subjects	Meta-bolite	Conc max ng/ml	Tmax h	AUC ng.h/ml
Shionoiri[140, 141]	Single dose 30 mg	EHT	DT	635	1.2	1859
			5-HOD	229	1.9	948
		CRF	DT	797	1.4	6400
			5-HOD	435	2.5	5068
Minamisawa[102]	Single dose 15 mg	EHT	DT	377	1.2	91
			5-HOD	170	2.6	47
		CRF	DT	477	1.0	211
			5-HOD	281	1.5	183
	15 mg daily for 7 days	CRF	DT	493	1.2	225
			5-HOD	378	1.6	364

For abbreviations, see Table 8-2.
EHT, essential hypertension; CRF, chronic renal failure; DT, deliprilat = delapril diacid; 5-HOD, 5-hydroxy delapril

15 mg $2\times$ daily in patients with mean creatinine clearance values of 37 ml/min/1.73m^2 led to increased values for the maximal concentration reached in the plasma (Cmax) and the area under the curve (Table 8-4). Therefore, dose reduction is required in renal failure. *In elderly patients*, delapril 15 mg twice daily was the approximate equivalent of captopril 25 mg three times daily.[3]

Outcome study. There appear to be no adequate outcome studies. In GLANT, delapril (n = 980) was compared with a dihydropyridine calcium blocker (n = 956) for 12 months, with cardiovascular and cerebrovascular end-points.[52] No differences were shown. The study was underpowered and too short.

ENALAPRIL

This compound was the first of the prodrug ACE inhibitors clinically available. Like others, it only becomes active after conversion to the active diacid form by metabolism. Enalaprilat, the resulting active compound, is excreted by the kidneys and has a considerably longer half-life than the parent. Thus the onset of action is delayed when compared with captopril, but enalapril is correspondingly longer acting. Like most other prodrugs, enalapril is non-sulfhydryl containing. Enalapril is the most widely tested ACE inhibitor in all degrees of heart failure.

Pharmacokinetics (Table 8-5). *Absorption* is rapid with peak concentrations of unchanged enalapril reached at about 1 hour and peak serum concentrations of enalaprilat reached after 3 to 4 hours. About 40% of oral enalapril becomes available as enalaprilat. Absorption is not altered by food;[157] however, enalapril-induced vasodilation may be enhanced by meals.[59] The chief site of metabolism, which

TABLE 8-5:   Enalapril. Some Pharmacokinetic Properties of
                   Enalaprilat

Author	Enalapril dose	Subjects	Conc max ng/ml	Tmax h	Elim T1/2	AUC ng.h/ml
Till[154]	10 mg orally	Normal volunteers	34	–	11*	–
Shio-noiri[132, 137]	10 mg	Hypertension	35	4	6	452
	10 mg	Hypertension	32	4	8	414
		Chronic RF	110	9	11	1708
Schwartz[131]	20 mg	Hypertension	about 60	5	–	865
	40 mg	Hypertension	about 80	5.5	2	1615
	5 mg	CHF	about 22	5	3.5	265
	10 mg	CHF	–	4.5	6	420

For abbreviations, see Table 8-2.
CHF, congestive heart failure; RF, renal failure; *From urine data.
Note other reports of terminal half-life of 30-35 hours.[85, 157]

occurs by de-esterification, is in the liver. *Plasma levels.* Following a single 20 mg dose the peak plasma concentration of enalaprilat is about 70 ng/ml at 2 to 4 hours after administration, dropping to about 20 ng/ml at 12 hours.[31] Values exceeding 10 ng/ml are required for adequate inhibition of plasma ACE activity in volunteers.[15] The maximum concentration of enalaprilat is linearly related to the enalapril dose but the area under the curve (AUC) is only closely related when the prolonged terminal phase is omitted in the calculation. *Plasma protein binding.* Less than 50% is bound to human protein with two binding sites, one with high affinity and low capacity which may represent the binding of enalaprilat to circulating ACE. It is thought that such binding accounts for the prolonged terminal phase of the plasma concentration profile. *Elimination, distribution and clearance.* The accumulation half-life is approximately 11 hours as calculated from urine data,[154] whereas the elimination half-life is approximately 6 hours as measured from plasma concentrations.[132] A very long terminal phase with a half-life of approximately 30 to 35 hours probably represents enalaprilat bound to circulating serum ACE.[2] Elimination is chiefly renal by glomerular filtration. However, 27% of an oral dose of enalapril can be recovered as fecal enalaprilat,[163] presumably the result of biliary excretion.

Pharmacodynamics. After a single 10 mg dose of enalapril given to patients with essential hypertension,[31] the peak enalaprilat concentration is reached between 2 and 8 hours at the same time that serum ACE activity is maximally depressed and the blood pressure falls most. Following the 10 mg dose, serum enalaprilat has reverted to normal at 24 hours.[31] and the blood pressure decrease is very much less than at 8 hours.[49] *Trough/peak ratios.* To obtain high ratios requires 10 mg twice daily rather than 20 mg once daily.[96] Trough/peak ratios are not given in the USA package insert.

Indications and doses. In *hypertension,* there is a dose-response relationship across the range of 2.5 to 40 mg once daily.[14] A mean single daily dose of 31 mg reduced blood pressure over 24 hours as shown by ambulatory blood pressure monitoring in 28 patients with hypertension and left ventricular hypertrophy.[54] Despite such evidence for once daily dosing, enalapril 10 mg 2× daily gives even better overall control than does 20 mg once daily.[96] The USA package insert recommends a starting dose of 5 mg once daily, going up to 40 mg once daily., adding a diuretic if needed. In some patients, the antihypertensive effect of enalapril decreases toward the end of the dosing interval, so that an increase in dosage or twice daily dosage should be considered.

In *congestive heart failure*, the standard protocol dose has been 10 mg 2× daily with mean doses of 16.7 mg in SOLVD-II, 18.4 mg in CONSENSUS-I, and 16.6 mg in SOLVD (Table 6-2). The dose range is 2.5 to 20 mg twice daily. Logically, but not based on evidence, the dose could be geared to the severity of heart failure. The initial test dose is 2.5 mg,[58] as recommended in the USA package insert. Even this low dose can, however, still cause significant prolonged hypotension (Fig 9-2). Therefore, again as recommended, the patient should be observed for at least two hours after the initial dose until the blood pressure has been stabilized for an additional hour. Even if there has been transient hypotension, careful dose titration may still proceed. Hypotension occurred in 14.8% of heart failure patients, and in about one-third was the cause of therapy withdrawal.[71]

In *asymptomatic left ventricular dysfunction*, the same dose schedule is followed as in heart failure, but the risk of hypotension is much less.

Concurrent disease and special situations. In *hypertension with microvascular angina*, enalapril reduced blood pressure and left ventricular mass, while improving angina.[103] In *acute myocardial infarction*, a study with early intravenous enalaprilat was terminated because of an adverse effect of drug-induced hypotension.[26] In the *elderly*, the area under the curve (AUC) is increased and the systemic clearance is reduced in proportion to the fall in creatinine clearance.[61] Thus, in elderly patients with normal renal function, enalapril in standard doses is an effective antihypertensive agent.[10] In *black subjects*, ACE inhibitors as a group are usually not recommended as monotherapy for hypertension, but enalapril works well in combination with a low-dose diuretic.[99] In *chronic renal failure*, the plasma concentrations of enalaprilat are very much higher, the area under the curve is very much greater, and the plasma half-life is prolonged.[137] The dose should be reduced by half when the creatinine clearance falls below 30 ml/min.[143] In *hepatic failure*, the appearance of enalaprilat in the plasma is reduced.[66] so that, if anything, the dose should be increased. In general, however, prodrug compounds are given in unchanged dose to patients with hepatic cirrhosis.

Combination therapy and drug interactions. These are the same as for all the other ACE inhibitors. Note the following: (1) increased efficacy when given with diuretics; (2) the capacity to combine with calcium antagonists in the therapy of hypertension; (3) the risk of hyperkalemia (especially in those with prior renal impairment or diabetes mellitus) with potassium-retaining diuretics or with potassium supplements; and (4) attenuation of the antihypertensive effect by non-steroidal anti-inflammatory drugs such as indomethacin. Note the negative interaction between enalapril and aspirin in CONSENSUS II (page 227).

Large outcome trials. In *heart failure,* enalapril is one of the best tested drugs, having been used in four major trials involving about 4,000 patients and all degrees of failure (Table 6-2). In 470 *diabetic hypertensives,* enalapril reduced the incidence of myocardial infarction (fatal and non-fatal) when compared with nisoldipine.[1]

FOSINOPRIL

Fosinopril is a long-acting prodrug with the active form being the diacid (fosinoprilat). Chemically, this compound differs from other ACE inhibitors chiefly in that it is a phosphinic acid.[33] It belongs to Class II (Fig 8-2). It is long-acting, highly protein bound, and has dual routes of excretion, hepatic and renal.[146] The latter, an unusual pharmacokinetic feature, separates it off into Class IIA. The result is that in chronic renal failure, the active fosinoprilat form accumulates less in the blood than does enalaprilat or lisi-

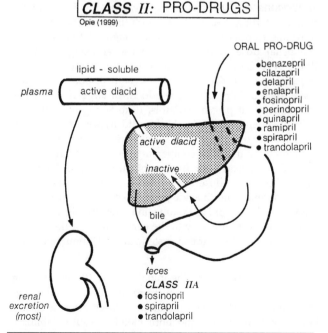

Figure 8-2. Class II. Pharmacokinetic patterns of prodrugs that are converted to active diacids and then excreted. The predominant pattern for most is renal excretion but Class IIA drugs, especially fosinopril, biliary and fecal excretion may be as important. Figure © LH Opie, 1999

nopril.[144] The reason is that the hepatic excretion of fosinoprilat increases as the renal elimination lessens.[64]

Pharmacokinetics. *Absorption, metabolism and elimination*
(Table 8-6). About one-third is absorbed after an oral dose
and metabolized in the liver and gut wall almost completely to the active diacid, fosinoprilat.[64] Fosinoprilat is excreted almost equally in urine and in the bile, hence
appearing in the feces. *Plasma levels, half-life and area under
the curve.* Following a single oral dose of 20 mg, the plasma
level at about 24 hours is 250 ng/ml of which about 99% is
bound to plasma proteins (Package insert). The plasma
terminal half-life is about 12 hours. The area under the
curve is not increased in renal failure because of the dual
renal and fecal elimination routes.

Pharmacodynamics. Inhibition of serum ACE in humans
is complete for 24 hours after a single dose of 80 mg fosinopril and after 20 mg the ACE activity returns slightly to
20% of baseline at 24 hours.[41] A single dose of 10 mg reduced blood pressure at 3 hours with a fall in peripheral
vascular resistance and a rise in plasma norepinephrine and
renin, together with a decreased aldosterone level.[113] After
12 weeks of administration, the fall in blood pressure was
less marked, but plasma epinephrine did not rise. Left ventricular mass fell by 11%. *Trough-peak ratios,* given in the
FDA-approved package insert, are 50–60% for the diastolic
response and 80% for the systolic response.

Indications and doses. In *hypertension,* the USA recommended starting dose is 10 mg, with the dose then adjusted
according to peak (2–6 hours) and trough (24 hrs) response.
The usual dose to obtain a response at trough is 20 to
40 mg once daily. If the trough response is inadequate, then
the dose may be divided. If the overall response is inadequate, then a diuretic may be added. In large clinical trials
with concurrent placebo controls, 10 to 80 mg was effective
when compared with placebo in mild hypertension.[7,116] In
550 patients, the effects of a stepwise increase of fosinopril
from 2.5 to 40 mg were compared with hydrochlorothiazide
5 to 37.5 mg, and with the combination in a factorial design.[116] Very low dose combinations gave such as 2.5 mg
fosinopril and 5 mg thiazide gave detectable blood pressure
reductions (–3.6 mmHg systolic and –1.6 mmHg diastolic).
Best results were found with the combination of the highest
doses of each (–15.1 mmHg systolic and –9.0 mmHg diastolic).

In *congestive heart failure,* the initial dose is 10 mg, or 5 mg
in those with moderate to severe renal failure, or after vigorous diuresis (USA package insert). Observe for at least 2
hours for hypotension and until blood pressure stabilizes.
Titrate up to 20–40 mg once daily. The once daily dosage is
the consequence of the only dosage used in clinical trials,
and "may not represent a known optimum dosage schedule" (USA package insert).

Concurrent diseases and special situations. In the *elderly*, the major reason for decreasing doses of other ACE inhibitors is renal impairment. In the case of fosinopril, no dosage adjustment is required. In *black subjects*, no specific studies have been reported. As for other ACE inhibitors, decreased anti-hypertensive efficacy may be expected (Chapter 3). In *renal failure*, no dosage adjustments are required because the plasma AUC remains the same (Table 8-6). During *dialysis* the clearance of fosinoprilat is minimal because of the high degree of binding to the plasma proteins.[143] In *hepatic failure*, the plasma AUC approximately doubles (USA package insert), but with normal renal function the dual paths of excretion should cope with an unchanged dose. With dual renal and hepatic failure, the dose must be reduced.

TABLE 8-6:   Fosinopril. Some Pharmacokinetic Properties of Fosinoprilat

Author	Fosinopril dose	Subjects	Conc max ng/ml	Tmax h	AUC ng.h/ml
Duchin[41]	20 mg	Young healthy	251	2.4	2000
Hui[64]	10 mg	Renal failure Mean CrCl 60 Mean CrCl 32 Mean CrCl 16	165 136 127	4.0 4.0 4.2	2135 2052 2405

For abbreviations, see Table 8-2
IV, intravenous; CrCl, creatinine clearance, ml/min.

Comparative studies. In a small study, captopril, lisinopril and fosinopril all reduced the blood pressure at mean doses of 113 mg, 47 mg and 52 mg daily, respectively.[178] Only fosinopril increased stroke volume, cardiac output, and filling parameters. The explanations could be (1) a lower systemic vascular resistance with a greater reflex adrenergic stimulation after fosinopril, or (2) a greater uptake of fosinoprilat into the myocardium, as favored by the author.

Drug combinations and interactions. These are similar to those of other ACE inhibitors. In addition, co-administration of antacids may impair absorption of fosinopril (USA package insert).

Outcome study. In acute myocardial infarction, in 142 thrombolysed patients within 9 hrs of the onset of symptoms, fosinopril was initiated at 5 mg and then increased to 20 mg once daily if the blood pressure permitted.[44] The drug was stopped at 3 months. After two years, the incidence of death and heart failure was reduced. These were secondary end-points, and the study needs to be repeated with larger numbers.

IMIDAPRIL

This agent, not yet widely registered, is a long acting, non-sulfhydryl ACE inhibitor, that is a prodrug and converted by the liver to active imidaprilat. It has been used in hypertension, heart failure and after myocardial infarction.[165] In a study over 3 months, high dose (10 mg once daily) was better at improving exercise than a low dose (2.5 mg). No outcome studies are available.

LISINOPRIL

Lisinopril is thus far the only clinically available representative of the type III class of non-metabolized and water-soluble ACE inhibitors (Fig 8-3). Thus, its salient pharmacokinetic features are that it has very low lipid solubility, does not undergo metabolism, and is largely excreted as such in the urine. In the USA, and several other countries, it appears to be the only ACE inhibitor with a triple license for hypertension, heart failure, and early phase myocardial infarction (within the first 24 hours). In the UK it is also licensed for diabetic nephropathy.

Pharmacokinetics. *Absorption.* This is slower than with other ACE inhibitors. After administration of 10 to 20 mg, peak plasma concentrations are reached at about 6 hours[73] or 7 hours (USA package insert). About 25% of lisinopril is absorbed. Food appears not to influence the bioavailability. *Metabolism.* Because the urinary recovery of an intravenous dose is essentially complete, it can be assumed that lisinopril does not undergo metabolism, in keeping with its very low lipophilicity. *Plasma levels.* After a single oral dose of 10 mg the serum lisinopril concentration is about 40 ng/ml in hypertensive patients with normal renal function

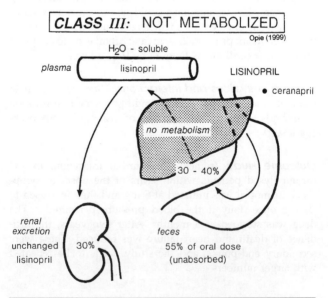

CLASS III: NOT METABOLIZED

Opie (1999)

H₂O - soluble
plasma — lisinopril — LISINOPRIL
● ceranapril
no metabolism
30 - 40%
renal excretion unchanged lisinopril 30%
feces 55% of oral dose (unabsorbed)

Figure 8-3. Class III. Pharmacokinetic patterns of lisinopril-like drugs that are water-soluble. At present the only compound clinically available is lisinopril. It undergoes no metabolism and is excreted unchanged in the urine. There is no plasma protein binding. That portion of the dose not absorbed is excreted in the feces. Figure © LH Opie, 1999

TABLE 8-7: Lisinopril. Some Pharmacokinetic Data

Author	Lisinopril dose	Subjects	Conc max ng/ml	Tmax h	Elim T1/2 h	AUC ng.h/ml
Cirillo[23]	20 mg	Young healthy	78	ND	ND	1380
		Elderly healthy	143	ND	ND	2379
Shionoiri[135]	10 mg single dose	Hypt, normal renal function	42	6	7	524
		Hypt, CRF	74	9	10	1109
Sica[144]	5 mg for 10 days	CRF Day 1	47	13	ND	816
		CRF Day 10	106	9	ND	2164

For abbreviations, See Table 8-2.
CRF, chronic renal failure; Hypt, hypertension; ND, no data.

(Table 8-7). *Plasma protein binding.* The drug is not at all bound to plasma proteins, being entirely water soluble.[53] *Elimination, distribution and clearance.* Elimination of the absorbed dose is by the kidneys without metabolism. Most of the drug is eliminated in the early phase with, however, a delayed terminal phase which is thought to represent binding to the angiotensin-converting enzyme.[73] The terminal half-life is 6.8 hours,[139] going up to 12 hours with multiple dosing (USA package insert).

Pharmacodynamics. *Duration of action* (Table 8-7). After a single 10 mg dose the inhibition of plasma ACE activity exceeds 80% at 4 hours, stays even higher until 5 hours, and then gradually declines to 20% at 24 hours.[101] In hypertensive patients, such a single dose reduces the blood pressure most over the 4 to 10 hours after the dose. With consecutive dosing the 24 hour blood pressure reduction is also significant.[139] In patients with congestive heart failure, single doses of 1.25 to 10 mg inhibit the renin-angiotensin system for at least 24 hours.[37] *Trough-peak ratio.* This is not given in the USA package insert, which states that the antihypertensive effect is substantially less at 24 hrs than at 6 hrs after dosing. In a careful study, the trough-peak ratio for a 20 mg dose (with if needed 12.5–25 mg hydrochlorothiazide) given for 12 months was 0.60.[110]

Indications and doses. In *hypertension*, the initial dose is 10 mg (5 mg if already on diuretic therapy). To achieve a full 24 hr response, the dose must usually be increased, according to the USA package insert. However, as with all ACE inhibitors, although the onset of antihypertensive effect is rapid, the full effect may take 2–4 weeks. In a randomized blinded parallel group study, lisinopril 10 mg reduced the diastolic blood pressure to 90 mmHg or below in 77% of the first group of patients, 20 mg was required in 48% of the second group of patients, and 40 mg in 14% of the third group of patients.[12] 80 mg daily gives a small additional BP reduction (Fig 3-8). If lisinopril alone does not give adequate control, then a diuretic such as 12.5 mg hydrochlorothiazide can be added. In hypertensives with *renal impairment*, there is an inverse correlation between the creatinine clearance and the area under the curve (AUC, Table 8-7). When the glomerular filtration rate falls below 30 ml/min, then the standard 10 mg initial dose must be reduced to 5 mg and when it falls below 10 ml/min (usually on dialysis), reduced to 2.5 mg (USA package insert).

In congestive heart failure, the usual starting dose is 5mg, working up to 20 mg once daily.[20,118] (USA package insert). With dose titration, the mean dose in patients mostly treated by both digoxin and furosemide, was 12 mg.[20] In the ATLAS study,[11] low dose (2.5–5.0 mg) was compared with high dose (about 35 mg). The higher dose gave a small non-significant reduction in all cause mortality, and a 12% reduction in the combined end point of mortality and hospitalization ($p = 0.002$). The initial dose of lisinopril should be reduced to 2.5 mg in those with hyponatremia (< 130 mEq/l), or a creatinine clearance below 30 ml/min or a serum creatinine above 3 mg/dl (USA package insert). After the initial dose, the patient should be observed for 6–8 hrs when peak blood pressure lowering occurs and until the BP is stable.

In acute myocardial infarction, lisinopril is indicated in hemodynamically stable patients within 24 hrs of the onset of symptoms. The initial dose is 5 mg (2.5 mg if systolic BP is 120 mmHg or less, or if there is renal failure), followed by 5 mg after 24 hrs, 10 mg after 48b hrs, and then 10 mg once daily. In GISSI-3,[51] lisinopril was continued for only 6 weeks. Despite increased hypotension (Table 9-1), mortality from persistent hypotension was less than in controls.[75] The greatest mortality reduction was (1) when lisinopril was combined with nitrate therapy, with a 17% reduction at 6 weeks; and (2) in diabetic patients, with a 32% reduction at 6 weeks, and 23% at 6 months.[177] *Renal function* needs attention in acute myocardial infarction. When the initial serum creatinine exceeds 2 mg/dl (177 μmol/l), then there should be caution. If during treatment the values reaches 3 mg/dl (266 μmol/l) or doubles, then lisinopril may have to be reduced in dose or stopped (USA package insert).

In diabetic nephropathy, the UK license is for use either in normotensive type 1 insulin-dependent diabetes.[43] or in hypertensive type 2 non-insulin diabetics.[106]

Special situations and concurrent disease. *In the elderly,* the rate of absorption of lisinopril is the same, but the maximum serum concentration and the area under the curve are higher, related to decreased renal function.[73] Dose increments need to made cautiously. In a number of fairly large trials, however, the lisinopril dose in elderly hypertensives has not been changed.[73] *In black subjects,* lisinopril is less antihypertensive than in non-blacks, even after addition of a diuretic.[115] *In obese hypertensives,* lisinopril reduces BP better than hydrochlorothiazide, while avoiding changes in blood sugar and serum potassium.[123] *Pre-existing renal impairment.* Lisinopril is excreted solely by the kidneys. As also emphasized in other USA package inserts for ACE inhibitors, "evaluation of patients with hypertension, heart failure, or myocardial infarction should always include assessment of renal function" (see previous sections). *In hepatic failure*, no dose adjustment is required as the drug is not metabolized by the liver. *In glucose intolerance*, lisinopril may be given without fear of increasing the defect.[139]

Large outcome trials. Lisinopril has been tested in (1) acute myocardial infarction within the first 24 hours in GISSI-3 with mortality reduction;[51] in (2) heart failure, in the dose-finding ATLAS study;[11] and in (3) the smaller EU-CLID.[43] study in insulin dependent diabetics, in which urinary albumin excretion rate was decreased. In STOP-2, an ACE inhibitor (lisinopril or enalapril) was compared with diuretics and/or beta-blockers in 6228 elderly hypertensives, in whom the all cause mortality was about 21 per 1000 patient years. The trial is being revealed in mid-June 1999. Preliminary indications are that the ACE inhibitor group did well in terms of hard outcome parameters.

PERINDOPRIL

This ACE inhibitor belongs to the category of ester prodrugs, being converted to the active form perindoprilat chiefly in the liver. Perindoprilat has a long pharmacological half-life. Perindopril has been particularly well studied, both experimentally and clinically, for its effects on the vascular changes in hypertension[8, 145, 153] and in ischemic heart disease.[176]

Pharmacokinetics. Absorption and metabolism (Table 8-8). After rapid absorption from the gastrointestinal tract, perindopril undergoes metabolism by two main pathways,

TABLE 8-8: PERINDOPRIL. SOME PHARMACOKINETIC PROPERTIES OF PERINDOPRILAT

Author	Perindopril dose	Subjects	Conc max ng/ml	Tmax h	AUC ng.h/ml
Lees[78]	4 mg IV	Normals	–	–	–
Lees[79]	8 mg orally	Normals	–	–	120
		Elderly normals	–	–	295
Drummer[38]	2 mg	Hypertension	2	6.5	–
	4 mg	Hypertension	6		
	8 mg	Hypertension	20		
Brown[16]	4 mg	Hypertension	15	3.6	252
Louis[86]	4 mg chronic dosing	Hypertension	15	2.5	143
Servier data	4 mg	Hypertension (H)	7	3.3	87
	4 mg	H; mild CRF	13	3.6	217
		H; severe CRF	33	12.0	1106
		Heart failure	5	8.2	181
Tsai[160]	8 mg	Mild cirrhosis	29	2.3	321

For abbreviations, see Table 8-2
CRF, chronic renal failure; H, hypertension; IV, intravenous

chiefly by cyclization (30% to 40%) to inactive forms, but 15% undergoes hydrolysis in the liver to form the active form, perindoprilat. Other relatively less important routes are excretion in the unchanged form (5%) and conjugation to a glucuronic acid conjugate (5%). *Elimination* of perindopril is chiefly by metabolic conversion, with renal excretion playing a small part.[156] Perindoprilat itself is eliminated in a biphasic manner, the free fraction rapidly eliminated by renal excretion with a half-life of only 1 hour and the bound fraction (bound to ACE) is eliminated much more slowly. Perindoprilat does not accumulate with repeat dosing reaching a state of equilibrium (formation versus elimination) in about 4 days. Such data suggest, as in the case of other ACE inhibitors with a long half-life, that the slow phase of elimination of the active drug results from tight binding to the active site of the enzyme or to other tissue sites. *Plasma concentration and kinetics*. The peak perindoprilat concentration is about 6 to 7 ng/ml, with a time to peak plasma concentration of about 3–7 hours, an elimination half life of 3–10 hrs (USA package insert), followed by a terminal half-life of 30 to 120 hours or even longer. The latter occurs with all long acting ACE inhibitors, and represents dissociation of perindoprilat from its body binding sites. The area under the plasma concentration-time curve is about 90 ng.h/ml. When considering peak and trough blood levels, the inhibitory effects on plasma ACE are similar, which is a desirable indication of sustained activity over 24 hours.[77] *Plasma binding and distribution.* The percentage binding of perindoprilat to plasma proteins is low, about 10–20%. The volume of distribution is about 9 to 10 liters following an intravenous dose. *Clearance.* This is almost entirely renal.

Pharmacodynamics. As expected, perindopril is active against animal models of hypertension and in human hypertension. Single oral doses of perindopril produce a dose-dependent inhibition of plasma ACE varying from 80% at peak values with a 2 mg dose to 95% with an 8 mg dose, whereas 24 hours after dosing the inhibition varies from 60% with the 2 mg dose to 79% with the 8 mg dose.[17] By contrast, in another study,[86] perindopril 4 to 8 mg produced about 45% inhibition of plasma ACE at 24 hours. Perindopril reduces left ventricular hypertrophy in humans.[55] *Vascular effects.* In animals and in humans, it favorably lessens the vascular alterations found in chronic hypertension,[153] while in humans it improves the compliance of the large blood vessels.[164] *Peak/trough levels.* These are given as 75 to 100% in the USA package insert.

Indications and doses. In *hypertension*, the majority of studies have used a single dose of 4 mg daily. In the USA package insert, the recommend initial dose is 4 mg daily, titrated to a usual dose of 4–8 mg once daily according to the blood pressure measured just before the next dose, with a maximum dose of 16 mg daily. Perindopril may be given twice daily, when the blood pressure falls by only 0.5 to 1.0 mmHg more than once daily dosing. In a parallel placebo

dose-response multicenter study over 16 weeks, the response curve flattened after 8 mg and a single daily dose
was as good as two.[21] In a second parallel placebo controlled study over 4 weeks, with automatic blood pressure
monitoring, the percentage of diastolic blood pressure readings still above 95 mmHg was 83% with placebo, 73% with
2 mg perindopril, 54% with 4 mg perindopril, and 42%
with 8 mg perindopril.[87] In a third study using conventional blood pressure recording techniques, in which
2 week treatment periods were used to compare perindopril
2 mg with perindopril 4 mg daily and with placebo, the
lower dose (2 mg) failed to reduce the blood pressure,
whereas 4 mg did.[88] Approximately 65% of the antihypertensive effect occurs within 10 days, 78% after 1 month,
and the full effect after 3 months.[76]

Congestive heart failure is a licensed indication in the UK and
in most (but not all) of the countries where it is marketed.
Perindopril 2–4 mg daily improved exercise tolerance by
27% versus 5% in placebo-treated subjects over 3 months.[97]
Background therapy was by a loop diuretic and, in about
half, also by digoxin. The delayed formation of perindoprilat with an increase of the area under the curve (Table 8-8)
means that the dose should be reduced by about half when
compared with that required for hypertension. An initial
dose of 2 mg seems safe,[91] providing a convenient one-step
titration to the standard dose of 4 mg once daily as recommended by the manufacturer.[151] In a dose of 2–4 mg daily,
plasma aldosterone decreased and angiotensin rose at 8
weeks, even though the BP did not fall when compared to
placebo.[90]

Special situations and concurrent disease. In the *elderly,*
the initial dose is still 4 mg for hypertension, but the maximum recommended dose is 8 mg (USA package insert). In
black subjects with hypertension, ACE inhibitors as a group
are about half as effective as in white subjects, but work
well in combination with a diuretic. In *renal failure,* there is
a reduction in the renal clearance of perindoprilat in proportion to the fall in creatinine clearance (Table 8-8). When
the clearance is reduced but still above 30 ml/min, the initial dose should be reduced by half from 4 mg to 2 mg
daily. With severe renal failure (clearance below 30 ml/
min), the safety and efficacy of perindopril has not been established (USA package insert). During *dialysis,* perindoprilat is effectively removed, probably because of its low
plasma protein binding.[143] In *hepatic failure and cirrhosis,*
plasma concentrations of perindoprilat are about 50%
higher than in controls (USA package insert), however
without any manufacturers' recommendations for dose
changes.

Side-effects and cautions. As with other ACE inhibitors,
the major problems relate to bilateral renal artery stenosis
(contraindicated), unilateral renal artery stenosis (relatively
contraindicated for long-term administration), and risk of
first-dose hypotension. However, in congestive heart failure
in elderly patients, taken off diuretics, there appears to be

relatively little risk of first-dose hypotension in response to an initial dose of 2 mg.[91,148]

Drug combinations and interactions. Perindopril can safely be combined with a diuretic with an enhanced antihypertensive effect.[16] In general, combination of any ACE inhibitor with a beta-blocker shows less than the expected additive antihypertensive response.[173] Further combination with calcium antagonists may increase antihypertensive effects. As in the case of all ACE inhibitors, combination with potassium supplements or potassium-sparing diuretics can lead to increased plasma potassium particularly in patients with renal failure.

Major outcome trials. In the PROGRESS trial, already all the aimed 6000 patients with a history of transient ischemic attacks (TIAs) or stroke have been recruited and will be followed for at least 4 years. The primary end point will be the total number of strokes.[119] Secondary end-points will include total cardiovascular events and deaths, and cognitive function. In the EUROPA trial, the object is to assess the effects of perindopril on outcome in patients with stable coronary artery disease, without clinical heart failure, with the primary combined end point being: total mortality, nonfatal acute myocardial infarction, unstable angina and cardiac arrest. 10,500 patients have been recruited and the trial will last for 3.5 years.[46]

QUINAPRIL

Quinapril belongs to the group of prodrugs that become active by conversion to the diacid metabolite, in this case quinaprilat. Quinapril is highly lipophilic, which may have some advantage for tissue penetration and for its effects on tissue renin-angiotensin systems.[63]

Pharmacokinetics. *Absorption* (Table 8-9). Quinapril is rapidly absorbed (approximately 60%) and its absorption not influenced by food intake. *Metabolism and plasma levels.* There is rapid hydrolysis of quinapril to quinaprilat, chiefly in the liver,[109] so that the peak plasma concentration of quinapril is achieved within 1 hour and the peak concentration

TABLE 8-9:   QUINAPRIL. SOME PHARMACOKINETIC PROPERTIES OF QUINAPRILAT

Author	Quina-pril dose	Subjects	Conc max ng/ml	Tmax h	Elim T1/2 h	Term T1/2 h	AUC* ng/h/ml
Olson[109]	Single dose 10 mg 40 mg	Normal volunteers	223 923	1.6 2.3	1.8 1.9	Not given	803 3386
FDA-approved package insert	Not stated	Not stated	Not given	Not given	2.0	25	Not given

For abbreviations, see Table 8-2. Term = terminal
*Total AUC

of quinaprilat about 2 hours after a single oral dose.[109] *Plasma protein binding.* This is very high, about 97%.[168] *Elimination and clearance.* Quinaprilat is excreted by the kidneys largely by tubular secretion.[143] The elimination half-life of quinaprilat is approximately 2 hours.[109]

Pharmacodynamics. It is proposed that the prolonged antihypertensive effect, exceeding the plasma half-life of quinaprilat, is because of *tissue binding* of quinaprilat. Thus, the dissociation time of quinaprilat from human atrial ACE was over 20-fold longer than that of enalaprilat.[69] *Trough/ peak ratios.* This is 50% according to the USA package insert.

Indications and doses. In *hypertension,* the dose recommended in the USA package insert is initially 10 mg/day up to a maximum of 80 mg/day. Dosage should be adjusted by measuring both the peak response (2–6 hrs after the dose) and the trough (before the next dose) when combined with a diuretic, the initial dose should be 5 mg/day (watching for hypotension). The dosage can be either once or twice daily; the latter gives a somewhat better effect although the difference is not clear cut.[48] Combination with a low dose diuretic further reduces the blood pressure while avoiding hypokalemia.[18] In *congestive heart failure,* the initial dose of 5 mg twice daily is titrated upwards to the usual maintenance dose of 10 to 20 mg twice daily (USA package insert). In a parallel placebo-controlled blinded study, a dose of 5 mg 2× daily did not significantly improve exercise time over 3 months of treatment, whereas 10 mg 2× daily and 20 mg 2× daily did so in a dose-response manner.[125] An improvement between 6 weeks and 3 months of therapy occurred only in the group given 40 mg daily. Symptomatic improvement has been found in a double-blind placebo controlled study (USA package insert). Mortality data are not available.

Special situations and concurrent diseases. In *elderly patients,* quinapril appears to be as effective in younger patients.[130] with an initial dose of 10 mg daily (USA package insert). In *black subjects,* ACE inhibitors as a group are usually not recommended as monotherapy for hypertension. However, quinapril may be more effective than expected.[168] In *renal failure,* the dose should be reduced in relation to the decrease in creatinine clearance, with 5 mg starting dose for clearances of 30–60 ml/min, and 2.5 mg for 10–30 ml/min (USA package insert). As for other ACE inhibitors, evaluation of patients with hypertension or heart failure should always include an assessment of renal function. In *liver disease,* conversion of quinapril to quinaprilat is delayed and the maximum quinaprilat concentration decreased.[168] Thus, the dose may need to be increased.

Drug interactions. As with other ACE inhibitors, diuretics and other antihypertensive drugs increase sensitivity to quinapril and the dose should therefore be reduced. Potassium-sparing diuretics or supplements may seriously elevate plasma potassium levels, especially in patients with renal impairment. A specific interaction is that between quinapril and tetracycline. When given simultaneously, the absorption of tetracycline is reduced by about one-third, possibly due to the high magnesium content of quinapril tablets (USA package insert).

Trials in coronary disease. TREND is not an outcome study, but showed that in normotensive patients with coronary artery disease, impaired endothelial function could be reversed by six months of therapy with quinapril, 40 mg once daily.[159] In QUIET, 1750 patients with coronary disease but normotensive and without lipidemia were under study.[120] The entry point was recent angioplasty or atherectomy. They then received quinapril 20 mg once daily for a minimum of 3 years. Trial end-points included sudden cardiac death, myocardial infarction, bypass surgery, angioplasty, hospitalization for unstable angina, angiographic progression or regression of atherosclerosis. However, none of these were altered. In the small QUO VADIS study, 18% of placebo vs 4% of patients given quinapril (40 mg daily) had serious ischemic events within one year of coronary bypass.[112]

RAMIPRIL

Ramipril is a prodrug that is converted to the active diacid, ramiprilat, which is long-acting. It has been particularly well studied in a large postinfarct trial, AIRE,[5] that has been continued for 5 years of follow up, AIREX.[6] It is also well studied in hypertension with left ventricular hypertrophy, where (1) it reduces the LVH better than atenolol,[4] and (2) some experimental and clinical evidence suggests that regression can be achieved in doses lower than those that decrease the blood pressure.[82]

Pharmacokinetics. *Absorption, metabolism, elimination* (Table 8-10). About 60% is absorbed. Ramipril is converted in the liver to ramiprilat, which is chiefly eliminated by the kidneys with a clearance of about 80—130 ml/min. There is also some fecal excretion.[155] *Plasma levels, half-life, and area under the curve.* These have been studied in hypertensive patients with normal renal function.[134] After 5 mg ramipril the peak plasma concentration reached is 18 ng/ml at 1.2 hours. On the other hand, the peak plasma concentration of ramiprilat is 4.7 ng/ml reached at 3.2 hours. The elimination half life on constant doses is 13–17 hrs, and the terminal half-life is > 50 hours (USA package insert). The area under the curve for ramiprilat is 87 ng.h/ml. Plasma protein binding is 56%.[155]

Pharmacodynamics. In normal volunteers, a 5 mg dose of ramipril can achieve nearly total and prolonged (48 hours) inhibition of plasma ACE activity.[166] The fall of systolic and diastolic blood pressure in hypertensive subjects reaches significance at 3 hours, with maximal values round about 5

TABLE 8-10: RAMIPRIL. SOME PHARMACOKINETIC PROPERTIES OF
RAMIPRILAT

Author	Ramipril dose	Subjects	Conc max ng/ml	Tmax h	AUC ng.h/ml
Meyer[98]	10 mg	Young healthy	33.6	2.1	217
		Elderly healthy	40.6	2.0	186
Witte[171]	10 mg	Hypt, healthy	24.0	3.0	414
Debusmann[32]	10 mg	Hypt, normal renal function	49.6	3.3	314
		Hypt, CRF	65.0	5.3	927
Shionoiri[134]	5 mg	Hypt, normal RF	4.7	3.2	87
	5 mg	Hypt, CRF	33.6	3.6	325

For abbreviations, See Table 8-2.
CRF, chronic renal failure; Hypt, hypertension; ND, no data; RF, renal
failure

to 12 hours, and is still detectable 24 to 48 hours after administration. Dose-effect relationships suggest that optimal
inhibition of ACE activity would require a dose of 10 mg.[77]
In a titration study comparing twice daily vs once daily
doses, two doses were better (USA package insert). *Peak-
trough ratios.* In the USA package insert, the ratio is 50–60%.

Indications and doses. In *hypertension,* in a double-blind
parallel-group placebo-controlled study, the supine diastolic
blood pressure dropped significantly when the ramipril
dose was 2.5 mg with greater falls at 5 and 10 mg.[166] The
USA package insert recommends an initial dose of 2.5 mg
with a dose range of 2.5 to 20 mg daily. In case of lack of
full effect at 24 hrs, the package insert recommends twice
daily dosing. Then, if needed, a diuretic is added. In *heart
failure post myocardial infarction*, in patients with signs of
congestion, the initial dose is 2.5 mg twice daily (1.25 mg if
hypotension is a problem), titrated up to 5 mg twice daily
as tolerated. In *congestive heart failure,* if the etiology is postinfarct, see above. Otherwise congestive heart failure is not
a licensed indication in the USA, but is in the UK and other
European countries. 5 mg of ramipril is the approximate
equivalent of 25 mg captopril 3× daily[93] with, however, a
much more prolonged action; the risk of severe prolonged
hypotension means that the starting dose should be 2.5 mg
or less.[35] Doses are usually based on those used in post infarct failure.

Special situations and concurrent disease. In *elderly patients*, circulating concentrations of ramiprilat were 20% to
100% higher even when serum creatinine was normal,
when compared with younger subjects.[50,98] Dose titration
should be careful. In *black subjects*, there have been no special studies on ramipril. In general, ACE inhibitors are not
recommended as monotherapy for hypertension, but work
well in combination with a diuretic or in a higher dose (see
trandolapril). *In patients with renal failure,* the area under the
curve of ramiprilat increases in relation to the fall in creati-

nine clearance.[134] Peak plasma levels are higher and decline more slowly.[32] A reduction to 25% of the normal dose is recommended when the clearance is below 40 ml/min/ $1.73m^2$ (serum creatinine approximately > 2.5 mg/dl, or > 220 μmol/l) (USA package insert). *In post infarct heart failure with renal impairment,* an initial dose of only 1.25 mg is required increasing to a maximum of 2.5 mg twice daily (USA package insert). In patients with *hepatic cirrhosis,* the dose is unchanged as is the case with other prodrug type ACE inhibitors.

Drug combinations and interactions. These resemble those for other ACE inhibitors including contraindication in the case of bilateral renal artery stenosis, relative contraindication with unilateral renal artery stenosis, while the major side-effects include cough and hypotension.

Large outcome trials. In early post-infarct heart failure,[5] ramipril was highly effective in an initial dose of 2.5 mg twice daily, started 2–9 days after the onset of infarction, and increasing to 5 mg twice daily in most patients. In AIREX, ramipril was continued for 42–59 months, and all cause mortality was reduced by an absolute amount of 11.4% with a relative risk reduction of 36%.[6] The authors calculate that there would be 114 additional survivors for 5 years by treating 1000 patients for an average of just over one year. In the relatively small REIN study on 97 patients, the incidence of end-stage renal failure was much lower in those allocated to ramipril in long term treatment of proteinuric non-diabetic nephropathy over 3 years.[122] In HOPE, 9333 high risk patients 55 years or older, ramipril (10 mg daily) or vitamin E (400 units per day) or placebo are being tested with endpoints cardiovascular deaths, stroke, and myocardial infarction.[62]

SPIRAPRIL

This drug belongs to Class II and is rapidly hydrolyzed to the active diacid, spiraprilat. Spiraprilat achieves the maximal blood concentration about 2 hours after oral administration to volunteers and disappears with a half-life of under 2 hours. Plasma ACE inhibition is found up to 6 hours after doses up to 0.3 mg/kg and 24 hours after 1 mg/kg. After rapid absorption, spirapril is transformed in the liver mainly to spiraprilat, which appears in the blood within 2 hours and then disappears with a relatively short half-life of about 2 hours or less. Elimination in rats and dogs is chiefly by the liver (biliary). Therefore, it should belong to Class IIA (Fig 8-2). Plasma ACE inhibition after a 12.5 mg dose lasts for 4 to 6 hours and after a 25 mg dose lasts for 6 to 8 hours.[126] In *hypertension,* spirapril 12 to 24 mg 1x daily reduced blood pressure as monotherapy in about half the patients; the average dose was 20 mg daily. In the remaining patients, combination with hydrochlorothiazide was usually effective.[19] In *left ventricular hypertrophy,* spirapril reduces left ventricular mass.[92,149]

TRANDOLAPRIL

This drug appears to be one of those with the longest duration of action. It has been studied in one positive post-infarct trial,[158] and is under study in a large prophylactic trial in those with coronary artery disease.[114]

Pharmacokinetics (Table 8-11). Trandolapril is converted to the active form, trandolaprilat, by hepatic metabolism. After fast absorption (40% to 60% of the oral dose) and high first-pass metabolism, trandolaprilat is rapidly formed and reaches peak plasma levels at 4–10 hours. Its binding to plasma proteins depends on the concentration, being 94% at low concentrations and 80% at higher concentrations. Approximately twice as much trandolaprilat is found in the feces as in the urine, suggesting a high rate of biliary elimination, so that the drug may belong to sub-Class IIA. After an initial fast half-life of about 3.5 hours, there is a prolonged terminal elimination phase as in the case of many other ACE inhibitors. The effective terminal half-life is given as 10 hrs in the USA package insert (but see Fig 8-4).

TABLE 8-11: TRANDOLAPRIL. SOME PHARMACOKINETIC PROPERTIES OF TRANDOLAPRILAT

Author	Tran-dolapril dose	Subjects	Conc max ng/ml	Tmax h	AUC ng.h/ml
Lenfant[80]	0.5 mg	Healthy	0.43	1.0	0.4
	1.0	males	0.86	0.5	0.95
	2.0		1.68	0.5	1.86
	4.0		3.32	0.5	0.91
Arner[9]	2.0	Young	7.5 (day 10)	1.0	82.3 (0–24 h)
		Elderly	8.4	0.5	96.8 (0–24 h)
Danielson[29]	2.0	Healthy	1.6 (day 10)	0.5	2.0
		CRF (31–80)	2.5 (day 10)	0.75	3.0
		CRF (7–30)	2.7 (day 10)	0.5	3.8

Young   = mean age 44 years;
elderly = mean age 69 years;
CRF   = chronic renal failure;
31–80   = creatinine clearance 31–80 ml/min/1.73 m^2;
7–30   = creatinine clearance 7–30 ml/min/1.73 m^2

Pharmacodynamics. In humans, after a single oral dose of 2 mg, there is rapid onset of ACE inhibition, starting at 30 minutes, with a peak at 2 to 4 hours and at 24 hours there is still 80% inhibition.[39] Doses of 0.5 to 8 mg for 10 days give a dose-dependent decrease of ACE activity.[39] *Persistence of antihypertensive action.* Despite the relatively short plasma half life, the antihypertensive effect takes 24–48 hrs to wear off (Fig 8-4). *Trough-peak ratio.* In the USA package insert, these are given as 0.5 to 0.9.

Dose and concurrent disease. *In hypertension,* 1 to 4 mg once daily reduced blood pressure effectively in 64% of pa-

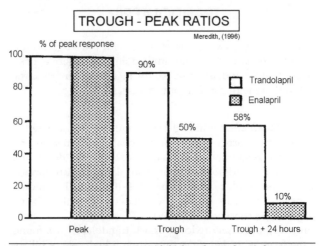

Figure 8-4. *A long-acting agent with high peak-trough ratio has a carry-over effect into the next 24 hours after a "missed" dose. Data from Mere-dith,[95] with permission of author and publisher. See also similar effects of perindopril.[150]*

tients in one study.[39] The initial dose is 1 mg daily in non-black patients and 2 mg daily in black patients (USA packet insert). Most patients will require 2–4 mg once daily. If once daily dosing at 4 mg is inadequate, twice daily dosing may be tried, or the agent combined with a diuretic. *In post-infarct heart failure* (USA license being applied for), the initial dose was 0.5 mg, then 1–4 mg once daily.[158] *In the elderly* with normal renal function, dose adjustment is not needed. *In chronic renal failure,* despite the predominant biliary excretion, there is some accumulation of trandolaprilat. The initial dose should be reduced to 0.5 mg daily when the creatinine clearance falls below 30 ml/min (USA package insert). *In hepatic cirrhosis,* the initial dose is likewise reduced to 0.5 mg.

Large outcome trials. In early (3 to 7 days) post-infarct left ventricular dysfunction, trandolapril gave very positive results in 876 patients in the TRACE (Trandolapril Cardiac Evaluation) study.[158] The drug is under test in PEACE, involving 8,100 patients and testing the hypothesis that patients with coronary disease but with normal LV function can be given protection from adverse outcome events.

ZOFENOPRIL

Its novel feature is that it would appear to be one of the very few compounds that is both a prodrug and contains a sulfhydryl group. It is especially able to inhabit cardiac ACE.[28] Owing to a relatively short duration of action of zofenoprilat, twice daily dosing is required. The dose in the SMILE study (Table 5-1) was 7.5 mg initially, then repeated after twelve hours, then doubled to a target of 30 mg twice daily. Over 48 weeks of follow up there was a 29% reduction in the risk of mortality.

SUMMARY

1. *Classification.* From the pharmacokinetic point of view, there are three classes of ACE inhibitors. Class I consists of captopril and allied agents, already in the active form but undergoing further metabolism. Class II has as its prototype enalapril, together with all the other agents that are metabolized to the active diacid form. Class IIA is a subclass with biliary excretion. The metabolite of fosinopril is excreted equally by the liver and kidney. This confers an advantage in renal failure when biliary excretion is increased. This advantage may also apply to benazepril, although the data are incomplete. Class III consists of lisinopril, a water-soluble drug not metabolized at all.

2. *Major indications.* These are hypertension, heart failure, early phase acute myocardial infarction, postinfarct left ventricular dysfunction, and diabetic nephropathy. However, even captopril, the gold standard drug, is registered for only four of these indications. At the other extreme, all are registered for use in hypertension. Each physician in each country should be aware of the registered approved indications in that country, and the approved doses. As none of the indications are thought to be a drug specific effect, but rather a class effect, pharmacokinetic and pharmacodynamic differences do become more important.

3. *Metabolism and frequency of dosing.* The majority of ACE inhibitors now available are Class II prodrugs, which must be converted to the active diacid that is then excreted by the kidneys. Dose reduction is usual in renal failure or in the elderly (except for fosinopril, see above). Of the prodrugs, some have longer half-lives than others, and in some the peak-trough ratios approach unity so that once daily dosing should be feasible. Because these agents bind to tissue ACE, from which they are released only slowly, it is difficult to extrapolate from the plasma half life to the frequency of dosing. Furthermore, trough peak ratios are open to criticism.

4. *Use in hypertension.* Of interest, although most of the ACE inhibitors may be given once daily according to the FDA-approved package inserts, yet the effect at 24 hours (trough) is often much less than the early peak effect, so that twice daily dosing may be needed for full effect. Addition of a diuretic in low dose also gives a better response, and is recommended especially in black patients.

5. *Captopril* is the only class I drug in frequent use. It has a longer therapeutic action than its rather short half-life would predict, in this case because it is found in the plasma in multiple forms and there may be an equilibrium between the bound and free forms. While captopril $2\times$ daily is often given for hypertension, in heart failure the drug should be given $3\times$ daily and in adequate doses.

6. *Enalapril* is the prototype of class II drugs. It is exceptionally well studied in all degrees of heart failure. Other class II drugs include benazepril, cilazepril, fosinopril, perindopril, quinapril, ramipril and trandolapril. Several of these have been well studied in specific situations, and some are involved in large outcome studies.

7. *Lisinopril* is the prototype of group III of drugs. It is entirely water-soluble, metabolized, and has, therefore, simple pharmacokinetic pattern with total renal excretion. In renal failure, corresponding dose adjustment is required.

8. *Differences between agents.* Despite the major chemical and pharmacokinetic differences between the drugs, they are all active in hypertension and most of them have been tested in heart failure, including postinfarct left ventricular dysfunction. Thus, different pharmacokinetic properties and durations of action may be among the factors influencing the choice of drug. In determining the doses, those used in large outcome trials can be regarded as being both efficacious and safe. However, use of high doses is not always tolerated nor obligatory.

REFERENCES

1. ABCD Study. Estacio RO, Jeffers BW, Hiatt WH, et al. The effect of nisoldipine as compared with enalapril on cardiovascular outcomes in patients with non-insulin-dependent diabetes and hypertension. N Engl J Med 1998;338:645–652.

2. Abrams WB, Davies RO, Gomez HJ. Clinical pharmacology of enalapril. J Hypertens 1984;2 (Suppl 2):31–36.

3. Acanfora D, Lanzillo T, Papa A, et al. Congestive heart failure in elderly patients: controlled study of delapril versus captopril. Am J Cardiol 1995;75:37F–43F.

4. Agabiti-Rosei E, Ambrosioni E, Palu CD, et al. On behalf of the RACE Study Group. ACE inhibitor ramipril is more effective than the β-blocker in reducing left ventricular mass in hypertension. Results of the RACE (Ramipril Cardioprotective Evaluation) study. J Hypertens 1995;13:1325–1334.

5. AIRE Study. The effect of ramipril on mortality and morbidity of survivors of acute myocardial infarction with clinical evidence of heart failure. Lancet 1993;342:821–828.

6. AIREX Study. Hall AS, Murray GD, Ball SG, et al. On behalf of the AIREX Study Investigators. Follow-up study of patients randomly allocated ramipril or placebo for heart failure after acute myocardial infarction: AIRE Extension (AIREX) Study. Lancet 1997;349:1493–1497.

7. Anderson RJ, Duchin KL, Gore RD, et al. Once-daily fosinopril in the treatment of hypertension. Hypertension 1991;17:636–642.

8. Antony I, Lerebours G, Nitenberg A. Angiotensin-converting enzyme inhibition restores flow-dependent and cold pressor test-induced dilations in coronary arteries in hypertensive patients. Circulation 1996;94:3115–3122.

9. Arner P, Wade A, Engfeldt P, et al. Pharmacokinetics and pharmacodynamics of trandolapril after repeated administration of 2 mg to young and elderly patients with mild-to-moderate hypertension. J Cardiovasc Pharmacol 1994;23 (Suppl 4):S44–S49.

10. Arr SM, Woollard ML, Fairhurst G, et al. Safety and efficacy of enalapril in essential hypertension in the elderly. Br J Clin Pharmacol 1985;20:279P–280P.

11. ATLAS Trial. Cohn JN. Assessment of Treatment with Lisinopril and Survival (ATLAS) Trial. Val-HeFT International Newsletter 1998;3:1.

12. Beevers DG, Blackwood RA, Garnham S, et al. Comparison of lisinopril vs atenolol for mild to moderate essential hypertension. Am J Cardiol 1991;67:59–62.

13. Bellet M, Sassano T, Guyenne P. Converting-enzyme inhibition buffers the counter-regulatory response to acute administration of nicardipine. Br J Clin Pharmacol 1987;24:465–472.

14. Bergstrand R, Herlitz H, Johansson S, et al. Effective dose range of enalapril in mild to moderate essential hypertension. Br J Clin Pharmacol 1985;19:605–611.

15. Biollaz J, Schelling J, Jacot des Combes B, et al. Enalapril maleate and a lysine analogue (MK-521) in normal volunteers; relationship between plasma drug levels and the renin angiotensin system. Br J Clin Pharmacol 1982;14:363–368.

16. Brown C, Backhouse C, Grippat J, et al. The effect of perindopril and hydrochlorothiazide alone and in combination on blood pressure and on the renin-angiotensin system in hypertensive subjects. Eur J Clin Pharmacol 1990;39:327–332.

17. Bussien JP, d'Amore TF, Perret L, et al. Single and repeated dosing of the converting enzyme inhibitor perindopril to normal subjects. Clin Pharmacol Therap 1986;39:554–558.

18. Canter D, Frank G, Knapp L, et al. Quinapril and hydrochlorothiazide combination for control of hypertension: assessment by factorial design. J Human Hypertens 1994;8:155–162.

19. Carlsen JE, Galloe A, Kober L, et al. Comparison of efficacy and tolerability of spirapril and nitrendipine in arterial hypertension. Drug Invest 1991;3:172–177.

20. Chalmers JP, West MJ, Cyran J, et al. Placebo-controlled study of lisinopril in congestive heart failure: A multicentre study. J Cardiovasc Pharmacol 1987;9 (Suppl 3):S89–S97.

21. Chrysant SG, McDonald RH, Wright JT, et al. For the Perindopril Study Group. Perindopril as monotherapy in hypertension: A multicenter comparison of two dosing regimens. Clin Pharmacol Ther 1993;53:479–484.

22. Circo A, Platania F, Mangiameli S, et al. Multicentre, randomized placebo-contolled, double-blind study of the safety and efficacy of oral delapril in patients with congestive heart failure. Am J Cardiol 1995;75:18F–24F.

23. Cirillo VJ, Till AE, Gomez HG, et al. Effect of age on lisinopril pharmacokinetics (Abstract). Clin Pharmacol Ther 1986;39:187.

24. Cody RJ, Schaer GL, Covit AB, et al. Captopril kinetics in chronic congestive heart failure. Clin Pharmacol Ther 1982;32:721–726.

25. Colfer HT, Ribner HS, Gradman A, et al. For the Benazapril Heart Failure Study Group. Effects of once-daily Benazapril therapy on exercise tolerance and manifestations of chronic congestive heart failure. Am J Cardiol 1992;70:354–358.

26. CONSENSUS II. Swedberg K, Held P, Kjekshus J, et al. Effects of the early administration of enalapril on mortality in patients with acute myocardial infarction. Results of the Co-operative Scandinavian Enalapril Survival Study II (CONSENSUS II). N Engl J Med 1992;327:678–684.

27. Creasey WA, Funke PT, McKinstry DN, et al. Pharmacokinetics of captopril in elderly healthy male volunteers. J Clin Pharmacol 1986;26:264–268.

28. Cushman DW, Wang FL, Fung WC, et al. Differentiation of angiotensin-converting enzyme (ACE) inhibitors by their selective inhibition of ACE in physiologically important target organs. Am J Hypertens 1989;2:294–306.

29. Danielson B, Querin S, LaRochelle P, et al. Pharmacokinetics and pharmacodynamics of trandolapril after repeated administration of 2 mg to patients with chronic renal failure and healthy control subjects. J Cardiovasc Pharmacol 1994;23 (Suppl 4):S50–S59.

30. Danser AHJ, Schalekamp MAD, Bax WA, et al. Angiotensin-converting enzyme in the human heart. effect of the deletion/insertion polymorphism. Circulation 1995;92:1387–1388.

31. Davies RO, Gomez JH, Irvin JD, et al. An overview of the clinical pharmacology of enalapril. Br J Clin Pharmacol 1984;18 (Suppl 2):215S–229S.

32. Debusmann ER, Pujadas JO, Lahn W, et al. Influence of renal function on the pharmacokinetics of ramipril (HOE 498). Am J Cardiol 1987;59:70D–78D.

33. DeForrest JM, Waldron TL, Harvey C, et al. Blood pressure lowering and renal hemodynamic effects of fosinopril in conscious animal models. J Cardiovasc Pharmacol 1990;16:139–146.

34. Deget F, Brogden RN. Cilazapril. A review of its pharmacodynamic and pharmacokinetic properties, and therapeutic potential in cardiovascular disease. Drugs 1991;41:799–820.

35. deGraeff P, Kingma JH, Dunselman PHJM, et al. Acute hemodynamic and hormonal effects of ramipril in chronic congestive heart failure and comparison with captopril. Am J Cardiol 1987;59:164D–170D.

36. DeLepeleire I, Van Hecken A, Verbesselt R, et al. Interaction between furosemide and the converting enzyme inhibitor benazepril in healthy volunteers. Eur J Clin Pharmacol 1988;34:465–468.

37. Dickstein A, Aarsland T, Woie L, et al. Acute hemodynamic and hormonal effects of lisinopril (MK-521) in congestive heart failure. Am Heart J 1986;112:121–129.

38. Drummer CH, Rowley K, Johnson H, et al. Metabolism and pharmacodynamics of angiotensin converting enzyme inhibitors with special reference to perindopril. In: Rand MR, Raper C, eds. Pharmacology. Amsterdam: Elsevier Science, 1987.

39. Duc LNC, Brunner HR. Trandolapril in hypertension: Overview of a new angiotensin-converting enzyme inhibitor. Am J Cardiol 1992;70:27D–34D.

40. Duchin KL, Singhvi SM, Willard DA, et al. Captopril kinetics. Clin Pharmacol Ther 1982;31:452–458.

41. Duchin KL, Wacklawski AP, Tu JI, et al. Pharmacokinetics, safety and pharmacologic effects of fosinopril sodium, an angiotensin-converting enzyme inhibitor in healthy subjects. J Clin Pharmacol 1991;31:58–64.

42. Elliott HL. Trough to peak ratio: current status and applicability. J Human Hypertens 1998;12:55–59.

43. EUCLID Study Group. Randomised placebo-controlled trial of lisinopril in normotensive patients with insulin-dependent diabetes and normoalbuminuria or microalbuminuria. Lancet 1997;349:1787–1792.

44. FAMIS Study. Borghi C, Marino P, Zardini P, et al. Post acute myocardial infarction. The Fosinopril in Acute Myocardial Infarction Study (FAMIS). Am J Hypertens 1997;10:247S–254S.

45. Fasanella d'Amore T, Bussein JB, Nussberger J, et al. Effects of single doses of the converting enzyme inhibitor cilazapril in normal volunteers. J Cardiovasc Pharmacol 1987;9:26–31.

46. Fox KM, Hendersen JR, Bertrand ME, et al. The European trial on reduction of cardiac events with perindopril in stable coronary artery disease (EUROPA). Eur Heart J 1998;19 (Suppl J):J52–J55.

47. Francis RJ, Brown AN, Kler L, et al. Pharmacokinetics of the converting enzyme inhibitor cilazapril in normal volunteers and the relationship to enzyme inhibition: development of a mathematical model. J Cardiovasc Pharmacol 1987;9:32–38.

48. Frank GJ, Knapp LE, Olson SC, et al. Overview of quinapril, a new ACE inhibitor. J Cardiovasc Pharmacol 1990;15 (Suppl 2):S14–S23.

49. Gavras H, Biollaz J, Waeber B, et al. Antihypertensive effect of the new oral angiotensin converting enzyme inhibitor MK-421. Lancet 1981;2:543–547.

50. Gilchrist WJ, Beard K, Manhem P, et al. Pharmacokinetics and effects on the renin angiotensin system of ramipril in elderly patients. Am J Cardiol 1987;59:28D–32D.

51. GISSI-3 Study Group. GISSI-3: effects of lisinopril and transdermal glyceryl trinitrate singly and together on 6-week mortality and ventricular function after acute myocardial infarction. Lancet 1994;343:1115–1122.

52. GLANT Study Group. A 12-month comparison of ACE inhibitor and Ca antagonist therapy in mild to moderate essential hypertension. Hypertens Res 1995;18:235–244.

53. Gomez HJ, Cirillo VJ, Moncloa F. The clinical pharmacology of lisinopril. J Cardiovasc Pharmacol 1987;9 (Suppl 3):527–534.

54. Gosse P, Roudaut R, Herrero G, et al. Beta-blockers vs angiotensin-converting enzyme inhibitors in hypertension: effects on left ventricular hypertrophy. J Cardiovasc Pharmacol 1990;16:S145–S150.

55. Grandi AM, Venco A, Barzizza A, et al. Double-blind comparison of perindopril and captopril in hypertension. Effects on left ventricular morphology and function. Am J Hypertens 1991;4:516–520.

56. Guntzel P, Kobrin I, Pasquier C, et al. The effect of cilazapril, a new angiotensin converting enzyme inhibitor, on peak and trough blood pressure measurements in hypertensive patients. J Cardiovasc Pharmacol 1991;17:8–12.

57. Guyene TT, Bellet M, Sassano P, et al. Crossover design for the dose determination of an angiotensin converting enzyme inhibitor in hypertension. J Hypertens 1989;7:1005–1012.

58. Hasford J, Busmann W-D, Delius W, et al. First dose hypotension with enalapril and prazosin in congestive heart failure. Int J Cardiol 1991;31:287–294.

59. Herrlin B, Sylven C, Nyquist O, et al. Short term haemodynamic effects of converting enzyme inhibition before and after eating in patients with moderate heart failure caused by dilated cardiomyopathy: a double-blind-study. Br Heart J 1990;63:26–31.

60. Himmelmann A, Hansson L, Hansson B-G, et al. Long-term renal preservation in essential hypertension. Angiotensin converting enzyme inhibition is superior to β-blockade. Am J Hypertens 1996;9:850–853.

61. Hockings N, Ajayi LAA, Reid JL. The effects of age on the pharmacokinetics and dynamics of the angiotensin converting enzyme inhibitors enalapril and enalaprilat. Br J Clin Pharmacol 1985;20:262P–263P.

62. HOPE Study Investigators. The HOPE (Heart Outcomes Prevention Evaluation) Study: The design of a large simple randomized trial of an angiotensin-converting enzyme inhibitor (ramipril) and vitamin E in patients at high risk of cardiovascular events. Can J Cardiol 1996;12:127–137.

63. Hornig B, Arakawa N, Haussmann D, et al. Differential effects of quinalaprilat and enalaprilat on endothelial function of conduit arteries in patients with chronic heart failure. Circulation 1998;98:2842–2848.

64. Hui KK, Duchin KL, Kripalani K, et al. Pharmacokinetics of fosinopril in patients with various degrees of renal function. Clin Pharmacol Ther 1991;49:457–467.

65. Jarrott B, Drummer O, Hooper R, et al. Pharmacokinetic properties of captopril after acute and chronic administration to hypertensive subjects. Am J Cardiol 1982;49:1547–1549.

66. Johnston CI, Jackson BJ, Larmour I, et al. Plasma enalapril levels and hormonal effects after short- and long-term administration in essential hypertension. Br J Clin Pharmacol 1984;18 (Suppl 2):233S–239S.

67. Johnston CI, Mendelsohn FAO, Cubela RB, et al. Inhibition of angiotensin converting enzyme (ACE) in plasma and tissues: studies ex vivo after administration of ACE inhibitors. J Hypertens 1988;6 (Suppl 3):S17–S22.

68. Kaiser G, Ackermann R, Sioufi A. Pharmacokinetics of a new angiotensin-converting enzyme inhibitor, benazepril hydrochloride, in special populations – part 1. Am Heart J 1989;117:747–751.

69. Kinoshita A, Urata H, Bumpus FM, et al. Measurement of angiotensin-1 converting enzyme inhibition in the heart. Circ Res 1993;73:51–60.

70. Kleinbloesem CH, Erb K, Essig J, et al. Haemodynamic and hormonal effects of cilazepril in comparison with propranolol in healthy subjects and in hypertensive patients. Br J Clin Pharmacol 1989;27:309S–315S.

71. Kostis JB, Shelton B, Gosselin G, et al. Adverse effects of enalapril in the studies of left ventricular dysfunction (SOLVD). SOLVD Investigators. Am Heart J 1996;131:350–355.

72. Kripalani KJ, McKinstry DN, Singhvi SM, et al. Disposition of captopril in normal subjects. Clin Pharmacol Ther 1980;27:636–641.

73. Lancaster SG, Todd PA. Lisinopril. A preliminary review of its pharmacodynamic and pharmacokinetic properties, and therapeutic use in hypertension and congestive heart failure. Drugs 1988;35:646–669.

74. Laragh JH. New angiotensin converting enzyme inhibitors. Their role in the management of hypertension. Am J Hypertens 1990;3:257S–265S.

75. Latini R, Avanzini F, Nicolao AD. GISSI-3 Investigators. Effects of lisinopril and nitroglycerin on blood pressure early after myocardial infarction: the GISSI-3 pilot study. Clin Pharmacol Ther 1994;56:680–692.

76. Leary WP, Reyes AJ, van der Byl K, et al. Time course of the hypotensive effect of the converting enzyme inhibitor perindopril. Curr Ther Res 1989;46:308–316.

77. Lees KR. The dose-response relationship with angiotensin-converting enzyme inhibitors: effects on blood pressure and biochemical parameters. J Hypertens 1992;10 (Suppl 5):S3-S11.

78. Lees KR, Green ST, Reid JL. Effects of intravenous S-9780, an angiotensin-converting enzyme inhibitor, in normotensive subjects. J Cardiovasc Pharmacol 1987;10:129–135.

79. Lees KR, Green ST, Reid JL. Influence of age on the pharmacokinetics and pharmacodynamics of perindopril. Clin Pharmacol Ther 1988;44:418–425.

80. Lenfant B, Mouren M, Bryce T, et al. Trandolapril: pharmacokinetics of single doses in healthy male volunteers. J Cardiovasc Pharmacol 1994;23 (Suppl 4):S38–S43.

81. Lewis AB, Chabot M. The effect of treatment with angiotensin-converting enzyme inhibitors on survival of pediatric patients with dilated cardiomyopathy. Pediatr Cardiol 1993;14:9–12.

82. Lievre M, Gueret P, Gayet C, et al. On behalf of the HYCAR Study Group. Ramipril-induced regression of left ventricular hypertrophy in treated hypertensive idividuals. Hypertension 1995;25:92–97.

83. Longhini C, Ansani L, Musacci GF, et al. The effect of captopril on peripheral hemodynamics in patients with essential hypertension: Comparison between oral and sublingual administration. Cardiovasc DrugsTher 1990;4:751–754.

84. Loock ME, Rossouw DS, Venter CP, et al. Benazepril and nifedipine alone and in combination for the treatment of essential hypertension in black patients (Abstract). Eur Heart J 1990;11:420.

85. Louis WJ, Conway EL, Krum H, et al. Comparison of the pharmacokinetics and pharmacodynamics of perindopril, cilazapril and enalapril. Clin Exp Pharmacol Physiol 1992;19 (Suppl 19):55–60.

86. Louis WJ, Workman BS, Conway EL, et al. Single-dose and steady-state pharmacokinetics and pharmacodynamics of perindopril in hypertensive subjects. J Cardiovasc Pharmacol 1992;20:505–511.

87. Luccioni R, Frances Y, Gass R, et al. Evaluation of the dose-effect relationship of a new ACE inhibitor (perindopril) by an automatic blood pressure recorder. Eur Heart J 1988;9:1131–1136.

88. Luccioni R, Frances Y, Gass R, et al. Evaluation of the dose-effect relationship of perindopril in the treatment of hypertension. Clin Exp Theory Pract 1989;A11 (Suppl II):521–534.

89. MacDonald NM, Elliott HL, Howie CA, et al. Age and the pharmacodynamics and pharmacokinetics of benazepril. Br J Clin Pharmacol 1988;27:707P–708P.

90. MacFadyen RJ, Barr CS, Sturrock ND, et al. Further evidence that chronic perindopril treatment maintains neurohormonal suppression but does not lower blood pressure in chronic cardiac failure. Br J Clin Pharmacol 1997;44:69–76.

91. MacFadyen RJ, Lees KR, Reid JL. Differences in first dose response to ACE inhibition in congestive cardiac failure – a placebo-controlled study. Br Heart J 1991;66:206–211.

92. Manolis AJ, Beldekos D, Handanis S, et al. Comparison of spirapril, isradipine, or combination in hypertensive patients with left ventricular hypertrophy. Am J Hypertens 1998;11:640–648.

93. Manthey J, Osterziel J, Rohrig N, et al. Ramipril and captopril in patients with heart failure: Effects of hemodynamics and vasoconstrictor systems. Am J Cardiol 1987;59:171D–175D.

94. Martell N, Gill B, Marin R, et al. Trough to peak ratio of once-daily lisinopril and twice-daily captopril in patients with essential hypertension. J Human Hypertens 1998;12:69–72.

95. Meredith PA. Implications of the links between hypertension and myocardial infarction for choice of drug therapy in patients with hypertension. Am Heart J 1996;132:222–228.

96. Meredith PA, Donnelly R, Elliott HL. Prediction of the antihypertensive response to enalapril. J Hypertens 1990;8:1085–1090.

97. Metcalfe M, Dargie HJ. Contribution of perindopril in the treatment of congestive heart failure. JAMA 1990;(Suppl):23–27.

98. Meyer BH, Muller O, Badian M, et al. Pharmacokinetics of ramipril in the elderly. Am J Cardiol 1987;59:33D–37D.

99. Middlemost SJ, Tager R, Davis J, et al. Effectiveness of enalapril in combination with low-dose hydrochlorothiazide versus enalapril alone for mild to moderate systemic hypertension in black patients. Am J Cardiol 1994;73:1092–1097.

100. Millar JA. Shortcomings in the trough to peak ratio as a guide to the dose interval for antihypertensive drugs. J Human Hypertens 1998;12:37–44.

101. Millar JA, Derkx FHM, McLean K, et al. Pharmacodynamics of converting enzyme inhibition: the cardiovascular endocrine and autonomic effects of MK421 (enalapril) and MK521. Br J Clin Pharmacol 1982;14:347–355.

102. Minamisawa K, Shionoiri H, Sugimoto K, et al. Depressor effects and pharmacokinetics of single and consecutive doses of delapril in hypertensive patients with normal or impaired renal function. Cardiovasc Drugs Ther 1990;4:1417–1424.

103. Motz W, Strauer BE. Improvement of coronary flow reserve after long-term therapy with enalapril. Hypertension 1996;27:1031–1038.

104. Myers MG. Trough-to-Peak Ratio and 24-hour blood pressure control. Am J Hypertens 1995;8:214–219.

105. Natoff IL, Nixon JS, Francis RJ, et al. Biological properties of the angiotensin-converting enzyme inhibitor cilazapril. J Cardiovasc Pharmacol 1985;7:569–580.

106. Nielsen FS, Rossing P, Gall M-A, et al. Impact of lisinopril and atenolol on kidney function in hypertensive NIDDM subjects with diabetes nephropathy. Diabetes 1994;43:110–1113.

107. Nussberger J, Fasanella d'Amore T, Porchet M, et al. Repeated administration of the converting enzyme inhibitor cilazapril to normal volunteers. J Cardiovasc Pharmacol 1987;9:39–44.

108. Ohman KP, Kagedal B, Larsson R, et al. Pharmacokinetics of captopril and its effects on blood pressure during acute and chronic administration in relation to food intake. J Cardiovasc Pharmacol 1985;7:S20–S24.

109. Olson SC, Horvath AM, Michniewicxz BD, et al. The clinical pharmacokentics of quinapril. Angiology 1989;40:351–359.

110. Omboni S, Fogari R, Palantini P, et al. For the SAMPLE Study Group. Reproducibility and clinical value of the trough-to-peak ratio of antihypertensive effect. Hypertension 1998;32:424–429.

111. Onoyama K, Hirakata H, Iseki K, et al. Blood concentration and urinary excretion of captopril (SQ 14,225) in patients with chronic renal failure. Hypertension 1981;3:456–459.

112. Oosterga M, Boors A, Veeger NJGM, et al. Beneficial effects of quinalapril on ischemia in coronary bypass surgery patients – one year clinical

follow-up of the QUO VADIS study (Abstract). Circulation 1998;98 (Suppl 1):I-636.

113. Oren S, Messerli FH, Grossman E, et al. Immediate and short-term cardiovascular effects of fosinopril, a new angiotensin-converting enzyme inhibitor, in patients with essential hypertension. J Am Coll Cardiol 1991;17:1183–1187.

114. PEACE Study. Pfeffer MA, Domanski M, Rosenberg Y, et al. Prevention of Events with Angiotensin-Converting Enzyme Inhibition (The PEACE Study Design). Am J Cardiol 1998;82:25H–30H.

115. Pool J, Gennari J, Goldstein R, et al. Controlled multicentre study of anti-hypertensive effects of lisinopril, hydrochlorothiazide and lisinopril plus hydrochlorothiazide in the treatment of 394 patients with mild to moderate essential hypertension. J Cardiovasc Pharmacol 1987;9:S36–S42.

116. Pool JL, Cushman WC, Saini RK, et al. Use of the factorial design and quadratic response surface models to evaluate the fosinopril and hydrochlorothiazide combination therapy in hypertension. Am J Hypertens 1997;10:117–123.

117. Pouleur H, Rousseau MF, Oakley C, et al. For the Xamoterol in Severe Heart Failure Study Group. Difference in mortality between patients treated with captopril or enalapril in the Xamoterol in Severe Heart Failure Study Group. Am J Cardiol 1991;68:71–74.

118. Powers ER, Chiaramida A, DeMaria AN, et al. A double-blind comparison of lisinopril with captopril in patients with symptomatic congestive heart failure. J Cardiovasc Pharmacol 1987;9 (Suppl 3):S82–S88.

119. PROGRESS Management Committee. PROGRESS: Perindopril Protection Against Recurrent Stroke Study: status in March 1997. J Human Hypertens 1998;12:627–629.

120. QUIET Trial. Cashin-Hemphill L, Holmvang G, Chan RC, et al. Angiotensin-converting enzyme inhibition as antiatherosclerotic therapy: no answer yet. Am J Cardiol 1999;83:43–47.

121. Razzetti R, Acerbi D. Pharmacokinetic and pharmacologic properties of delapril, a lipophilic nonsulfhydryl angiotensin-converting enzyme inhibitor. Am J Cardiol 1995;75:7F–12F.

122. REIN Study. Ruggenenti P, Perna A, Gherardi G, et al. On behalf of the Gruppo Italiano di Studi Epidemiologici in Nefrologia (GISEN) Study. Renal function and requirements for dialysis in chronic nephropathy patients on long-term ramipril: REIN follow up trial. Lancet 1998;352:1252–1256.

123. Reisin E, Weir MR, Falkner B, et al. For the Treatment in Obese Patients with Hypertension (TROPHY) Study Group. Lisinopril versus hydrochlorothiazide in obese hypertensive patients. Hypertension 1997;30 (Part I):140–145.

124. Richer C, Giroux B, Plouin P, et al. Captopril: pharmacokinetics, antihypertensive and biological effects in hypertensive patients. Br J Clin Pharmacol 1984;17:243–250.

125. Riegger G. Effects of quinapril on exercise tolerance in patients with mild to moderate heart failure. Eur Heart J 1991:705–711.

126. Salvetti A. Newer ACE inhibitors: A look at the future. Drugs 1990;40:800–828.

127. Salvetti A, Pedrinelli R, Magagna A, et al. Influence of food on acute and chronic effects of captopril in essential hypertensive patients. J Cardiovasc Pharmacol 1985;7:S25–S29.

128. SAVE Study. Pfeffer MA, Braunwald E, et al. Effect of captopril on mortality and morbidity in patients with left ventricular dysfunction after myocardial infarction. Results of the Survival and Ventricular Enlargement trial. N Eng J Med 1992;327:669–677.

129. Schaller M, Nussberger J, Waeber B, et al. Haemodynamic and pharmacological effects of the converting enzyme inhibitor benazepril HCl in normal volunteers. Eur J Clin Pharmacol 1985;28:267–272.

130. Schnaper HW. Use of quinapril in the elderly patient. Am J Hypertens 1990;3:278S–282S.

131. Schwartz JB, Taylor A, Abernethy D, et al. Pharmacokinetics and pharmacodynamics of enalapril in patients with congestive heart failure and patients with hypertension. J Cardiovasc Pharmacol 1985;7:767–776.

132. Shionoiri H, Gotoh E, Miyazaki N, et al. Serum concentration and effects of a single dose of enalapril maleate in patients with essential hypertension. Jpn Circ J 1985;49:46–51.

133. Shionoiri H, Gotoh E, Takagi N, et al. Antihypertensive effects and pharmacokinetics of single and consecutive doses of cilazapril in hypertensive patients with normal and impaired renal function. J Cardiovasc Pharmacol 1988;11:242–249.

134. Shionoiri H, Ikeda Y, Kimura K, et al. Pharmacodynamics and pharmacokinetics of single-dose ramipril in hypertensive patients with various degrees of renal function. Curr Ther Res 1986;40:74–85.

135. Shionoiri H, Minamisawa K, Ueda S, et al. Pharmacokinetics and antihypertensive effects of lisinopril in hypertensive patients with normal and impaired renal function. J Cardiovasc Pharmacol 1990;16:594–600.

136. Shionoiri H, Miyazaki N, Ochiai H, et al. The effects of twice daily captopril and once daily enalapril on ambulatory intraarterial blood pressure in essential hypertension. Clin Exp Theory Pract 1987;A9:599–603.

137. Shionoiri H, Miyazaki N, Yasuda G, et al. Blood concetration and urinary excretion of enalapril in patients with chronic renal failure. Jpn J Nephrol 1985;27:1291–1297.

138. Shionoiri H, Miyazaki N, Yasuda G, et al. Pharmacokinetics and antihypertensive effects of single and consecutive dosing of alacepril (DU-1219) in patients with severe hypertension. Cur Ther Res 1985;38:537–547.

139. Shionoiri H, Ueda S, Gotoh E, et al. Glucose and lipid metabolism during long-term lisinopril therapy in hypertensive patients. J Cardiovasc Pharmacol 1990;16:905–909.

140. Shionoiri H, Yasuda G, Abe Y, et al. Pharmacokinetics and acute effect of the renin-angiotensin system of delapril in patients with chronic renal failure. Clin Nephrol 1987;27:65–70.

141. Shionoiri H, Yasuda G, Ikeda A, et al. Pharmacokinetics and depressor effect of delapril in patients with essential hypertension. Clin Pharmacol Ther 1987;41:74–79.

142. Shionoiri H, Yasuda G, Sugimoto K, et al. The antihypertensive effect and the pharmacokinetic profile of captopril retard (CS-522-R) in patients with essential hypertension. Jpn J Nephrol 1986;28:73–78.

143. Sica DA. Kinetics of angiotensin-converting enzyme inhibitors in renal failure. J Cardiovasc Pharmacol 1992;20 (Suppl 10):S13–S20.

144. Sica DA, Cutler RE, Parmer RJ, et al. Comparison of the steady-state pharmacokinetics of fosinopril, lisinopril and enalapril in patients with chronic and renal insufficiency. Clin Pharmacokinet 1991;20:420–427.

145. Sihm I, Schroeder AP, Aalkjaer C, et al. Normalization of structural cardiovascular changes during antihypertensive treatment with a regimen based on the ACE-inhibitor perindopril. Blood Pressure 1995;4:241–248.

146. Singhvi SM, Kuchin KL, Morrison RA, et al. Disposition of fosinopril sodium in healthy subjects. Br J Clin Pharmacol 1988;27:9–15.

147. Smith EF, Egan JW, Goodman FR, et al. Effects of two nonsulfhydryl angiotensin-converting enzyme inhibitors, benazeprilat and abutapril, on myocardial damage and left ventricular hypertrophy following coronary artery occlusion in the rat. Pharmacology 1988;37:254–263.

148. Squire IB, MacFayden RJ, Reid JL, et al. Differing early blood pressure and renin-angiotensin system responses to the first dose of angiotensin-converting enzyme inhibitors in congestive heart failure. J Cardiovasc Pharmacol 1996;27:657–666.

149. Steensgaard F, Kober L, Torp-Pedersen C, et al. Effect of a new ACE inhibitor, spirapril, and nitrendipine on left ventricular mass and function in essential hypertension (Abstract). Eur Heart J 1990;11:420.

150. Tan KW, Leenen FHH. Persistence of anti-hypertensive effect after missed dose of perindopril (Abstract). Can J Cardiol 1998;184 (Suppl F):149.

151. Task Force of the Working Group on Heart Failure of the European Society of Cardiology. The treatment of heart failure. Eur Heart J 1997;18:736–753.

152. Thind GS. Angiotensin converting enzyme inhibitors: Compariative structure, pharmacokinetics, and pharmacodynamics. Cardiovasc Drugs Ther 1990;4:199–206.

153. Thybo NK, Stephens N, Cooper A, et al. Effect of antihypertensive treatment on small arteries of patients with previously untreated essential hypertension. Hypertension 1995;25:474–481.

154. Till AE, Gomez HJ, Hichens M, et al. Pharmacokinetics of repeated oral doses of enalpril maleate (MK-421) in normal volunteers. Biopharmaceutics and Drug Disposition 1984;5:273–280.

155. Todd PA, Benfield P. Ramipril. A review of its pharmacological properties and therapeutic efficacy in cardiovascular disorders. Drugs 1990;1:110–135.

156. Todd PA, Fitton A. Perindopril – a review of its pharmacological properties and therapeutic use in cardiovascular disorders. Drugs 1991; 42:90–114.

157. Todd PA, Heel RC. Enalapril. A review of its pharmacological properties, and therapeutic use in hypertension and congestive heart failure. Drugs 1986;31:198–248.

158. TRACE Study. Kover L, Torp-Pedersen C, Carson JE, et al. A clinical trial of the angiotensin-converting-enzyme inhibitor trandolapril in patients with left ventricular dysfunction after myocardial infarction. N Engl J Med 1995;333:1670–1676.

159. TREND Study. Mancini GB, Henry GC, Macaya C, et al. Angiotensin-converting enzyme inhibition with quinapril improves endothelial vasomotor dysfunction in patients with coronary artery disease. The TREND

(Trial on Reversing Endothelial Dysfunction) Study. Circulation 1996;94:258–265.

160. Tsai HH, Lees KR, Howden CW, et al. The pharmacokinetics and pharmacodynamics of perindopril in patients with hepatic cirrhosis. Br J Clin Pharmacol 1989;28:53–59.

161. Ueda S, Meredith PA, Morton JJ, et al. ACE (I/D) genotype as a predictor of the magnitude and duration of the response to an ACE inhibitor drug (enalaprilat) in humans. Circulation 1998;98:2148–2153.

162. UKPDS Study. UK Prospective Diabetes Study Group. Efficacy of atenolol and captopril in reducing risk of macrovascular and microvascular complications in type 2 diabetes: UKPDS 39. BMJ 1998;317:713–20.

163. Ulm EH, Hichens H, Gomez HJ, et al. Enalapril maleate and a lysine analogue (MK-521): disposition in man. Br J Clin Pharmacol 1982;14:357–362.

164. Van Bortel L, Kool MJ, Struijker Boudier HA. Effects of antihypertensive agents on local arterial distensibility and compliance. Hypertension 1995;26:531–534.

165. van Veldhuisen DJ, Genth-Zotz S, Brouwer J, et al. High- versus low-dose ACE inhibition in chronic heart failure. A double-blind, placebo-controlled study of imidapril. J Am Coll Cardiol 1998;32:1811–1818.

166. Vasmant D, Bender N. The renin-angiotensin system and ramipril, a new converting enzyme inhibitor. J Cardiovasc Pharmacol 1989;14 (Suppl 4):S46–S52.

167. Veterans Administration Cooperative Study Group on Antihypertensive Agents. Captopril: evaluation of low doses, twice-daily doses and the addition of diuretic for the treatment of mild to moderate hypertension. Clin Sci 1982;14:127–131.

168. Wadworth AN, Brogden RN. Quinapril. A review of its pharmacological properties, and therapeutic efficacy in cardioascular disorders. Drugs 1991;41:378–399.

169. Wellstein A, Essig J, Belz GG. Inhibition of angiotensin-I response by cilazapril and its time course in normal volunteers. Clin Pharmacol Ther 1987;41:639–644.

170. Whalen JJ. Definition of the effective dose of the converting enzyme inhibitor benazepril. Am Heart J 1989;117:728–734.

171. Witte PU, Irmisch R, Hajdu P, et al. Pharmacokinetics and pharmacodynamics of a novel orally active angiotensin converting enzume inhibitor (HOE 498) in healthy subjects. Eur J Clin Pharmacol 1984;27:577–581.

172. Wu RA, Kailasam MT, Cervenka JH, et al. Does liphophilicity of angiotensin converting enzyme inhibitors selectively influence autonomic neural function in human hypertension? J Hypertens 1994;12:1243–1247.

173. Zanchetti A, Desche P. Perindopril: first-line treatment for hypertension. Clin Exper Therapy Pract 1989;A11:555–573.

174. Zannad F, Bernaud CM, Fay R. For the General Physicians Investigators' Group. Double-blind, randomized, multicentre comparison of the effects of amlodipine and perindopril on 24 h therapeutic coverage and beyond in patients with mild to moderate hypertension. J Hypertens 1999;17:137–146.

175. Zannad F, Matzinger A, Larche J. Trough/peak ratios of once daily angiotensin converting enzyme inhibitors and calcium antagonists. Am J Hypertens 1996;9:633–643.

176. Zhuo JL, Froomes P, Casley D, et al. Perindopril chronically inhibits angiotensin-converting enzyme in both the endothelium and adventitia of the internal mammary artery in patients with ischemic heart disease. Circulation 1997;96:174–182.

177. Zuanetti G, Latini R, Maggioni AP, et al. Effect of ACE inhibitor lisinopril on mortality in diabetic patients with acute myocardial infarction. Circulation 1997;96:4239–4245.

178. Zusman RM. Left ventricular hypertrophy and performance: Therapeutic options among the angiotensin-converting enzyme inhibitors. J Cardiovasc Pharmacol 1992;20 (Suppl 10):S21–S28.

CHAPTER 9

ACE Inhibitors: Safety, side-effects and contraindications

"Long-term use of ACE inhibitors may protect against cancer. The status of this finding is . . . that of hypothesis generation; randomised controlled trials are needed."
(Lever et al, 1998)

SAFETY

Present demands are for drugs that work not only on short-term end points such as blood pressure, but also safely achieve an improvement in morbidity and mortality. While there are excellent data on the overall safety of ACE inhibitors in heart failure, the same cannot be said of hypertension. To assess safety, there has to be the absence of significant adverse effects when the drug is used with due regard for its known contraindications. Renal failure when ACE inhibitors are used for bilateral renal artery stenosis is not an issue of safety but of ignorance and negligence. Evidence for safety comes form a variety of sources, including observational studies (case-control, cohort), randomized controlled trials and meta-analyses of such trials. In the case of hypertension, there are as yet no randomized controlled trials that have been published in detail, so that two sets of observational data are important. First, in a retrospective study[1] on *cardiovascular outcomes* in hypertensive patients, ACE inhibitors gave an almost significant trend to a 56% improvement in outcome (Odds ratio, 0.44; CI 0.19–1.01). Second, in a retrospective cohort study, the relative *risk of cancer* was significantly reduced by about 30% when compared with all other antihypertensive drugs, none of which had any association with cancer, whether positive nor negative.[30] Some basic science data also suggest that ACE inhibitors inhibit tumor growth.[54] In this study all-cause mortality was unchanged in those receiving ACE inhibitors, but increased in those receiving other antihypertensives. Prospective randomized studies are required to assess the possibility that ACE inhibitors give improved safety when compared with other antihypertensives. The CAPP study shows that captopril given only once or twice daily is less effective than beta-blocker and/or diuretic therapy in stroke prevention, but better at avoiding the development of diabetes.

Ratio of benefit to harm in heart failure. A new model allows the calculation of the benefits versus risk of ACE inhibitors in heart failure, based on the data of the SAVE study. In that study, the chief treatment related adverse effects were cough, taste abnormally, dizziness or hypotension. Yet therapy is very effective and reduction in mortality can be achieved without side effects after treating only 24 patients.[38] After treating 38 patients, the practitioner would encounter a patient with a side effect that would require a "management decision". Yet nearly 200 patients would have to be treated before encountering one case in which side effects were found without a mortality benefit. This makes ACE inhibition, even with captopril, a very safe form of therapy in heart failure with a high ratio of benefit to harm.

SIDE EFFECTS

Currently the ACE inhibitors are regarded as a rather safe category of drugs with only occasional side-effects (Fig 9-1), although with serious risk to the fetus if given during the second or third trimesters of pregnancy. The most common side effect, apart from coughing, is hypotension, and the most serious angioedema (Table 9-1).

Captopril side effects. Initially the godfather ACE inhibitor, captopril, was thought to have such serious side-effects that it could only be used in exceptional circumstances. Near-fatal neutropenia, serious renal disease with increased proteinuria, as well as less lethal side-effects such as skin rashes, loss of taste (ageusia), and angioedema, came to be recognized. Most of these serious side-effects of captopril appear to be dose-related and at the doses currently used, neutropenia, for example, is hardly an issue, although there

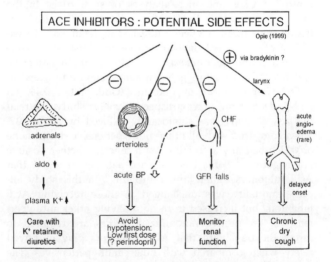

Figure 9-1. *Potential side-effects of ACE inhibitors include cough, hypotension and renal impairment. To avoid hypotension, a low first test dose is usually given (see Fig. 9-2). CHF, congestive heart failure; aldo, aldosterone; GFR, glomuerular filtration rate. Fig. © LH Opie*

TABLE 9-1. SIDE-EFFECTS OF ACE INHIBITORS IN HEART FAILURE, AS FOUND WITH ENALAPRIL IN 6797 PATIENTS IN THE SOLVD STUDY.

Side-effect	Enalapril group	Control group	P value
Hypotension	14.8%	7.1%	P < 0.0001
Azotemia	3.8%	1.6%	P < 0.0001
Cough	5.0%	2.0%	P < 0.0001
Fatigue	5.8%	3.5%	P < 0.0001
Hyperkalemia	1.2%	0.4%	P = 0.0002
Angioedema	0.4%	0.1%	P < 0.05%
Withdrawal from drug	15.2%	8.6%	P < 0.0001
Total side effects	28.1%	16.0%	P < 0.0001

For further details see Kostis.[27]

are still warnings in the package inserts. On the other hand, angioedema remains a truly serious although rare risk, and a class side-effect. Strangely enough, the possession of the SH-group once thought to be so harmful and the cause of several of the serious side-effects including neutropenia, may theoretically benefit by free radical scavenging.

Angioedema. Although rare, when it does occur this reaction can be near-fatal or even fatal. The USA package insert for all ACE inhibitors warns that subcutaneous epinephrine and measures to keep the airways patent must be at hand to relieve vocal cord edema. The true incidence is not known but could be 1 per 3000 patients per week,[28] or about 0.4% vs 0.1% as in controls.[27] Classically there is subcutaneous edema of the face, tongue, pharynx and glottis. It usually follows the first dose or else develops within 48 hours of starting therapy.[12] In a large Swedish study, 77% of cases occurred within 3 weeks of starting the drug.[21] Sometimes a parenteral antihistaminic is incorrectly given, although histamine is not part of the signal cascade. Lesser degrees of the same phenomenon may occur after a delay, sometimes thought to be up to several years. Black American are more susceptible, showing that there is a genetic component to the etiology. The mechanism of the angioedema involves bradykinin, with increased circulating levels.[41] This does not mean that angioedema can not rarely occur with the AT-1 receptor blockers. The USA package inserts for losartan and valsartan give angioedema as a rare side effect, and yet do not high-light the potential need for subcutaneous epinephrine, so that a change to an AT-1 blocker may be made but with caution. Because it seems that angioedema is rarer with AT-1 blockers than with ACE inhibitors (no exact comparative data), the mechanism of the effect may be different, or the AT-1 blockers perhaps generate much lesser amounts of bradykinin. Changing from one ACE inhibitor to another can not help.

Cough. This, probably the most common and literally the most irritating side-effect of ACE inhibitors, is thought to occur in a variable percentage of the population from about

3% to 22%. In one retrospective study, the incidence was 43%,[47] whereas in a very large open-label general practice study it was 9.7%, leading to withdrawal in only 3.3%.[44] Much depends on the method used to detect cough.[57] Not all patients are susceptible; rather it seems that there is a specific subgroup in whom ACE inhibitors increase the sensitivity of the cough reflex.[39] "The cough usually starts with a tickling sensation in the throat and is persistent, dry and on occasions severe enough to cause vomiting."[57] It seems as if the incidence of cough may have been grossly underestimated in some earlier studies, and it is not even commented on in the "quality of life" study by Croog et al,[8] nor is it sufficiently frequently commented on in post-marketing surveys.[57] The incidence is greater in women than in men, and the onset of this side-effect may be delayed for up to 24 months after the onset of ACE inhibitor therapy.[56] Using a visual analog scale in a carefully controlled study, enalapril (mean daily dose 33 mg) had an incidence of associated cough of 29% versus 10% in nifedipine-treated patients, so that the excess incidence associated with enalapril was 19%.[56] In the same study, the incidence of cough assessed by spontaneous reporting was only 6%.

The mechanism remains poorly understood, but appears to be related to prostaglandin formation,[40] which in itself is thought to follow increased bradykinin activity. The next step may be induction of cyclo-oxygenase-2 (COX-2) by bradykinin, leading to formation of thromboxane-B$_2$.[26] A new proposal is that cough relief follows inhibition of thromboxane synthase by the highly effective but still investigational antiplatelet agent, picotamide.[37]

Treatment (Table 9-2). How should the cough be dealt with? The simplest is to persuade the patient to stay on the ACE inhibitor, as the cough may wane over 4 months in about half the cases.[47] A clinical impression is that switching from one ACE inhibitor to another may sometimes benefit, a practice that is supported by imperfect evidence.[7,15,29] While the addition of *sulindac* (200 mg daily) in two doses will limit the symptom of cough and inhibit the cough reflex,[40] the effect on blood pressure control may not be desirable. Sulindac, a non-steroidal anti-inflammatory, may theoretically impair blood pressure control in patients treated by ACE inhibitors. Also, sulindac has a small risk of peptic ulcers. Therefore, it is of interest that *inhaled sodium cromoglycate* gave benefit in an isolated case report.[25] In hypertensive patients, a dihydropyridine calcium blocker such as nifedipine may give relief but is not as good as indomethacin.[14] Depending on the underlying disease for which the ACE inhibitor is given, the option of drug withdrawal and changing to another agent such as an AT-1 blocker, may be considered (Table 9-2).

Hypotension and ACE inhibitor therapy. Hypotension is a feared complication, reported both in patients with congestive heart failure (Fig 9-2) and also in severe hypertension, especially in those with high-renin values.[45] Patients at risk include those with severe renal artery stenosis[55] or

TABLE 9-2: How to Handle an ACE Inhibitor Cough

Basic Diagnosis	Policy options	Rationale	Reference
Heart failure	Persuade patient to keep on	– track record of ACEi in reducing mortality – cough may become less – cough may reflect LV failure	Ch 6, Reisin[47]
	Sodium cromoglycate	anti-asthmatic that acts by suppressing inflammatory mediators	Keogh[25]
	Sulindac	non-steroidal anti-inflammatory; but risk of Na retention	McEwan[40]
	Change to AT-1 blocker	losartan tested in the elderly	ELITE[10]
Hypertension	Any of above	no outcome data for ACE inhibitors or AT-1 blockers	Ch 3
	Change to AT-1 blocker	losartan may decrease incidence of cough to placebo levels*	USA package insert
	Add Ca blocker	mechanism unknown	Fogari[14]
Hypertension with heart failure	As for heart failure	track record of ACEi in reducing mortality in HF	JNC VI[24]
Hypertension with diabetic nephropathy	As for heart failure	track record of ACEi in diabetic nephropathy	JNC VI[24]

*although some degree of cough has been reported
ACEi = ACE inhibitor; HF = heart failure

severe heart failure, especially if treated by high doses of diuretics. Patients over the age of 60 years are at greater risk, presumably because of impaired circulatory reflexes. The *mechanism* seems to involve venodilation.[4] The absence of a compensatory tachycardia suggests, in part, a parasympathomimetic action,[55] resembling vasovagal syncope.

Incidence of hypotension. Careful evaluation of the patient and the use of low test doses of ACE inhibitors can substantially reduce the incidence of excess hypotension. In an out-patient setting, it is possible to give 6.25 mg captopril to patients, to observe the blood pressure for one or two hours, and then to go ahead with higher doses. A fall of mean blood pressure of more than 30% can be expected in 3% to 4% of patients.[45] In hospital practice, a large prospective study on 599 patients with moderately severe congestive heart failure (chiefly New York Heart Association Classes II and III) showed that only three experienced severe hypotension in response to an initial dose of enalapril 2.5 mg, the maximum fall being 4 to 5 hrs post dose.[20]

Differences between ACE inhibitors. In a comparative placebo-controlled study, the possible hypotensive effects of captopril (6.25 mg), enalapril (2.5 mg), and perindopril (2 mg) were compared in unselected elderly patients with congestive heart failure.[34] Diuretic therapy had been withdrawn for 24–48 hours. Captopril produced early hypotension, maximal at 1.5 hours, whereas enalapril decreased blood pressure maximally 4 to 5 hours after the dose, an effect still manifest at 10 hours (Fig 9-2). Surprisingly, perindopril did not decrease the blood pressure when compared with control. Because both perindopril and enalapril equally inhibited plasma ACE activity, the possibility was raised that changes in tissue and not plasma ACE were responsible for differences in the degree of hypotension resulting from these two agents. In a follow-up study, again in elderly patients but this time over 8 weeks and with sustained diuretic therapy, perindopril 2–4 mg was able to inhibit plasma ACE activity without any more hypotension than with placebo.[33] If the absence of first-dose hypotension with perindopril is confirmed in a larger series including younger patients and both genders, this agent could become the drug of choice for the initial therapy of congestive heart failure. Why perindopril differs from captopril and enalapril is not clear, because the active form, perindoprilat, decreases blood pressure as much as enalaprilat.[35] Hypothetically, the parent drug, perindopril, interacts with the active diacid, perindoprilat, to delay the effect of the latter on tissue ACE activity.

Temporary exaggeration of renal failure. Renal failure as a class effect of ACE inhibitors is completely different from captopril-induced kidney damage (see Chapter 4). Found most commonly in heart failure and profoundly in the case of bilateral renal artery stenosis, the mechanism is that ACE inhibition removes efferent glomerular arteriolar tone and thereby decreases the glomerular filtration rate. In the presence of bilateral renal artery stenosis, renal blood flow is fixed and compensation cannot occur. Sometimes a similar phenomenon occurs in the presence of unilateral renal artery stenosis especially when in a single kidney. In patients with severe congestive heart failure where the

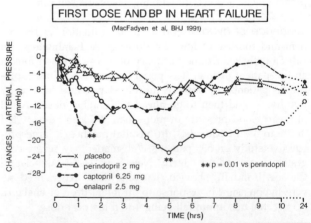

Figure 9-2. Effect of placebo, perindopril (2 mg), captopril (6.25 mg), and enalapril (2.5 mg) on blood pressure (BP) of elderly patients with congestive heart failure in a double-blind randomized paralled group study. Diuretic therapy had been withdrawn for 24 to 48 hours. Note similar fall of blood pressure with placebo and perindopril. Despite dissimilar effects on blood pressure, perindopril and enalapril produced similar degrees of inhibition of plasma ACE activity. Reproduced from MacFayden et al,[34] with permission.

renal perfusion is bilaterally decreased, again a similar phenomenon can occur because of excess hypotension.[43] Thus the introduction of an ACE inhibitor may be followed by increasing blood urea and creatinine values which, if serious, would require reduction of the ACE inhibitor, as well as a temporary lessening of the diuretic dosage. The mechanism of the renal impairment can be related to the degree of arterial hypotension,[9] as also confirmed in CONSENSUS-I.[31]

Practical policy in severe congestive heart failure where renal function is already limited by poor renal blood flow, it may be a difficult decision to know whether or not to introduce ACE inhibitor therapy. The danger of exaggeration of the heart failure must be balanced against the possible benefit from an improved cardiac output and decreased renal affer-ent arteriolar vasoconstriction resulting from ACE inhibitor therapy. Problems can be expected especially when the glo-merular filtration is already low and the renin-angiotensin axis highly stimulated.[31] The best policy is to reduce the diuretic dose temporarily and to add the ACE inhibitor in very low doses and to work up, watching blood pressure, plasma creatinine and urea. Provided that hypotension is avoided, it makes no difference whether a long or short-act-ing ACE inhibitor is used.[42]

Pre-existing renal failure. Sometimes ACE inhibitor ther-apy can precipitate temporary acute on chronic renal fail-ure.[53] The presumed mechanism is either the hypotensive effect or a reduction in efferent glomerular arteriolar tone. As indicated in Ch 4, a pre-existing serum creatinine above a certain value is often regarded as a contraindication to ACE inhibitor therapy, although many experienced physi-cians would still proceed cautiously while watching renal function.

Hyperkalemia. Because ACE inhibitors act to inhibit the release of aldosterone, they tend to increase plasma potas-sium. Hence, combination with potassium supplement ther-apy or potassium-containing diuretics may lead to hyperkalemia[3] especially in the presence of pre-existing renal failure. Such combination therapy should therefore generally be avoided. For example, in the management of hypertension, it is not appropriate to combine an ACE inhi-bitor with either hydrochlorothiazide-triamterene (Dyazide) or with hydrochlorothiazide-amiloride (Moduretic) unless the measured plasma potassium is low. Yet the RALES study[46] (Ch 6, p 141) has shown that in selected patients with clinically severe heart failure, low dose spironolactone (25 mg daily) can be added to prior therapy by a diuretic and an ACE inhibitor with striking outcome benefits.

Aplastic anemia. There are single case reports, suggesting that captopril, enalapril and lisinopril[19] can cause or be as-sociated with aplastic anemia. Note the therapeutic use of ACE inhibitors to suppress post-renal transplant erythrocy-tosis.[36]

SIDE-EFFECTS INITIALLY DESCRIBED
WITH HIGH-DOSE CAPTOPRIL

Neutropenia. Although most firmly linked to the use of
high-dose captopril, it is of interest that the FDA-approved
package inserts for non-sulfhydryl-containing agents, such
as enalapril and quinapril, also mention the risk of neutropenia. Thus, there is a suggestion (but no proof) that such
effects may be in part a class side-effect. It should be considered that the incidence of neutropenia is extremely low
and that the reported cases linking this condition to drugs
such as enalapril are very few indeed and could have arisen
by chance. Nonetheless, these conditions are listed in the
package insert and attention must be paid to the possibility
that there could also be very rare side-effects of non-sulfhydryl-containing ACE inhibitors. *Proteinuria.* Proteinuria occurs in about 1% of patients receiving captopril, especially
in the presence of pre-existing renal disease or high doses
of captopril (more than 150 mg/day).[23] *Impaired taste and
buccal ulcers.* Impaired taste is dose-related and was reported to occur in 2 to 7% of patients treated by captopril.
Although it is still found, it now seems rare with the low
doses of captopril currently used. Both apthous and tongue
ulcers have occurred. *Scalded mouth syndrome.* This very rare
syndrome is described as being similar to scalding by very
hot coffee or pizza. It is not specific to captopril and has
been found with enalapril and lisinopril.[48] It seems not to
be related to impaired taste. *Immune-based side-effects.*
Should any of the above side-effects, thought to be immune-based, occur during captopril therapy, it would make
sense cautiously to change to one of the nonsulfhydryl-containing agents. However, there is no assurance that the alternate agent would be totally free from any such side-
effect, although commonsense would argue the case. In an
interesting court decision in the United States, the manufacturers of nonsulfhydryl-containing agents without a significant incidence of any of the above side-effects were unable
to refute the claims made by the manufacturers of captopril
that there were, in fact, no true differences in the side-effect
profiles of the two types of agents. The USA package inserts for drugs other than captopril suggest that neutropenia and renal damage might still occur, so the issue
remains open.

Precautions with high-dose captopril. Because the side-
effects thought to be immune-based were largely found in
patients with either collagen vascular disease or already
taking other drugs likely to alter the immune response, it
may still be sensible as a caution that all patients who may
need high doses of captopril should have a pre-captopril
renal evaluation, test for nuclear antibodies, and a white
cell count. In practice, many physicians dispense with these
precautions.

Overdose with ACE inhibitors. Several suicide attempts
have been reported with prominent hypotension and some-

times oliguria.[22] Therapy consists of intravenous fluids, vaso-constrictors, calcium infusions, and atropine. When these have failed, an angiotensin infusion may be required.[22]

CONTRAINDICATIONS TO ACE INHIBITORS

Renal. From the possible renal complications, it follows that bilateral renal artery stenosis is a contraindication to the use of ACE inhibitors, as is unilateral renal artery stenosis in a solitary kidney. Severe congestive heart failure with much decreased glomerular filtration rate or elevated serum creatinine is a relative contraindication, as already outlined under side-effects.

Pre-existing hypotension as a contraindication. In heart failure, no exclusion levels are given, neither in the proto-cols of the large studies nor in the package inserts. In acute myocardial infarction, several studies exclude those with initial systolic levels below 100 mmHg. In CONSENSUS II,[6] exclusion values of 100/60 mmHg were later changed to 105/65 mmHg on the recommendation of the safety committee. With lisinopril, one of the few ACE inbhitors licensed for use in the first 24 h of myocardial infarction in the USA, no exclusion criteria are given, but the drug should be withdrawn if the systolic BP falls below 90 mmHg for more than one hour.

Aortic stenosis and severe obstructive cardiomyo-pathy. ACE inhibitors acting as afterload reducing agents can increase the pressure gradient across the aortic valve or across the obstructed septum. ACE inhibitor therapy is therefore contraindicated in these conditions unless very carefully given under close supervision, for example if inoperable aortic stenosis is accompanied by left ventricular failure.[16]

Pregnancy: prominent warning in USA. There is now sound and solid evidence that ACE inhibitors given to the mother during the second and third trimesters of pregnancy are *embryopathic* and can result in severe fetal and neonatal problems, including renal failure, face or skull deformities, and pulmonary hypoplasia.[2, 11, 18] The Food and Drug Administration in the USA now requires a boxed warning on the package. A similar severe warning exists for the AT-1 blockers. Pharmacists will place a sticker on the prescription bottle reading: "If you become pregnant, consult your doctor promptly about switching to a different drug." The FDA[11] and Brent and Beckman[2] state that there is no risk to the fetus from ACE inhibitors given only during the first trimester. Hanssens et al,[18] however, review a few studies in which captopril and enalapril were stopped before 16 weeks of pregnancy, yet with adverse fetal or neonatal problems.

RELATIVE CONTRAINDICATIONS

Chronic cough. Because of the erratic incidence of cough as a side-effect of ACE inhibitor therapy, patients already coughing prior to the use of such agents should be treated with care. If the seriousness of the coughing augments during ACE inhibitor therapy, then the drug should be stopped, tailed off or changed (see Table 9-2). *Asthma or bronchospasm are* rarely precipitated though not specific contraindications to ACE inhibitor therapy.[32]

Severe congestive heart failure, pre-existing hypotension, hyponatremia or co-existing angina. Each of these may be followed by adverse effects in response to standard doses of ACE inhibitors. For the first two situations, initiation of therapy with half the standard dose is appropriate with careful monitoring. In a group of 18 severely ill patients with congestive heart failure and angina, deterioration in angina after ACE inhibition was probably caused by failure of the blood pressure to increase during exercise.[5] This adverse effect could be seen as a manifestation of ACE inhibitor-induced hypotension. Such severely ill patients need to be treated with great care and caution. Surgical evaluation of the angina is required.

Hemodynamically stable acute coronary syndromes are not a contraindication. In the SOLVD studies[49] (Table 6-2) on less severely ill patients, most with heart failure of ischemic origin, and about one-third with current angina, enalapril benefited the group as a whole and lessened the development of unstable angina. Thus, in less critically ill patients also with congestive heart failure and angina, the ACE inhibitors can be used beneficially.

QUALITY OF LIFE

The landmark "quality of life" study by Croog et al[8] showed that patients taking captopril felt better than patients taking equieffective antihypertensive doses of methyldopa or propranolol. In particular, captopril-treated patients had fewer nervous system complaints, performed better sexually, and had a higher general well-being score. While it is by no means certain that captopril brought down the blood pressure (because there was no placebo group), this study nonetheless made a profound impact on the choice of an antihypertensive drug to such an extent that all antihypertensive agents now have to be evaluated for their effect on the "quality of life". Subsequently, an important study by Steiner et al[50] showed that the quality of life with captopril, enalapril, and atenolol was essentially similar and better than that on propranolol. A reasonable hypothesis is that propranolol and methyldopa, centrally acting agents at least in part, have adverse effects on the quality of life, whereas the other agents do not. For example, the quality of life on enalapril is in reality no better than on placebo,[52] although there may be subsets of feelings in which enalapril benefits.[50]

Captopril vs enalapril. Thus, it came as a surprise that Testa et al,[51] on the basis of a large prospective study, proposed that captopril gave a better quality of life than enalapril. The absence of concurrent blood pressure and quality of life data, and full details of the exact doses used means that this study is difficult to assess, especially when compared to the Steiner study,[50] also on large groups of patients. In the latter study, captopril improved a depressed mood when compared with atenolol or propranolol, whereas enalapril gave a better (not worse) index of general health than captopril.

SEXUAL DYSFUNCTION

In these days of Viagra, it is difficult to avoid the effect of anti-hypertensive agents and of ACE inhibitors on sexual function. The common perception is that antihypertensive drugs, as a group, promote sexual dysfunction and specifically, impotence in males. Often it is forgotten that age and systolic hypertension both predispose to sexual dysfunction,[17] the presumed mechanism being endothelial damage with decreased release of vasodilatory nitric oxide. In middle-aged subjects with mild hypertension, therapy with life style advice plus one of five drugs (enalapril, doxasozin, acebutolol, amlodipine and chlorthalidone) did not, in general, cause erectile dysfunction. A clear exception was the diuretic, which even in the low doses used (15 mg daily), increased impotence from 8.1% to 17.1% after 2 years of follow up.[17]

ACE inhibitors are generally thought not to cause erectile problems, whereas beta-blockers are often suspect (despite the negative data for acebutolol cited above). Lisinopril (20 mg daily) and atenolol (100 mg daily) were compared in a cross over study, with the incidence of successful sexual intercourse as the end point. At first, both agents had inhibitory effects, but with prolonged therapy, lisinopril reverted to near normal function.[13] Thus atenolol caused chronic and lisinopril only temporary sexual problems.

SUMMARY

1. *Major side-effects.* In practice, the two major side-effects associated with ACE inhibitor therapy are cough and hypotension. The latter can be a major problem in the management of congestive heart failure. Hypotension may be lessened by the use of low initial test doses and by reduction of the diuretic dose. There is evidence that the type of ACE inhibitor used may be important in avoiding first-dose hypotension.

2. The *incidence of cough* seems to be increasing in recent reports using more subtle means such as visual analog

analysis to detect it. The onset of cough may be delayed for up to 24 months after the start of ACE inhibitor therapy. The simplest policy is to wait to see whether the cough spontaneously passes over, which occurs in about half the patients. Then, addition of sulindac or inhaled sodium cromoglycate or a dihydropyridine calcium blocker may help.

3. *Contraindications to ACE inhibitor therapy* include bilateral renal artery stenosis, unilateral renal artery stenosis in a solitary kidney, significant aortic stenosis, severe obstructive cardiomyopathy, and pregnancy or risk thereof. Pre-existing chronic cough is a relative contraindication.

REFERENCES

1. Alderman MH, Cohen H, Roque R, et al. Effect of long-acting and short-acting calcium antagonists on cardiovascular outcomes in hypertensive patients. Lancet 1997;349:594–598.

2. Brent RL, Beckman DA. Angiotensin-converting enzyme inhibitors, an embryopathic class of drugs with unique properties: information for clinical teratology counselors. Teratology 1991;43:543–546.

3. Burnakis T, Mioduch H. Combined therapy with captopril and potassium supplementation. A potential for hyperkalemia. Arch Intern Med 1984;144:2371–2372.

4. Capewell S, Capewell A. "First dose" hypotension and venodilation. Br J Clin Pharmacol 1991;31:213–215.

5. Cleland JGF, Henderson E, McLenachan J, et al. Effect of captopril, an angiotensin-converting enzyme inhibitor, in patients with angina pectoris and heart failure. J Am Coll Cardiol 1991;17:733–739.

6. CONSENSUS II. Swedberg K, Held P, Kjekshus J, et al. Effects of the early administration of enalapril on mortality in patients with acute myocardial infarction. Results of the Co-operative Scandinavian Enalapril Survival Study II (CONSENSUS II). N Engl J Med 1992;327:678–684.

7. Coulter DM, Edwards IR. Effect of captopril, an angiotensin-converting enzyme inhibitor, in patients with angina pectoris and heart failure. J Am Coll Cardiol 1987;17:733–739.

8. Croog S, Levine S, Testa M, et al. The effect of antihypertensive therapy on the quality of life. N Eng J Med 1986;314:1657–1664.

9. Crozier IG, Ikram H, Nicholls G, et al. Acute hemodynamic, hormonal and electrolyte effects of ramipril in severe congestive heart failure. Am J Cardiol 1987;59:155D–163D.

10. ELITE Study, Pitt B, Segal R, Martinez FA, et al. On behalf of the ELITE Study Investigators. Randomised trial of losartan versus captopril in patients over 65 with heart failure (Evaluation of Losartan in the Elderly Study, ELITE). Lancet 1997;349:747–752.

11. FDA. (Food and Drug Administration). Pregnancy warnings strengthened on ACE inhibitors. Health and Human Services News 1992, March; 13.

12. Ferner RE, Simpson JM, Rawlins MD. Effects of intradermal bradykinin after inhibition of angiotensin converting enzyme. Br Med J 1987;294:1119–1120.

13. Fogari R, Zoppi A, Corradi L, Mugellini A, et al. Sexual function in hypertensive males treated with lisinopril or atenolol. A cross-over study. Am J Hypertens 1998;11:1244–1247.

14. Fogari R, Zoppi A, Tettamanti F, et al. Effects of nifedipine and indomethacin on cough induced by angiotensin-converting enzyme inhibitors: a double-blind, randomized, cross-over study. J Cardiovasc Pharmacol 1992;19:670–673.

15. Goldszer RC, Lilly LS, Solomon HS. Prevalence of cough during angiotensin-converting enzyme inhibitor therapy. Am J Med 1988;85:887.

16. Grace AA, Brooks NH, Schofield PM. Beneficial effects of angiotensin-converting enzyme inhibition in severe symptomatic aortic stenosis (Abstract). Circulation 1991;84 (Suppl II0:II-46).

17. Grimm RH, Grandits GA, Prineas RJ, et al. Long-term effects on sexual function of five antihypertensive drugs and nutritional hygienic treatment in hypertensive men and women. Treatment of Mild Hypertension Study (TOMHS). Hypertension 1997;29:8–14.

18. Hanssens M, Keirse M, Vankelcom F, et al. Fetal and neonatal effects of treatment with angiotensin-converting enzyme inhibitors in pregnancy. Obstet Gynecol 1991;31:128–135.

19. Harris BD, Ludlow ST, Really JET. Fatal aplastic anaemia associated with lisinopril. Lancet 1995;346:247–248.

20. Hasford J, Busmann W-D, Delius W, et al. First dose hypotension with enalapril and prazosin in congestive heart failure. Int J Cardiol 1991;31:287–294.

21. Hedner T, Samuelsson O, Lunde H, et al. Angio-oedema in relation to treatment with angiotensin-converting enzyme inhibitors. Br Med J 1992;304:941–946.

22. Jackson T, Corke C, Agar J. Enalapril overdose treated with angiotensin infusion. Lancet 1993;31:703.

23. Jenkins AC, Deslinski GR, Tadross SS, et al. Captopril in hypertension: seven years later. J Cardiovasc Pharmacol 1985;7:S96–S101.

24. JNC VI. Joint National Committee on Prevention, Detection, Evaluation and Treatment of High Blood Pressure. The Sixth Report of the Joint National Committee on Prevention, Detection, Evaluation and Treatment of High Blood Pressure. Arch Intern Med 1997;157:2413–2446.

25. Keogh A. Sodium cromoglycate prophylaxis for angiotensin-converting enzyme inhibitor cough. Lancet 1993;341:560.

26. Knox AJ, Pang L. Tackling ACE inhibitor cough (Letter). Lancet 1997;350:814.

27. Kostis JB, Shelton B, Gosselin G, et al. Adverse effects of enalapril in the studies of left venricular dysfunction (SOLVD). SOLVD Investigators. Am Heart J 1996;131:350–355.

28. Lapostolle F, Barron SW, Bekka R, et al. Lingual angioedema after perindopril use. Am J Cardiol 1998;81:523.

29. Lees KR, Reid JC, Scott MG, et al. Captopril versus perindopril: a double-blind study in essential hypertension. J Human Hypertens 1989; 3:17–22.

30. Lever AF, Hole DJ, Gillis CR, et al. Do inhibitors of angiotensin-I-converting enzyme protect against risk of cancer? Lancet 1998;352:179–184.

31. Ljungman S, Kjekshus J, Swedberg K. For the CONSENSUS Trial Group. Renal function in severe congestive heart failure during treatment with enalapril. The Cooperative North Scandinavian Enalapril Survival Study (CONSENSUS). Am J Cardiol 1992;70:479–487.

32. Lunde H, Hedner T, Samuelsson O, et al. Dyspnoea, asthma and bronchospasm in relation to treatment with angiotensin-converting enzyme inhibitors. Br Med J 1994;308:18–21.

33. MacFadyen RJ, Barr CS, Sturrock ND, et al. Further evidence that chronic perindopril treatment maintains neurohormonal suppression but does not lower blood pressure in chronic cardiac failure. Br J Clin Pharmacol 1997;44:69–76.

34. MacFadyen RJ, Lees KR, Reid JL. Differences in first dose response to ACE inhibition in congestive cardiac failure – a placebo-controlled study. Br Heart J 1991;66:206–211.

35. MacFadyen RJ, Lees KR, Reid JL. Double blind controlled study of low dose intravenous perindoprilat or enalaprilat infusion in elderly patients with heart failure. Br Heart J 1993;69:293–297.

36. MacGregor MS, Rowe PA, Watson MA, et al. Treatment of postrenal transplant erythrocytosis. Nephron 1996;75:517–521.

37. Malini PL, Strocchi E, Zanardi M, et al. Thromboxane antagonism and cough induced by angiotensin-converting-enzyme inhibitor. Lancet 1997;350:15–15.

38. Mancini GBJ, Schulzer M. Reporting risks and benefits of therapy by use of the concepts of unqualified success and unmitigated failure. Applications to highly cited trials in cardiovascular medicine. Circulation 1999;99:377–383.

39. McEwan JR, Choudry N, Street R, et al. Change in cough reflex after treatment with enalapril and ramipril. Br Med J 1989;299:13–16.

40. McEwan JR, Choudry NB, Fuller RW. The effect of sulindac on the abnormal cough reflex assicated with dry cough. J Pharmacol Exp Ther 1990;255:161–164.

41. Nussberger J, Cugno M, Amstutz C, et al. Plasma bradykinin in angio-oedema. Lancet 1998;351:1693–1697.

42. Osterziel KJ, Dietz R, Harder K, et al. Comparison of captopril with enalapril in the treatment of heart failure: influence on hemodynamics and measures of renal function. Cardiovasc Drugs Ther 1992;6:173–180.

43. Pierpont GP, Francis GS, Cohn JN. Effect of captopril on renal function in patients with congestive heart failure. Br Heart J 1981;46:522–527.

44. Poggi L, Renucci J-F, Denolle T. Treatement of essential hypertension in general practice: An open-label study of 47,351 French hypertensive pa-

tients treated for one year with perindopril. Can J Cardiol 1994;10:21D–24D.

45. Postma CT, Dennesen PJW, de Boo T, et al. First dose hypotension after captopril: can it be predicted? A study of 240 patients. J Human Hypertens 1992;6:205–209.

46. RALES Study. Spironolactone for heart failure. Inpharma 1998;1168:12.

47. Reisin L, Schneeweiss A. Complete spontaneous remission of cough induced by ACE inhibitors during chronic therapy in hypertensive patients. J Human Hypertens 1992;6:333–335.

48. Savino LB, Haushalter NM. Lisonopril-induced "scaled mouth syndrome". Ann Pharmacother 1992;26:1381–1382.

49. SOLVD Investigators. Effect of enalapril on mortality and the development of heart failure in asymptomatic patients with reduced left ventricular ejection fractions. New Engl J Med 1992;327:685–691.

50. Steiner SS, Friedhoff AJ, Wilson BL, et al. Antihypertensive therapy and quality of life: a comparison of atenolol, captopril, enalapril and propranolol. J Human Hypertens 1990;4:217–225.

51. Testa MA, Anderson RB, Nackley JF, et al. The Quality of Life Hypertension Study Group. Quality of life and antihypertensive therapy in men. A comparison of captopril with enalapril. New Engl J Med 1993;328:907–913.

52. TOMH Study. Treatment of Mild Hypertension Research Group (TOMH). The treatment of mild hypertension study. A randomized, placebo-controlled trial of a nutritional-hygenic regimen along with various drug monotherapies. Arch Intern Med 1991;151:1413–1423.

53. Verbeelen DL, de Boel S. Reversible acute on chronic renal failure during captopril treatment. Br Med J 1984;289:20–21.

54. Volpert OV, Ward WF, Lingen MW, et al. Captopril inhibitors angiogenesis and slows the growth of experimental tumors in rats. J Clin Invest 1996;98:671–679.

55. Webster J. Angiotensin converting enzyme inhibitors in the clinic: first-dose hypotension. J Hypertens 1987;5 (Suppl: S27–S30).

56. Yeo WW, MacLean D, Richardson PJ, et al. Cough and enalapril: assesment by spontaneous reporting and visual analogue scale under double-blind conditions. Br J Clin Pharmacol 1991;31:356–359.

57. Yeo WW, Ramsay LE. Persistent dry cough with enalapril: incidence depends on method used. J Human Hypertens 1990;4:517–520.

CHAPTER 10

ACE Inhibitors: Drug combinations and interactions

Increasing use of ACE inhibitors has led to consideration of possible combinations with other antihypertensive agents, such as beta-blockers, diuretics, calcium antagonists, and more recently with AT-1 receptor blockers. The combination of ACE inhibitors with diuretics is well established and that with calcium antagonists is coming to be accepted practice. Combination with beta-blockers or AT-1 blockers is not yet, however, into the realm of standard practice.

AT-1 RECEPTOR BLOCKERS

Of the various mechanisms whereby ACE inhibitors could exert their beneficial effect, inhibition of formation of angiotensin II (A-II) is thought to be of major importance. Another benefit lies in depressed levels of aldosterone. Nonetheless, levels of A-II and of aldosterone may rebound ("escape") during chronic treatment with ACE inhibitors. A-II is thought to exert most or all of its vascular and cardiac effects, and on release of aldosterone, by acting on AT-1 receptors. Thus it is logical to hypothesize that addition of an AT-1 receptor blocker such as losartan could interact beneficially and additively with ACE inhibition. There are a number of such studies to suggest benefit of combined renin-angiotensin blockade.

1. In the early postinfarct period, a pilot study showed that the combination of captopril and losartan gave better BP reduction, but with unchanged values of plasma norepinephrine and angiotensin II.[15] The latter finding is of interest, because normally AT-1 receptor blockade is accompanied by a rise in plasma A-II. In some circumstances stimulation of the unopposed AT-2 receptor might be considered harmful. Therefore maintenance of normal levels could be an advantage.
2. In the Val-Heft trial, a large mortality study with valsartan in heart failure, almost all the patients already received an ACE inhibitor and a diuretic. Therefore this trial will show whether there is further mortality benefit with the addition of the AT-1 blocker.
3. Regarding blood pressure, enalapril and losartan have additive effects on blood pressure and plasma renin in

sodium-deprived normotensive subjects.[5] Detailed studies in hypertensives still need to be done.

4. In advanced heart failure, losartan improves exercise capacity when added to maximal doses of ACE inhibitors.[20A]

BETA-BLOCKERS

In hypertension, based on experience with captopril, it has been commonly thought that beta-blockade added to ACE inhibition might not be an optimal combination because beta-blockade probably acts in part by renin-angiotensin suppression. ACE inhibitors decrease the renin-angiotensin axis through inhibition of the angiotensin converting enzyme, and beta-blockers act on the same axis by inhibition of renin release. Thus, beta-blockade is associated with substantially decreased plasma renin levels in those already treated by an ACE inhibitor and/or a diuretic.[23] Nonetheless, the addition of beta-blockers to the ACE inhibitor captopril is less effectively antihypertensive than diuretic addition.[38] In those already treated by amlodipine and lisinopril, a diuretic is more effective than a beta-blocker as a third agent.[3] It is therefore somewhat surprising that a detailed study adding propranolol to the ACE inhibitor cilazapril showed an additive antihypertensive effect.[7] With cilazapril, the peripheral vascular resistance fell and the cardiac output rose; opposite changes were found with propranolol and, with the combination, there was no change in either parameter. Clearly, further studies are required on larger populations and with 24 hour BP recording.

In heart failure, this combination is likely to be used more and more. Both agents decrease mortality. ACE inhibitors are as effective in reducing mortality or even more so in patients receiving beta-blockers, as in a retrospective observational analysis of the SAVE study,[43] and as also shown in the Flather-Yusuf meta-analysis.[18]

DIURETICS

Advantages of an ACE Inhibitor plus Diuretic. In the therapy of hypertension, the blood pressure lowering capacity of diuretics is limited by a *reactive hyperreninemia* (Fig 10-1). Therefore, the combination with ACE inhibitor therapy becomes logical and the response rate to the combination is high, possibly up to 80%.[14] Taking a standard dose of an ACE inhibitor, for example 5 mg ramipril, and doubling it, is less effective in reducing the blood pressure than adding a diuretic, hydrochlorothiazide 25 mg daily.[21] Second, in *black hypertensives,* often held to be a low-renin group, the response to ACE inhibition alone is poor but the sensitivity is restored by combination with a diuretic.[44] Third, *secondary hyperaldosteronism* is lessened by ACE inhibitors, which decrease the effect of angiotensin II in releasing aldosterone, with a consequent tendency to potassium retention. Thiazide diuretics, on the other hand, promote

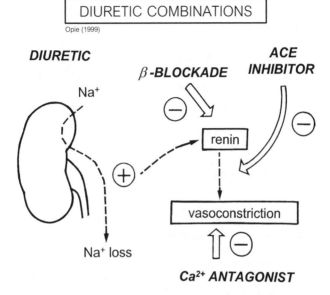

| DIURETIC COMBINATIONS |
| Opie (1999) |

Figure 10-1. Theoretical basis for beneficial interaction between diuretics and ACE inhibitors in the therapy of hypertension. Figure © LH Opie, 1999

potassium loss. Specifically, hydrochlorothiazide 25 mg decreased the mean potassium concentration by 0.47 mmol/L, whereas the addition of ramipril 2.5 to 10 mg almost eliminated the fall.[35] Fourth, the *metabolic effects of thiazide diuretics* in increasing blood uric acid and blood sugar are diminished by concurrent therapy with ACE inhibitors.[45] Fifth, in heart failure, the *natriuresis of diuretics* is potentiated by ACE inhibitors. Conversely, addition of diuretics to ACE inhibitor therapy lessens the dose of ACE inhibitor required.

Disadvantages of the combination ACE inhibitor-diuretic. First, when there is marked salt retention, as in heart or renal failure, there tends to be a considerable reactive hyperreninemia, so that the addition of the ACE inhibitor can cause a serious *hypotensive first-dose effect*. This problem can be overcome by giving a very low first dose of the ACE inhibitor as a test dose, for example 6.25 mg of captopril. Second, the addition of an ACE inhibitor to a diuretic may *decrease the glomerular filtration rate* with an increase in the plasma creatinine level. This is particularly so in patients with resistant heart failure,[11] or in those with severe hypertension and a fixed renal vascular resistance as in the case of bilateral renal artery stenosis. Thus, patients with severe congestive heart failure need monitoring of serum creatinine for some days after the addition of ACE inhibitor therapy and careful dose titration. Third, when combined with potassium-sparing diuretics or potassium supplements, there is danger of *hyperkalemia*.[39] The ideal diuretic to be combined with an ACE inhibitor should not have any potassium-retaining qualities nor have any built-in or added potassium supplementation.[9] A standard combination for hypertension could be the usual dose of the ACE inhibitor together with 12.5 mg hydrochlorothiazide daily.

Interaction between ACE inhibitors and loop diuretics. *Captopril – furosemide.* There appears to be a specific inhibitory effect of captopril on the diuretic action of furosemide,[40] not shared by ramipril nor enalapril. The mechanism is that captopril interferes with the renal tubular excretion of furosemide. It is this negative interaction that may explain why captopril 1 mg allows a greater diuresis than captopril 25 mg when combined with furosemide.[31] Thus, if these agents are given together in standard doses, the times of administration should be spaced.

Beneficial interaction of ACE inhibitor with spironolactone. Low doses of captopril have been successfully combined with furosemide and with spironolactone in patients with severe heart failure,[12] despite potential hyperkalemia. This combination may be particularly useful when captopril causes excess hypotension and the dose must be limited.

RALES study. As discussed (Chapter 6, page 141), the addition of low-dose spironolactone to prior therapy by standard dose ACE inhibitor and a loop diuretic gave a marked improvement in mortality in class III – IV heart failure with only a modest rise in plasma potassium. The benefit should not automatically apply to patients with renal impairment and therefore at greater risk of hyperkalemia.

CALCIUM ANTAGONISTS

Since the initial report by Guazzi et al,[19] the combination ACE inhibitor/calcium antagonist has been widely used (Fig 10-2). Calcium antagonists, being vasodilators, tend to increase plasma renin and therefore combination with an ACE inhibitor is theoretically sound. Second, ACE inhibitors are better at reducing the blood pressure than calcium antagonists in the lower hypertensive ranges, whereas the reverse is the case in more severe hypertension.[22] Furthermore, calcium antagonists of the nifedipine group (dihydropyridines) tend to have a diuretic effect which, again, should combine well with ACE inhibition. Of considerable interest is that diuresis and natriuresis can be invoked by the addition of the calcium antagonist isradipine to captopril.[27] Because the efficacy of ACE inhibitors is so dependent on the sodium status (Fig 3-3), combining an ACE inhibitor with a calcium antagonist may theoretically have the same improved hypotensive effect as adding a diuretic. More definitive studies are required to clarify this issue.

In the therapy of *hypertension,* amlodipine and lisinopril have additive effects.[3] When this combination is insufficient to control the BP, the further addition of a diuretic is more effective than a beta-blocker.[3] Also of interest is the lessening of the tachycardia induced by felodipine during concur-

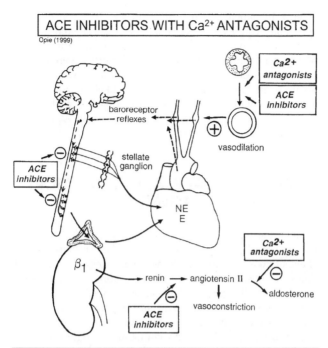

Figure 10-2. Mechanisms for additive arteriolar dilation induced by calcium antagonists and ACE inhibitors. The latter inhibit two consequences of acute vasodilation: (1) the reflex baroreceptor stimulation and (2) the indirect activation of the renin-angiotensin system. Fig copyright © LH Opie.

rent ACE inhibitor therapy by ramipril,[6] in keeping with the proposed sympatho-inhibitory effect of ACE inhibitors. In *hypertensive left ventricular hypertrophy*, the BP reducing effects of the combination of spirapril and isradipine were only modestly better than isradipine alone, and there appeared to be no additive effects on the LV mass.[28] In *hypertension with chronic renal failure*, the combination of nitrendipine and cilazapril reduced blood pressure more than either agent alone.[25] In *diabetic hypertensive nephropathy* with microalbuminuria, the combination of verapamil with either cilazapril or lisinopril lessens microalbuminuria more than either agent alone, and apparently does so independent of blood pressure changes (see Chapter 11).

NITRATES

ACE inhibitors appear to limit the development of nitrate tolerance (Fig 5-3).

DIGOXIN

Despite earlier data suggesting that captopril increases serum digoxin by about one-quarter,[10] a further study showed no effect of captopril on digoxin kinetics.[29] Also, neither ramipril nor lisinopril altered digoxin levels in volunteers,[16,30] nor did perindopril alter digoxin levels or kinetics in patients with heart failure.[42] To reconcile these apparently conflicting data, it should be considered that the study of Cleland et al.[10] was conducted on patients with severe heart failure, whereas the other studies were on normal volunteers or on patients with mild heart failure. In severe heart failure, captopril is more likely to cause renal impairment with a secondary rise in digoxin levels. Thus, in considering the possible interaction between ACE inhibitors and digoxin, it is important to monitor renal function.

NON-STEROIDAL ANTI-INFLAMMATORY AGENTS

In hypertension, it is known that non-steroidal anti-inflammatory drugs (NSAIDs) can blunt the antihypertensive effect of most agents, including ACE inhibitors (Fig 10-3). The mechanism may include lessened formation of vasodilatory prostaglandins.[46] These agents do not all have the same effects and indomethacin and naproxen appear more consistently to cause a blood pressure increase than sulindac or ibuprofen.[33] Indomethacin (50 mg 2x daily) added to ACE inhibitor therapy in several double-blind trials variably lessened the antihypertensive effect by 3% to 34%.[1,34]

Whereas the effects of NSAIDs in interfering with the control of blood pressure are now well accepted, it is generally less well known that these agents can interfere with the hemodynamic status in congestive heart failure. Acute administration of indomethacin decreased cardiac index, increased left ventricular filling pressure, and increased arterial pressure and systemic vascular resistance in patients with congestive heart failure and hyponatremia.[17] The

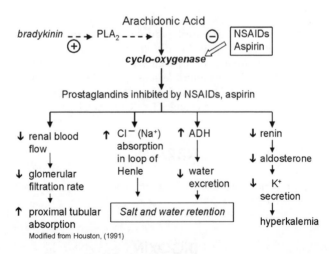

Figure 10-3. Proposed mechanism whereby NSAIDs block cyclo-oxygenase pathway and thereby inhibit formation of vasodilatory prostaglandins. Ultimately salt and water retention decreases the effects of almost all antihypertensives. In addition, NSAIDs decrease renin and aldosterone through an entirely different mechanism. PLA_2 = phospholipase A_2. Modified from Houston,[24] with permission.

effects of the NSAIDs in lowering renin and decreasing aldosterone can be dissociated from effects on the blood pressure.[24] More detailed studies of the interactions between NSAIDs and ACE inhibitors are required.

ASPIRIN

When aspirin (325 – 350 mg) was combined with enalapril (10 mg daily), in a short term study, the ACE inhibitor was much less vasodilatory and the left ventricular filling pressure no longer improved.[20,37] Thus, not only NSAIDs but aspirin may also impair the hemodynamic effect of ACE inhibition in heart failure. When, however, lower doses of aspirin are used, then there was little or no hemodynamic interaction.[41] In the CONSENSUS II study, in which intravenous enalaprilat was given within 24 h of the onset of AMI, there was a trend to a negative interaction of enalapril and aspirin.[32] In the AIRE study, in which ramipril gave mortality benefit to post-infarct patients with heart failure, about 85% of patients were also receiving an unstated dose of aspirin.[2] In a meta-analysis on large post-infarct trials, mortality reduction was similar at about 25% in those not receiving, and in those receiving aspirin at a baseline.[18] In a recent preliminary oral presentation, Dr Eric Topol retrospectively examined the combination of aspirin-ACE inhibitor in the large GUSTO thrombolysis study and in the smaller EPILOG angioplasty study. He reported adverse interactions with a two to three times increase in mortality in patients taking both. However, the problem of this observational study is that the drug combination could have been selected for sicker patients with a worse prognosis.

Therefore, taking these observations together, no general rules can be made. Overall, there is evidence for a negative interaction. In patients with systolic heart failure, the meta-analysis suggests that the combination is safe,[19] but the aspirin dose should be kept low especially in those with serious hemodynamic problems. In patients without systolic heart failure, but receiving ACE inhibitors and aspirin, the replacement of aspirin by ticlopidine or clopidogrel may be considered.

TICLOPIDINE AND CLOPIDOGREL

Ticlopidine inhibits the activation of the GPIIb/IIIa platelet receptor, and therefore differs in its mechanisms from aspirin, which impairs synthesis of vasodilatory prostaglandins. Spaulding et al.[37] reasoned that ACE inhibitors could better be combined with ticlopidine than with aspirin. Short term enalapril gave better peripheral vasodilation when combined with ticlopidine 500 mg daily than with aspirin 325 mg daily. *Clopidogrel* is another antiplatelet agent that acts by inhibition of ADP-promoted platelet adhesion, therefore also differing in its mode of action from aspirin. It should also give better vasodilation than aspirin, but the prospective studies are still missing. Whereas ticlopidine may cause neutropenia, clopidogrel does not.

LITHIUM

ACE inhibitors may increase blood lithium levels and the risk of toxicity, according to USA package inserts. In normal volunteers, however, lithium levels rose in only one of nine subjects after the addition of enalapril.[13] Conceivably, in patients with renal impairment, the ACE inhibitors are more likely to increase lithium levels.

PROBENECID

Many of the ACE inhibitors are organic acids and therefore excreted both by glomerular filtration and renal tubular secretion. Probenecid decreases the excretion of captopril and leads to higher blood levels.[36] This possible interaction presumably holds for all ACE inhibitors that are organic acids (and most of them are). An exception is the relatively new ACE inhibitor, fosinopril, which is a sodium salt and another recent ACE inhibitor, zofenopril, which is a calcium salt.[26]

POSSIBLE INTERACTION WITH DIABETIC THERAPY

ACE inhibitors are thought to improve insulin sensitivity (Chapter 11). Hence, in patients with type II diabetes receiving oral anti-diabetic therapy, there is the risk of additive effects of ACE inhibitor therapy leading to symptomatic hypoglycemia.[4] The mechanism could include a reduction in glomerular function induced by ACE inhibitor therapy.[8] Although these findings are controversial, it is appropriate to recheck blood sugar levels whenever ACE inhibitors are added to oral hypoglycemics.

SUMMARY

1. *Combination with other antihypertensive drugs.* ACE inhibitors have been combined with virtually all other classes of antihypertensive drugs, especially with diuretics. A new combination, only being explored, is that of an ACE inhibitor and an AT-1 receptor blocker.

2. *In heart failure,* ACE inhibitors blunt the hypokalemic effect of standard diuretics so that potassium-retaining diuretics should only be used if indicated, to avoid hyperkalemia. An exception is in heart failure patients with normal renal function, in whom the addition of low dose spironolactone gives added mortality benefit.

3.   *Captopril* interferes with the diuretic effect of furose-mide in healthy volunteers and captopril also increases serum digoxin. Neither of these effects appear to be shared by some of the other ACE inhibitors.

4.   *Non-steroidal anti-inflammatory agents* lessen the anti-hypertensive effect of ACE inhibitors; indomethacin appears to be particularly potent in this regard. Not only is the antihypertensive effect of ACE inhibitors blunted by NSAIDs, but the beneficial effect in heart failure may be overcome.

5.   *Aspirin.* Although standard dose aspirin (325–350mg per day) impairs the vasodilatory effects of ACE inhi-bition in patients with heart failure, a meta-analysis of post infarct patients shows that the taking of aspirin does not annul the reduction in mortality. Observa-tional studies, however, suggest an increased mortality with the combination, so that the issue is still open. Low dose aspirin seems a practical step.

REFERENCES

1. Abdel-Haq B, Magagna A, Favilla S, et al. Hemodynamic and humoral interactions between perindopril and indomethacin in essential hyperten-sive subjects. J Cardiovasc Pharmacol 1991;18 (Suppl 1):S33–S36.

2. AIRE Study. The effect of ramipril on mortality and morbidity of surviv-ors of acute myocardial infarction with clinical evidence of heart failure. Lancet 1993;342:821–828.

3. Antonios T, Cappuccio F, Markandu N, et al. A diuretic is more effective than a β-blocker in hypertensive patients not controlled on amlodipine and lisinopril. Hypertension 1996;27:1325–1328.

4. Arauz-Pacheco C, Ramirez LC, Rios JM, et al. Hypoglycemia induced by angiotensin-converting enzyme inhibitors in patients with non-insulin dependent diabetes receiving sulfonylurea therapy. Am J Med 1990;89:811–813.

5. Azizi M, Guyene T-T, Chatellier G, et al. Additive effects of losartan and enalapril on blood pressure and plasma active renin. Hypertension 1997;29:634–640.

6. Bainbridge AD, MacFadyen RJ, Lees KR, et al. A study of the acute phar-macodynamic interaction of ramipril and felodipine in normotensive subjects. Br J Clin Pharmacol 1991;31:148–153.

7. Belz GG, Breithaupt K, Erb K, et al. Influence of the angiotensin-convert-ing enzyme inhibitor cilazapril, the beta-blocker propranolol and their combination on haemodynamics in hypertension. J Hypertens 1989; 7:817–824.

8. Buller GK, Perazella M. ACE inhibitor-induced hypoglycemia. Am J Med 1991;91:104–105.

9. Burnakis T, Mioduch H. Combined therapy with captopril and potas-sium supplementation. A potential for hyperkalemia. Arch Intern Med 1984;144:2371–2372.

10. Cleland JG, Dargie HJ, Pettigrew A, et al. The effects of captopril on serum digoxin and urinary urea and digoxin clearances in patients with congestive heart failure. Am Heart J 1986;112:130–135.

11. Cleland JGF, Gillen G, Dargie HJ. The effects of frusemide and angio-tensin-converting enzyme inhibitors and their combination on cardiac and renal haemodynamics in heart failure. Eur Heart J 1988;9:132–141.

12. Dahlstrom U, Karlsson E. Captopril and spironolactone therapy for refractory congestive heart failure. Am J Cardiol 1993;71:29A–33A.

13. DasGupta K, Jefferson JW, Koban KA, et al. The effect of enalapril on serum lithium levels in healthy men. J Clin Psychiatry 1992;53:398–400.

14. Degaute J-P, Leeman M, Desche P. Long-term acceptability of perindo-pril: European Multicenter Trial on 858 patients. Am J Med 1992;Suppl 4B:84S–89S.

15. Di Pasquale P, Bucca V, Scalzo S, et al. Safety, tolerability and neuro-hormonal changes of the combination captopril plus losartan in the early postinfarction period: A pilot study. Cardiovasc Drugs Ther 1998;12:211–216.

16. Doering W, Maass L, Irmisch R, et al. Pharmacokinetic interaction study with ramipril and digoxin in healthy volunteers. Am J Cardiol 1987;59:60D–64D.

17. Dzau VJ, Packer M, Lilly LS, et al. Prostaglandins in severe congestive heart failure: relation to activation of the renin-angiotensin system and hyponatremia. N Engl J Med 1984;310:347–352.

18. Flather MD, Yusuf S, Kober L, et al. Systematic overview of individual patient data from the large randomized trials of long term ACE inhibition or therapy in patients with heart failure or left ventricular dysfunction following myocardial infarction. Submitted for publication 1999.

19. Guazzi MD, Cesare ND, Galli C. Calcium-channel blockade with nifedipine and angiotensin converting enzyme inhibition with captopril in the therapy of patients with severe primary hypertension. Circulation 1984;70:279–284.

20. Hall D, Zeitler H, Rudolph W. Counteraction of the vasodilator effects of enalapril by aspirin in severe heart failure. J Am Coll Cardiol 1992;20:1549–1555.

20A Hamroth G, Katz SD, Mancini D, et al. Addition of angiotensin II receptor blockade to maximal angiotensin-converting enzyme inhibition improves exercise capacity in patients with severe congestive heart failure. Circulation 1999;99:990–992.

21. Heidbreder D, Froer K-L, Breitstadt A, et al. Combination of ramipril and hydrochlorothiazide in the treatment of mild to moderate hypertension: Part 1 – a double-blind, comparative, multicenter study in nonresponders to ramipril monotherapy. Clin Cardiol 1992;15:904–910.

22. Herpin D, Vaisse B, Pitiot M, et al. Comparison of angiotensin-converting enzyme inhibitors and calcium antagonists in the treatment of mild to moderate systemic hypertension, according to baseline ambulatory blood pressure level. Am J Cardiol 1992;69:923–926.

23. Holmer SR, Hense H-W, Danser AHJ, et al. β adrenergic blockers lower renin in patients treated with ACE inhibitors and diuretics. Heart 1998;80:45-48.

24. Houston MC. Nonsteroidal anti-inflammatory drugs and antihypertensives. Am J Med 1991;90(suppl 5A):42S–47S.

25. Kloke JH, Huysmans F, Wentzel J, et al. Antihypertensive effects of nitrendipine and cilazapril alone, and in combination in hypertensive patients with chronic renal failure. J Human Hypertens 1989;2:289S–296S.

26. Kostis JB. Angiotensin-converting enzyme inhibitors. Emerging differences and new compounds. Am J Hypertens 1989;2:57-64.

27. Krusell LR, Sihm I, Jespersen LT, et al. Combined actions of isradipine and captopril on renal function in hypertension. J Human Hypertens 1992;6:401–407.

28. Manolis AJ, Beldekos D, Handanis S, et al. Comparison of spirapril, isradipine, or combination in hypertensive patients with left ventricular hypertrophy. Am J Hypertens 1998;11:640–648.

29. Miyakawa T, Shionoiri H, Takasaki I, et al. The effect of captopril on pharmacokinetics of digoxin in patients with mild congestive heart failure. J Cardiovasc Pharmacol 1991;17:576–581.

30. Morris FP, Tamrazian S, Marks C, et al. An acute pharmacokinetic study of the potential interaction of lisinopril and digoxin in normal volunteers. Br J Clin Pharmacol 1985;20:281P–282P.

31. Motwani J, Fenwick M, Morton J, et al. Furosemide-induced natriuresis is augmented by ultra-low dose captopril but not by standard doses of captopril in chronic heart failure. Circulation 1992;86:439–445.

32. Nguyen KN, Aursnes I, Kjekhus J. Interaction between enalapril and aspirin on mortality after acute myocardial infarction: subgroups analysis of the Cooperative New Scandinavian Enalapril Survival Study II (CONSENSUS II). Am J Cardiol 1997;79:115–119.

33. Pope JE, Anderson JJ, Felson DT. A meta-analysis of the effects of nonsteroidal anti-inflammatory drugs on blood pressure. Arch Intern Med 1993;153:477–484.

34. Salvetti A. Newer ACE inhibitors. A look at the future. Drugs 1990;40:800–828.

35. Scholze J. For the East Germany Collaborative Trial Group. Short report: ramipril and hydrochlorothiazide combination therapy in hypertension: a clinical trial of factorial design. J Hypertens 1993;11:217–221.

36. Singhvi SM, Duchin KL, Willard DA, et al. Renal handling of captopril: effect of probenecid. Clin Pharmacol Ther 1982;32:182–189.

37. Spaulding C, Charbonnier B, Cohen-Solal A, et al. Acute hemodynamic interaction of aspirin and ticlopidine with enalapril. Circulation 1998;98:757–765.

38. Staesen J, Fagard R, Lijnen P, et al. A double-blind comparison between propranolol and bendroflumethiazide in captopril treated resistant hypertensive patients. Am Heart J 1983; 106:321–328.

39. Textor SC, Bravo EL, Fouad FM, et al. Hyperkalemia in azotemic patients during angiotensin-converting enzyme inhibition and aldosterone reduction with captopril. Am J Med 1982;73:719–725.

40. Toussaint C, Masselink A, Gentges A, et al. Interference of different ACE inhibitors with the diuretic action of furosemide and hydrochlorothiazide. Klin Wochenschr 1989;67:1138–1146.

41. Van Wijngaarden, Smit AJ, de Graeff PA, et al. Effects of acetylsalicyclic acid on peripheral hemodynamics in patients with chronic heart failure treated with angiotensin-converting enzyme inhibitors. J Cardiovasc Pharmacol 1994;23:240–245.

42. Vandenburg MJ, Stephens J, Resplandy G, et al. Digoxin pharmacokinetics and perindopril in heart failure patients. J Clin Pharmacol 1993;33:146–149.

43. Vantrimpont P, Rouleau JL, Wun C-C, et al. Additive beneficial effects of β-blockers to angiotensin converting enzyme inhibitors in the survival and ventricular enlargement (SAVE) study. JACC 1997;29:229–236.

44. Veterans Administration Cooperative Study Group on Antihypertensive Agents. Captopril: evaluation of low doses, twice-daily doses and the addition of diuretic for the treatment of mild to moderate hypertension. Clin Sci 1982;14:127–131.

45. Weinberger M. Comparison of captopril and hydrochlorothiazide alone and in combination in mild to moderate essential hypertension. Br J Clin Pharmacol 1982;14:127–131.

46. Witzgall H, Hirsch F, Scherer B, et al. Acute haemodynamic and hormonal effects of captopril are diminished by indomethacin. Clin Sci 1982;62:611-615.

Metabolic cardiovascular syndrome. Diabetic complications

The outstanding efficacy of ACE inhibitors in congestive heart failure and their prophylactic potential against post-infarct complications has now been extended to proof of protection against the renal complications of diabetes mellitus. Protection against diabetic retinopathy also seems possible. Furthermore, if ACE inhibitors could improve glucose tolerance or avoid atheroma in the early phases of this disease, then these agents could truly improve the outlook of early diabetics or pre-diabetics. Such prophylactic benefit could bring hope that pre-diabetics could be rescued from the devastating effects of overt clinical diabetes. An ongoing issue is the extent to which protection against vascular diabetic complications is the result of superior blood pressure reduction, or due to specific vascular protection.

The metabolic cardiovascular syndrome. The association of insulin resistance with hypertension is well established.[10,17,23,26] *The hypothesis is that insulin resistance is clinically manifest as a pentad – obesity, non-insulin-dependent diabetes mellitus, hypertension, arteriosclerosis, and blood lipid disturbances* (Fig 11-1). Alternatively, the name Syndrome X has been proposed.[66] This new name does not appeal to cardiologists who already regard Syndrome X as angina pectoris not associated with coronary artery disease. Better names are the metabolic cardiovascular syndrome[3] or the insulin-resistance syndrome.[16] It is *central obesity* that is specifically a cardiovascular risk.[15] Such obesity is also associated with higher insulin levels and elevated concentrations and turnover of blood free fatty acids,[38] which supports the hypothesis proposed (Fig 11-2). The diagnosis of central obesity can usually be made by inspection, while sometimes an abdominal CT scan is required. The concept of *insulin resistance* is undoubtedly an important advance in conceptual thinking, because it explains the commonly found clinical association between obesity and hypertension, at least in white patients. In other population groups, such as the Pima Indians and American blacks, there appears to be no relation between insulin resistance and hypertension.[68] Therefore, important genetic considerations are also involved.

Blood lipids and insulin resistance. Whether insulin resistance

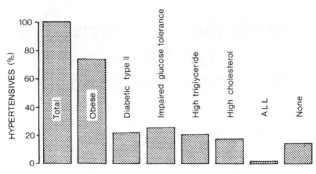

Figure 11-1. *The metabolic pentad thought to exist in hypertension is composed of obesity, type II diabetes, impaired glucose tolerance, high blood triglyceride levels, and high blood cholesterol levels. Of these, obesity is by far the most common. Data from Ferrannini et al.[24] with permission of the author and the Journal of Hypertension.*

by itself is sufficient to explain all the features of the clinical pentad seems unlikely. In contrast to the high incidence of insulin resistance in essential hypertension, the actual incidence of overt blood lipid disorders (dyslipidemia) is only about 12%, so that other factors, possibly genetic, may be involved in the association.[25] When, however, the distribution of LDL particles is considered, then at the same total level, pre-diabetics have more of the harmful small particles than non-diabetics.[5] Therapy of overt lipidemias is by a statin such as pravastatin.[30]

INSULIN AND ATHEROGENESIS

Insulin insensitivity and dyslipidemia in diabetes mellitus. Diabetes mellitus is a well established risk factor for ischemic heart disease and for acute myocardial infarction, as well as for stroke. Diabetes is also known to be associated with an increased incidence of an atherogenic blood lipid profile. Excess of circulating insulin is an early lesion in pre-diabetes and in insulin resistance (Fig 11-2). Insulin is potentially atherogenic through at least two mechanisms. First, insulin excess and the lack of tissue metabolic effects of insulin, as found in non-insulin-dependent diabetes mellitus, is associated with hypertriglyceridemia, with an increased very low density lipoprotein, and with a corresponding decrease in the high density lipoprotein.[29] Although total LDL is not affected, the particles are smaller in size than normal,[5] and therefore more atherogenic (possibly easier penetration of the endothelium). One of the results is an increase in the highly atherogenic apolipoprotein E.[16] The mechanism for the fall in plasma high-density lipoprotein (HDL) levels may be due to an increase in the rate of breakdown of HDL secondary to defects in carbohydrate metabolism.[29] In non-diabetics, hyperinsuline-

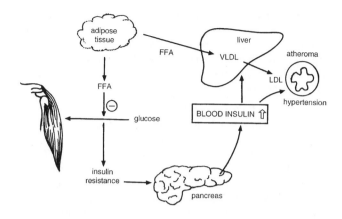

Figure 11-2. *Proposed sequence of events leading to insulin resistance; based on inhibition of uptake of glucose by circulating free fatty acids (FFA). See also Martin et al.[49] VLDL, very low density lipoproteins. Fig. © LH Opie, 1999*

mia is associated with hypertension, at least in white patients, and is positively correlated with triglyceride levels.[31]

Insulin as growth factor. In addition to effects on the blood lipid profile, insulin may directly be involved in atherogenesis by acting as a growth factor,[81] and as a stimulant to lipid synthesis in the arterial wall.[58,80,82] Insulin promotes proliferation of vascular smooth muscle cells, and stimulates synthesis of connective tissue,[17] two processes that are integral components of the atherogenic process.

Insulin as risk factor. Links between insulin and atherosclerosis, as described in diabetic patients, also exist in healthy persons in whom there is an association between hyperinsulinemia and coronary artery disease.[20,88] Thus excess circulating insulin may be the basic factor in the promotion of atherosclerosis in diabetics, and resistance to its effects may explain the association of impaired glucose tolerance and coronary artery disease found in the large study on Whitehall civil servants in London.[27]

Mechanism of insulin resistance: the glucose-fatty acid cycle. The proposed explanations for the origin of insulin resistance are many and varied. One simple proposal is based on a modification of the *glucose-fatty acid cycle* of Randle et al.[65] In 1961 several workers, including our group,[75] showed that circulating free fatty acids could inhibit the uptake of glucose by muscle. Therefore myocytes could become resistant to the normal effects of insulin in increasing the transport of glucose inwards. As a consequence, the pancreas would be called on to secrete more insulin. The result would be the combination of a high circulating insulin and resistance to its effects, as commonly found in prediabetes or obese diabetics.[49] Obesity itself predisposes to higher than normal fasting levels of free fatty acids (next section). Exercise promotes uptake of glucose by muscle[59] so that lack of exercise predisposes to lower rates of glucose disposal. Prolonged demand on the pancreas to continue to produce insulin may eventually lead to pancreatic exhaustion and late low insulin levels. Fatty acid suppression could be therapeutic.[44]

Obesity and blood free fatty acids (FFA). The mechanism whereby hyperglycemia is produced in Type II diabetes is thought to be by loss of the normal ability of insulin to suppress release of free fatty acids from adipose tissue.[66] Consequently, the abnormally high blood FFA levels are thought to stimulate formation of glucose in the liver (gluconeogenesis). Furthermore, increased FFA levels can stimulate insulin secretion.[8] Fasting plasma FFA are higher in obese than in lean subjects.[60] Hence the abnormalities of plasma FFA may link central obesity, hyperinsulinism, and non-insulin dependent diabetes mellitus.[9,38]

INSULIN RESISTANCE AND HYPERTENSION

There is good evidence linking insulin resistance to hypertension. First, in an Israeli study on 2475 randomly selected subjects, 83% of hypertensives were either obese or had impaired glucose tolerance.[53] Post-glucose insulin levels were increased as follows: 12 mU/L for hypertension alone, 47 mU/L for obesity alone, 52 mU/L for those with abnormal glucose tolerance alone, and 124 mU/L for the combination of all three. Similarly, in the large San Antonio study, hyperinsulinemia positively correlated with blood pressure.[31] Second, Ferrannini et al.[23] directly measured insulin sensitivity with the euglycemic clamp technique – the amount of glucose that had to be infused to prevent the blood glucose from falling during a constant infusion of insulin (Fig 11-3). The quantity of glucose infused equals the rate of disposal of glucose by the whole body, provided that there is no endogenous production of glucose. The latter was allowed for by measurements of isotopic dilution. In moderately severe hypertension, insulin-induced glucose uptake was markedly impaired (Fig 11-3). Conversely, when insulin sensitivity is restored to muscles by therapy with metformin in non-diabetic patients with hypertension, then fasting insulin levels fall and so does the blood pressure.[16]

Mechanism linking insulin to hypertension. This problem remains unclarified despite many postulates.[17] One proposal is that insulin enhances adrenergic activity.[77] When, however, insulin was chronically infused into dogs over 7 days, plasma catecholamine levels did not change.[33] Secondly, insulin may act on membrane pumps in vascular smooth muscle cells to increase cell sodium and calcium, thereby sensitizing the cells to vasoconstrictive stimuli.[16] Thirdly, and most attractive to the present author, the AT-1 vascular receptor may be the site of insulin action. Insulin

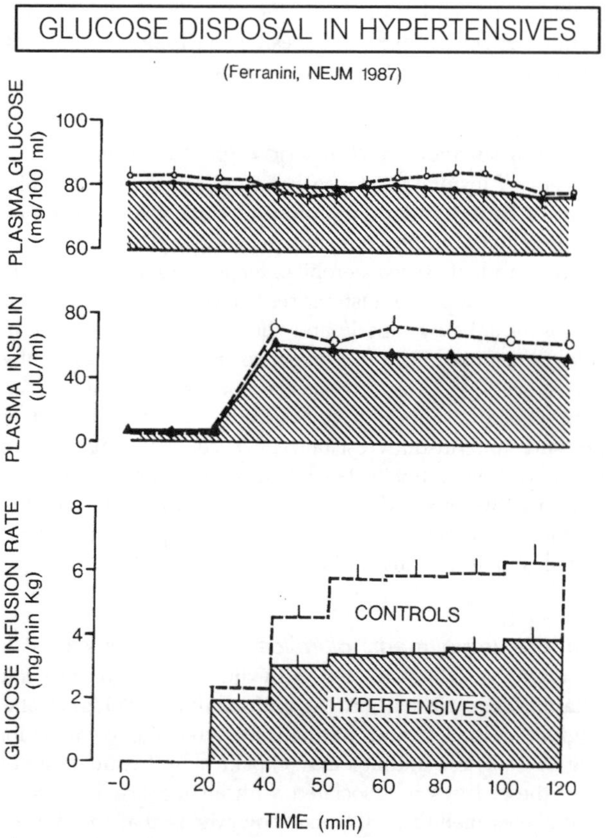

Figure 11-3. In hypertensive patients infused with insulin, less glucose must concurrently be infused to keep the plasma glucose level the same (top panel). Therefore, there is decreased glucose disposal in the hypertensive subjects. For further details, see Ferrannini et al.[23] Modified from original data with permission of authors and New England Journal of Medicine.

upregulates the vascular expression of this receptor, thereby predisposing to an angiotensin-mediated increase in vascular resistance.[57]

Reservations to the hypothesis linking insulin resistance to hypertension. First, the hypothesis linking insulin resistance to hypertension does not hold in black American subjects nor in Pima Indians, suggesting that the link is not directly between insulin and hypertension but rather may involve a genetic association.[68] This lack of association is not likely to be limited to American blacks because in the South African Bantu the insulin response to an oral glucose load is only 50% of that found in whites.[67] Second, there are hypertensive patients in whom the relation between fasting serum insulin and glucose does not suggest hyperinsulinemia.[52] Third, insulin also has vasodilator besides vasoconstrictor properties.[2] A further proposal is that insulin resistance is the result rather than the cause of the abnormalities of circulatory control found in skeletal muscle in hypertension. Nonetheless, the concept of this syndrome provides a useful framework for thought in linking non-insulin-dependent diabetes, obesity, dyslipidemias, and hypertension as risk factors for atherosclerosis.

Insulin resistance and therapy for hypertension. The concept of insulin resistance has implications for the treatment of hypertension. First, non-pharmacological treatment can potentially improve insulin sensitivity. Thus, weight reduction and increased aerobic exercise should both act favorably to improve insulin resistance. Exercise increases glucose uptake by muscle and should, therefore, reduce insulin resistance (Fig 11-2). Exercise training is also antihypertensive.[39, 42] Thus aerobic exercise and weight loss are both effective, although not additive, in reducing blood pressure and insulin resistance.[18] Second, because insulin resistance seems not to be linked to hypertension in black subjects, this aspect does not warrant special consideration in their treatment. Third, certain antihypertensive drugs further impair insulin resistance.

Glucose impairment, diuretics and beta-blockers. In hypertensive whites treated with diuretics or diuretics and beta-blockers, plasma glucose and insulin were higher after a glucose load.[83] and particularly after the combination (Fig 11-4). These findings may explain why treatment involving these drugs is associated with an increased incidence of diabetes mellitus.[78] Of note however is that the diuretic doses used in those days were often high or even very high, which in an observational study were associated with increased mortality.[83] Even a beta-blocker alone can impair glucose uptake and increase very low density lipoprotein as well as decreasing high density lipoprotein levels (HDL) in hypertensives.[63] Other types of drugs, namely the ACE inhibitors, calcium antagonists and alpha-blockers, are likely to have neutral or beneficial effects on the insulin status.[47,73,74] Thus, changing from a beta-blocker to an ACE inhibitor may improve insulin resistance in a subset of hypertensives with marked insulin resistance.[7]

ACE inhibition vs thiazide therapy. In 50 patients with mild hypertension,[63] captopril improved glucose disposal, whereas the thiazide impaired it. Furthermore, the thiazide increased serum cholesterol and low density lipoprotein levels, as well as triglyceride levels. In contrast, captopril had none of these potentially deleterious effects. ACE inhibition also lessened the hypokalemic effects of insulin, thereby leading to improved glucose tolerance in non-diabetic hypertensives.[70] Hypothetically, the ACE inhibitor could be beneficial for those patients at risk of diabetes mellitus and/or coronary artery disease and the thiazide could be harmful. This attractive hypothesis receives support from the CAPP study,[13] in which captopril was compared with conventional antihypertensive therapy by a beta-blocker or a diuretic. In this study, captopril reduced the risk of development of diabetes.

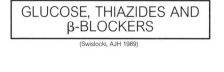

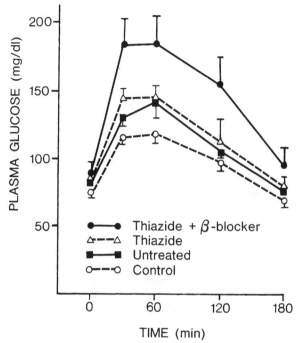

Figure 11-4. In response to an oral glucose load, the plasma glucose rises very much higher in patients receiving thiazide and beta-blocker therapy than in controls. Note that untreated hypertensive subjects have values intermediate between the controls and those with impaired glucose tolerance. Thiazide-treated patients likewise have mild degrees of impairment of glucose tolerance. Reprinted by permission of Elsevier Science Publishing Co from Swislocki et al.[83]

DIABETES MELLITUS AND HYPERTENSION

Definitions of diabetes mellitus and impaired fasting glucose. The presence of diabetes profoundly increases the cardiovascular risk, in a large part by the adverse combination of diabetes and hypertension (Fig 11-5). Thus, the prediction charts of the British joint committees[12] and several other bodies such as the combined European Societies of Cardiology, Hypertension and Atherosclerosis[84] are divided into those who have diabetes and those who do not. But, what is diabetes? Recently, the diagnosis has been simplified. In the USA, the new guidelines take a consistently elevated fasting blood glucose of 110 up to 125 mg/dl (6.1 to 6.9 mmol/l) as an impaired fasting glucose, and higher values as diabetes mellitus.[22] Similar are the new proposals of the World Health Organization expert committee,[1] diagnosing diabetes a fasting plasma glucose of 7 mmol/l or more, with values of 6.1 mmol/l but below 7.0 mmol/l, as im-

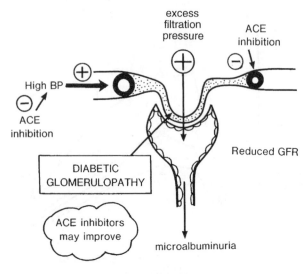

Figure 11-5. When diabetes is combined with hypertension, then in addition to the diabetic glomerulopathy there is excess intraglomerular filtration pressure so that the microalbuminuria can become a marked proteinuria (nephrotic kidney of Kimmelstiel-Wilson). Fig. © LH Opie, 1999

paired fasting glycemia (IFG). If the two hour glucose is also abnormal in a glucose tolerance test, being above 11.1 mmol/l, then there is impaired glucose tolerance (IGT). However, the major aim is simplification, and the new reliance is on the fasting glucose values, rather than on the glucose tolerance curve, which becomes less important than before.

ACE inhibitor therapy in hypertensive type 1 diabetes with nephropathy. Hypertension usually reflects diabetic nephropathy, and "almost all patients with type 1 diabetes and overt nephropathy, are hypertensive".[12] Here nephropathy is defined by the British Committees as dipstick proteinuria or urine protein loss > 200 mg per 24 hrs.[12] Blood pressure increases as the urinary albumin loss increases. Are there specific advantages for ACE inhibition? Three persuasive studies show that ACE inhibition can fundamentally change the course of Type I diabetic renal disease.

Progression of microalbuminuria to overt disease. Captopril (50 mg 2× daily) was given to 67 normotensive insulin-dependent diabetics (Type I) over 2 years. It decreased the rate of progression to overt proteinuria and prevented the glomerular filtration rate from falling.[45]

Progression of microalbuminuria to clinical proteinuria. Captopril given over 2 years to those with an initial protein loss of at least 200 μg/min had the probability of progression diminished.[87] However, the BP did fall by 3 to 7 mmHg, raising the possibility of a hypotensive mechanism.

Reduction of hard end-points. In this major trial on 409 patients over 3 years, the end-points were death, dialysis or renal transplantation (Fig 11-6).[46] The patients were Type I diabetics with proteinuria and had an increased serum creatinine and retinopathy. Captopril (25 mg 3× daily) decreased the risk of reaching each of the end-points by about half. Captopril also induced remission much more frequently than did placebo.[35]

ACE inhibitor therapy in normotensive type 1 diabetes with nephropathy. Logically, if the diabetic damage to the glomerular capillaries were sufficiently severe, then added hypertension would not be required to cause intraglomerular hypertension and hyperfiltration of albumin (Fig 11-5). An important hypothesis is that ACE inhibition could specifically decrease the glomerular permeability to proteins by lessening the size of the selective pores.[54]

In a study from Parving's group,[51] on 21 normotensive type 1 diabetics followed for 4 years, captopril in an initial dose of 25 mg daily increased to 100 mg daily, reduced microalbuminuria when compared with 23 controls, and only untreated patients developed overt clinical diabetic nephropathy. It was claimed that the blood pressure was virtually unchanged, yet the 24 hour blood pressure profiles revealed clearly lower values for the captopril treated group than for the other group, so a primary hypotensive mechanism with reduced intraglomerular pressure still cannot be excluded. Hence the data of the EUCLID study are of interest. Here lisinopril was given over 24 months to

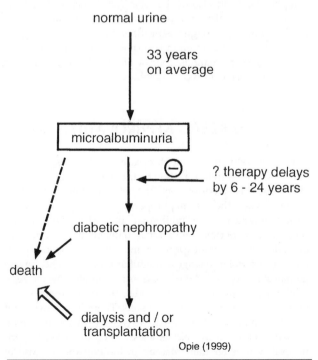

Figure 11-6. Model of progression of diabetic renal disease and possible benefits of antihypertensive treatment by an ACE inhibitor, according to Borch-Johnsen et al.[11] Fig. © LH Opie, 1999

type 1 diabetics with microalbuminuria, defined as a urinary albumin excretion of at least 20 µg/min (about 30 mg per day, see Table 4-1).[21] The final treatment difference was 38.5 µg/min less in the lisinopril group. There was even a decrease in those with normal urine albumin values at the start. There was a small fall in blood pressure (3 mmHg, initially 122/79 mmHg) thought not to be significant.

Renoprotection by ACE inhibitors. The above studies in type 1 diabetics, in both hypertensives and normotensives, suggest that ACE inhibitors are renoprotective in type 1 diabetics. Yet there must be strict control of blood pressure, to values of below 130/80 mmHg or even 125/75 mmHg if there is proteinuria.[12] To achieve such low values, will almost certainly need multiple drug therapy, which should include an ACE inhibitor titrated to maximal does.

Type 2 diabetes with hypertension. In this type of diabetes, hypertension is very common, at about 40%, is closely related to obesity, and may not indicate nephropathy.[12] Strict reduction of the blood pressure, by either ACE inhibitor therapy or beta-blockade both improves microalbuminuria and hypertension, whereas a diuretic does not change the protein loss even though the blood pressure falls as much with the diuretic as with enalapril or atenolol.[79] In the large and long UK prospective study over 9 years, either captopril or atenolol with other agents added in thereafter, could equally achieve very vigorous control the blood pressure, with a major reduction of macrovascular complications and also of retinopathy.[86] Other studies have shown that a calcium blocker-based regime can also be used, but here the diagnosis of diabetes was not exactly defined.[36,85] Thus the first aim in a diabetic hypertensive must be to achieve meticulous control of the blood pressure, to the same levels as in type 1 diabetes.

DIABETIC NEPHROPATHY

Thus it is evident that nephropathy in diabetes can exist apart from hypertension, though these are often associated. When there is hypertension, that must be very vigorously treated. When there is nephropathy, that too needs active treatment, and an ACE inhibitor is the agent of first choice (Fig 11-7). Experimentally, renal damage in hypertensive diabetic rats that overexpress renin, includes tubular degeneration, arteriolar changes, medullary fibrosis and severe glomerulosclerosis.[40] All of these are attenuated by the ACE inhibitor perindopril. In this model, the tissue renin-angiotensin system is markedly activated. There is however, not yet clear evidence that similar activation occurs in human diabetic nephropathy. Nonetheless, over three years perindopril was better than placebo in limiting the increase in thickness of glomerular basement membrane in diabetics, with however a few mmHg drop in BP in the perindopril group.[55]

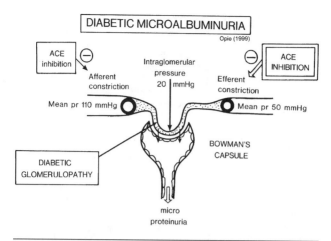

Figure 11-7. In diabetic microalbuminuria without hypertension, the problem is that of diabetic glomerular disease (glomerulopathy), so that the same intraglomerular pressure as normal causes loss of protein into the urine. Fig. © LH Opie, 1999

DIABETIC RETINOPATHY

There is a strong association between diabetic nephropathy, retinopathy, and neuropathy. Hypertension is a common risk factor for each of these, and the mechanisms may involve hypertensive microvascular dysfunction. Thus vigorous treatment of hypertension in type 2 diabetics in the UK prospective trial over 9 years, led to decreased retinopathy as judged by reduced retinal photocoagulation.[86] However, even in normotensive type 1 diabetics, with little or no nephropathy, lisinopril decreased the progression of retinopathy.[14] Thus there appears to be a specific benefit of ACE inhibitors on diabetic microvascular disease, as also suggested by the effect of perindopril on retinal blood flow over one year.[62]

DIABETIC NEUROPATHY

On the hypothesis that the microvascular lesions are similar in neuropathy and retinopathy, the ACE inhibitor trandolapril was given to normotensive diabetics, type 1 or 2, for 12 months, with improved nerve conduction.[48]

THE TICKING CLOCK HYPOTHESIS

To put observations on diabetic microalbuminuria into perspective, requires mention of the "ticking clock hypothesis". Based on an 8-year follow-up of 614 non-diabetic Mexican Americans in the San Antonio Heart Study, it appears that an atherogenic pattern of risk factors for coronary disease preceded the development of diabetes.[32] In such patients, the clock for atherosclerosis is hypothetically set in motion early in life by a constellation of genetic and environmental factors, including those regulating insulin secretion and sen-

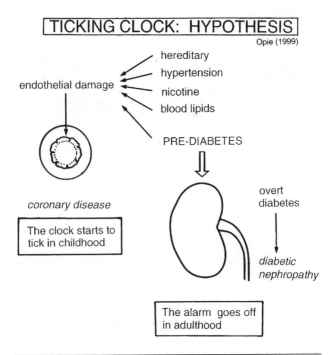

Figure 11-8. The ticking clock hypothesis wheeby the clock-regulating the development of coronary disease starts to tick long before the development of overt diabetes and nephropathy.[16,32] Fig. © LH Opie, 1999

sitivity (Fig 11-8). Conversely, the clock for microvascular complications, including nephropathy, starts to tick much later in life with the onset of overt hyperglycemia.[16] Therefore, the real challenge is not how to control the hyperglycemia and nephropathy, but (1) to prevent the development of overt diabetes in pre-diabetics, and (2) to promote a lifestyle counteracting the effects of insulin resistance. Prominent among the latter aims should be increased exercise, control of obesity, and a diet high in complex carbohydrates. Whether, in addition, ACE inhibition may play a preventative role is still a fascinating speculation.

THE DIABETIC HEART

The diabetic heart remains an outstanding challenge. Diabetes is a prime risk factor for coronary heart disease and for increased mortality. When the diabetic patient develops acute myocardial infarction, the prognosis is worse than in the non-diabetic, both in the early phase and in the post-infarct development of heart failure.[4] The mechanism of this diabetes-associated adverse prognosis is probably multi-factorial. First, there is increased macrovascular disease and the whole atherosclerotic process is accelerated. Secondly, there is also increased microvascular disease, even in the absence of large vessel disease. Thirdly, there is augmented collagen formation and fibrosis. Fourthly, there is a greater thrombotic tendency. Fifthly, there may be a metabolic cardiomyopathy.

Management of acute myocardial infarction (AMI) in diabetics. First, it must be recalled that diabetes is a metabolic disease, and that a key problem is the impaired glucose uptake by muscle including the myocardium. Because of this metabolic problem, and because glucose is a protective fuel for the ischemic cells, it is important that steps be taken to ensure that the patient with non-insulin dependent diabetes (type II) should not be left on oral antidiabetics. AMI is an acute stress reaction, in which high circulating free fatty acid levels inhibit the uptake and metabolism of glucose. There is acute insulin resistance. In addition, oral anti-diabetic agents may prevent opening of the protective ATP-dependent potassium channel.[28] Thus oral anti-diabetic agents should be stopped in the early phase of AMI and replaced by insulin.[28] The patients should be placed on intravenous insulin and covered by glucose, as in the DIGAMI study.[19] Follow up should also be by insulin-based therapy for three months or more. Such therapy reduces mortality at one year.

Second, ACE inhibitors should be given in the acute phase of myocardial infarction. "The diabetic patient may have far more to gain than the non-diabetic" Nesto stated in an important editorial.[56] In the GISSI-3 study, in which lisinopril was given prophylactically, the major benefit was in diabetics.[89] Just when to start the ACE inhibitor is not clear. Of note, in GISSI III, the best results were obtained by the combination of an ACE inhibitor with nitrate therapy, started within 24 hours of the onset of symptoms, but this observation was not specifically made in the diabetic population.

Third, all other standard procedures for patients with AMI need to be followed: relief of pain, early aspirin, early thrombolysis (with heparin if tissue plasminogen activator is used), and also early intravenous beta blockade. Logically, the beta blockade should be given as urgently as possible, because the catecholamine stress[76] is maximal in the first few hours. Beta blockade should also help to alleviate the insulin resistance, though there are no trial data on this point.

In the postinfarct follow-period, protection by beta-blockade and aspirin is standard. Although not formally tested, beta-blockade seems to benefit diabetics even more than non-diabetics.[41] Heart failure is a special risk in diabetics[37] and the early use of ACE inhibition makes good sense. Additionally, there may be the need for revascularization. Coronary bypass surgery carries a much better prognosis than does angioplasty (PTCA).[6] The reasons are not well understood but could be related to the exaggerated intimal hyperplasia of the diabetic arterial wall.[43]

AGEING

Last but not least in the list of metabolic challenges facing the ACE inhibitors is ageing. Theories of ageing are many[50] and include formation of free radicals. In highly select

experimental conditions, ACE inhibitors reduce the generation of free radicals.[72] Ageing is accompanied by increased
fibrosis and other structural changes, especially in the
cardiovascular system.[69] ACE inhibitors could theoretically
protect against such changes.[34, 71] Of greater immediate
application is the prevention of systolic hypertension in the
elderly.

Ageing and systolic hypertension. Loss of compliance of
the major arteries is an excellent explanation for systolic hypertension. Thus a 35% decrease in compliance causes a
15% increase in systolic blood pressure and a 12% decrease
in the diastolic blood pressure, while the mean pressure
and cardiac output stay unchanged.[64] When the loss of
compliance goes up to 63%, then the systolic pressure rises
by 18% and the diastolic pressure falls by 24%, again with
no changes in the overall mean blood pressure. In the latter
situation, the cardiac output falls because the reduced compliance increases the afterload, compliance being one important component of the afterload, the other being the
peripheral vascular resistance. Thus an increasing loss of arterial compliance represents an increasing load to the left
ventricle and will increase the systolic blood pressure and
decrease the diastolic blood pressure. The fact that the diastolic blood pressure is often normal or slightly high in elderly patients cannot be explained by a pure loss of arterial
compliance.[64] Rather, a further process such as that suggested in the hypothesis shown in Figure 3-7, to increase
peripheral vascular resistance, would adequately explain
the relative increase of diastolic blood pressure associated
with systolic hypertension.

Ageing and insulin resistance. As in younger patients,
ACE inhibition improved insulin resistance in elderly hypertensives.[61] The drugs tested were captopril, enalapril,
quinapril, ramipril and lisinopril.

SUMMARY

1. *The metabolic cardiovascular syndrome.* Links between
    central obesity, hypertension, insulin insensitivity, and
    diabetes mellitus are outlined. Prolonged elevations fo
    blood free fatty acids levels may be crucial, acting on
    the glucose-fatty acid cycle.

2. *In early diabetic nephropathy*, increasing evidence sug-
    gests that ACE inhibitors are beneficial against the
    microalbuminuria. In insulin-dependent diabetics, ACE
    inhibition reduced hard end-points such as death,
    transplantation or dialysis.

3. *Long-term outcome studies* in Type II (non-insulin-
    dependent) diabetes show the major benefit of very
    tight blood pressure control by an ACE inhibitor or by
    a beta-blocker. Smaller and shorter trials suggest bene-
    fit of ACE inhibition in the control of diabetic retinopa-
    thy and neuropathy. A recent intriguing suggestion is

that ACE inhibitors may be able to control some aspects of the ageing process.

REFERENCES

1. Alberti KGMM, Zimmer P. For the WHO Consultation. Definition, diagnosis and classification of diabetes mellitus and its complications. Part I: Diagnosis and clarification of diabetes mellitus. Provisional report of a WHO consultation. Diabet med 1998;15:539–553.

2. Anderson E, Mark A. The vasodilator action of insulin. Implications for the insulin hypothesis of hypertension. Hypertension 1993;21:136–141.

3. Arnesen H. Introduction: the metabolic cardiovascular syndrome. J Cadiovasc Pharmacol 1992;20 (Suppl 8):S1–S4.

4. Aronson D, Rayfield EJ, Chesebro JH. Mechanisms determining course and outcome of diabetic patients who have had acute myocardial infarction. Ann Intern Med 1997;126:296–306.

5. Austin MA, Mykkanen L, Kuusisto J, et al. Prospective study of small LDLs as a risk factor for non-insulin dependent diabetes mellitus in elderly men and women. Circulation 1995;92:1770–1778.

6. BARI Investigators. Influence of diabetes on 5-year mortality and morbidity in a randomized trial comparing CABG and PTCA in patients with multivessel disease. Circulation 1997;96:1761–1769.

7. Berntorp K, Lindgarde F, Matiasson I. Long-term effects on insulin sensitivity and sodium transport in glucose-intolerant hypertensive subjects when beta-blockade is replaced by captopril treatment. J Human Hypertens 1992;6:291–198.

8. Boden G. Role of fatty acids in the pathogensis of insulin resistance and NIDDM. Diabetes 1996;45:3–10.

9. Boden WE. "Maimed Myocardium": Incomplete, delayed functional recovery late after reperfusion following acute myocardial infarction. In: Yellon DM, Rahmitoola SH, Opie LH, eds. New Ischemic Syndromes. New York: Lippincott-Raven, 1997.

10. Bonora E, Zavaroni I, Pezzarossa A, et al. Relationship between blood pressure and plasma insulin in non-obese and obese non-diabetic subjects. Diabetelogia 1987;30:719–723.

11. Borch-Johnsen K, Wenzel H, Viberti G, et al. Is screening and intervention for microalbuminuria worthwhile in patients with insulin dependent diabetes? Br Med J 1993;306:1722–1723.

12. British Committees. British Cardiac Society, British Hyperlipidaemia Association, British Hypertension Society endorsed by the British Diabetic Association. Joint British recommendations on prevention of coronary heart disease in clinical practice. Heart 1998;80 (Suppl 2):S1–S29.

13. CAPP Study Group. Hansson L, Lindholm LH, Niskanen L, et al. Effect of angiotensin-converting-enzyme inhibition compared with conventional therapy on cardiovascular morbidity and mortality in hypertension: the Captopril Prevention Project (CAPPP) randomised trial. Lancet 1999;353:611–616.

14. Chaturvedi N, Sjolie A-K, Stephenson JM, et al. for the EUCLID Study Group. Effect of lisinopril on progression of retinopathy in normotensive people with type 1 diabetes. Lancet 1998;351:28–31.

15. Daniels SR, Morrison JA, Sprecher DL, et al. Association of body fat distribution and cardiovascular risk factors in children and adolescents. Circulation 1999;99:541–545.

16. DeFronzo RA. Insulin resistance, hyperinsulinemia, and coronary artery disease: a complex metabolic web. J Cardiovasc Pharmacol 1992;20 (Suppl 11):S1–S16.

17. DeFronzo RA, Ferrannini E. Insulin resistance. A multifaceted syndrome responsible for NIDDM, obesity, hypertension, dilipidemia, and atherosclerotic cardiovascular disease. Diabetes Care 1991;14:173–194.

18. Dengel DD, Galecki AT, Hagberg JM, et al. The independent and combined effects of weight loss and aerobic exercise on blood pressure and oral glucose tolerance in older men. Am H Hypertens 1998;11:1405–1412.

19. DIGAMI Study. Malmberg K, Ryden L, Efendic S, et al. Randomized trial of insulin-glucose infusion followed by subcutaneous insulin treatment in diabetic patients with acute myocardial infarction (DIGAMI Study): Effects on mortality at 1 year. JACC 1995;26:57–65.

20. Ducimetiere P, Eschwege L, Papoz L, et al. Relationship of plasma insulin levels to the incidence of myocardial infarction and coronary aftery disease mortality in a middle-aged population. Diabetologia 1980;19:205–210.

21. EUCLID Study Group. Randomised placebo-controlled trial of lisinopril in normotensive patients with insulin-dependent diabetes and normoalbuminuria or microalbuminuria. Lancet 1997;349:1787–1792.

22. Expert Committee. Report of the Expert Committee on the Diagnosis and Classification of Diabetes Mellitus. Diabetes Care 1997;20:1183–1197.

23. Ferrannini E, Buzzigoli G, Bonadonna R, et al. Insulin resistance in essential hypertension. New Engl J Med 1987;317:350–357.

24. Ferrannini E, Haffner SM, Stern MP. Insulin sensitivity and hypertension. J Hypertens 1990;8 (Suppl 7):S169–S173.

25. Foster DW. Insulin resistance – a secret killer? N Engl J Med 1989;320:733–734.

26. Fournier AM, Gadia MT, Kubusly DB, et al. Blood pressure, insulin and glycemia in nondiabetic subjects. Am J Med 1986;80:861–864.

27. Fuller J, Shipley M, Rose G, et al. Coronary-heart-disease risk and impaired glucose tolerance. Lancet 1980;1:1373–1376.

28. Garratt KN, Brady PA, Hassiner NL, et al. Sulfonylurea drugs increase early mortality in patients with diabetes mellitus after direct angioplasty for acute myocardial infarction. J Am Coll Cardiol 1999;33:119–124.

29. Golay A, Sech L, Shi M-Z, et al. High density lipoprotein (HDL) metabolism in non-insulin-dependent diabetes mellitus: measurement of HDL turnover using tritiated HDL. J Clin Endorcinol Metab 1987;65:512–518.

30. Goldberg RB, Mellies MJ, Sacks FM, et al. Cardiovascular events and their reduction with pravastatin in diabetic and glucose-intolerant myocardial infarction survivors with average cholesterol levels. Subgroup analysis of the Cholesterol and Recurrent Events (CARE) Trial. Circulation 1998;98:2513–2519.

31. Haffner SM, Fong D, Hazuda HP, et al. Hyperinsulinemia, upper body adiposity and cardiovascular risk factors in non-diabetics. Metabolism 1988;37:338–345.

32. Haffner SM, Stern MP, Hazuda HP, et al. Cardiovascular risk factors in confirmed prediabetic individuals. Does the clock for coronary artery disease start ticking before the onset of clinical diabetes? JAMA 1990;263:2893–2898.

33. Hall J, Brands M, Kivlighn S, et al. Chronic hyperinsulinemia and blood pressure. Interaction with catecholamines? Hypertension 1990;15:519–527.

34. Harris M. Do ACE inhibitors delay symptoms of aging? Inpharma 1993;898:5.

35. Hebert L, Bain R, Cattran D, et al. Remission (RM) of nephrotic-range proteinuria (NRP) in Type I diabetes: experience of the NIH multicentre controlled trial (T) of captopril (CAP) therapy in diabetic nephropathy (DN) (abstr). J Am Soc Nephrol 1993;4:303.

36. HOT Study. Hansson L, Zanchetti A, Carruthers SG, et al. Effects of intensive blood-pressure lowering and low-dose aspirin in patients with hypertension: principal results of the Hypertension Optimal Treatment (HOT) randomised trial. Lancet 1998;351:1755–1762.

37. Jaffe AS, Spadaro JJ, Schechtman K, et al. Increased congestive heart failure after myocardial infarction of modest extent in diabetes with diabetes mellitus. Am Heart J 1984;108:31–37.

38. Jensen MD, Haymond MW, Rizza RA, et al. Influence of body fat distribution on free fatty acid metabolism in obesity. J Clin Invest 1989;83:1168–1173.

39. Kelemen M, Effron M, Valenti S, et al. Exercise training combined with antihypertensive drug therapy. JAMA 1990;263:2766–2711.

40. Kelly DJ, Wilkinson-Berka JL, Allen TJ, et al. A new model of diabetic nephropathy with progressive renal impairment in the transgenic (mRen-2)27 rat (TGR). Kidney International 1998;54:343–352.

41. Kjekshus J, Gilpin E, Cali G, et al. Diabetic patients and beta-blockers after acute myocardial infarction. Eur Heart J 1990;11:43–50.

42. Kokkinos PF, Narayan P, Colleran JA, et al. Effects of regular exercise on blood pressure and left ventricular hypertrophy in African-American men with servere hypertension. N Engl J Med 1995;333:1462–1467.

43. Kornowski R, Mintz GS, Kent KM, et al. Increased restenosis in diabetes mellitus after coronary interventions is due to exaggerated intimal hyperplasia. Circulation 1997;95:1366–1369.

44. Kumar S, Durrington P, Bhatnagar I. Suppression of non-esterified fatty acids to treat type A insulin resistance syndrome. Lancet 1994;343:1073–1074.

45. Laffel L, Gans D, McGill J. Captopril decreases the rate of progression of renal disease in normotensive, insulin-dependent diabetes mellitus (DDM) patients with microalbuminuria (abstr). J Am Soc Nephrol 1993;4:304.

46. Lewis E, Hunsicker L, Bain R, et al. For the Collaborative Study Group. The effect of angiotensin-converting enzyme inhibition on diabetic nephropathy. N Engl J Med 1993;329:1456–1462.

47. Lithell H. Effect of antihypertensive drugs on insulin, glucose, and lipid metabolism. Diabetes Care 1991;14:203–209.

48. Malik RA, Williamson S, Abbott C, et al. Effect of angiotensin-converting-enzyme (ACE) inhibitor trandolapril on human diabetic neuropathy: randomised double-blind controlled trial. Lancet 1998;352:1978–1981.

49. Martin B, Warram J, Krolewski A, et al. Role of glucose and insulin resistance in development of type 2 diabetes mellitus: results of a 25-year follow-up study. Lancet 1992;340:925–929.

50. Martin G, Danner D, Holbrook N. Aging - causes and defenses. Ann Rev Med 1993;44:419–429.

51. Mathiesen E, Hommel E, Giese J, et al. Efficacy of captopril in postponing nephropathy in normotensive insulin dependent diabetic patients with microalbuminuria. Br Med J 1991;303:81–87.

52. Mbanya J-C, Thomas T, Wilkinson R, et al. Hypertension and hyperinsulinemia: a relation in diabetes but not essential hypertension. Lancet 1988;1733–734.

53. Modan M, Halkin H, Almog S, et al. Hyperinsulinemia. A link between hypertension, obesity and glucose intolerance. J Clin Invest 1985;75:809–817.

54. Morelli E, Loon N, Meyer T, et al. Effects of converting-enzyme inhibition on barrier function in diabetic glomerulopathy. Diabetes 1990;39:76–82.

55. Nankervis A, Nicholls K, Kilmartin G, et al. Effects of perindopril on renal histomorphometry in diabetic subjects with microalbuminuria: a 3-year placebo-controlled biopsy study. Metabolism 1998;47 (Suppl 1):12–15.

56. Nesto RW, Zarich S. Acute myocardial infarction in diabetes mellitus. Lessons learned from ACE inhibitors. Circulation 1998;97:12–15.

57. Nickenig G, Roling J, Strehlow K, et al. Insulin induces upregulation of vascular AT_1 receptor gene expression by postranscriptional mechanisms. Circulation 1998;98:2543–2460.

58. Opie L. Lipid metabolism of the heart and arteries in relation to ischaemic heart disease. Lancet 1973;1:192–195.

59. Opie LH, Mansford KRL, Owen P. Effects of increased heart work on glycolysis and adenine nucleotides in the perfused heart of normal and diabetic rats. Biochem J 1971;124:475–490.

60. Opie LH, Walfish PG. Plasma free fatty acid concentrations in obesity. N Engl J Med 1963;268:757–760.

61. Paolisso G, Bambardella A, Verza M, et al. ACE inhibition improves insulin-senstivity in aged insulin-resistant hypertensive patients. J Human Hypertens 1992;6:175–179.

62. Patel V, Rassam SMB, Chan HC, et al. Effect of angiotensin-converting enzyme inhibition with perindopril and β-blockade with atenolol on retinal blood flow in hypertensive diabetic subjects. Metabolism 1998;47 (Suppl 1):38–33.

63. Pollare T, Lithell H, Berne C. A comparison of the effects of hydrochlorothiazide and captopril on glucose and lipid metabolism in patients with hypertension. N Eng J Med 1989;321:868–873.

64. Randall OS, Bos GCvd, Westerhof N. Systemic compliance: does it play a role in the genesis of essential hypertension? Cardiovasc Res 1984;18:455–462.

65. Randle PJ, Garland PB, Hales CN, et al. The glucose fatty acid cycle: its role in insulin sensitivity and the metabolic disturbances of diabetes mellitus. Lancet 1963;April 13:785–789.

66. Reaven GM. Banting Lecture 1988: role of insulin resistance in human disease. Diabetes 1988;37:1595–1607.

67. Rubenstein AH, Seftel HC, Miller K, et al. Metabolic response to oral glucose in healthy South African White, Indian and African subjects. Br Med J 1969:1 748–751.

68. Saad MF, Lillioja S, Hyoma BL, et al. Racial differences in the relation between blood pressure and insulin resistance. N Engl J Med 1991;324:733–739.

69. Safar M. Ageing and its effects on the cardiovascular system. Drugs 1990;39 (Suppl 1):1–8.

70. Santoro D, Natali A, Palombo C, et al. Effects of chronic angiotensin-converting enzyme inhibition on glucose tolerance and insulin sensitivity in essential hypertension. Hypertension 1992;20:181–191.

71. Schwartzkopff B, Boerrigter G, Brehm MU, et al. Regression of interstitial fibrosis by chronic treatment with ACE-inhibitors in patients with hypertensive heart disease (Abstract). Circulation 1998;98 (Suppl 1):I-792.

72. Sharma M, Buettner G, Kerber R. Angiotensin-converting enzyme inhibitors reduce free radical generation during post-ischemic reperfusion of canine myocardium: a real-time study by electron spin resonance spectroscopy (abstr). J Am Coll Cardiol 1993;410A:949-42.

73. Sheu W, Swislocki A, Hoffman B, et al. Comparison of the effects of atenolol and nifedipine on glucose, insulin, and lipid metabolism in patients with hypertension. Am J Hypertens 1991;4:199–205.

74. Shieh S, Sheu W, Fuh S, et al. Glucose insulin and lipid metabolism in doxazosin-treated patients with hypertension. Am J Hypertens 1992;5:827–831.

75. Shipp J, Opie L, Challoner D. Fatty acid and glucose metabolism in the perfused heart. Nature 1961;189:1018–1019.

76. Shu CC, Hoffman WE, Thomas C, et al. Sympathetic activity enhances glucose-related ischemic injury in the rat. Anesthesiology 1993;78:1120–1125.

77. Siani A, Strazzullo P, Giorgione N, et al. Insulin-induced increase in heart rate and its prevention by propranolol. Eu J Clin Pharmacol 1990;38:393–395.

78. Skarfors E, Lithell H, Selinus I, et al. Do antihypertensive drugs precipitate diabetes in predisposed men? Br Med J 1989;298:1147–1152.

79. Stornello M, Valvo E, Scapellato L. Comparative effects of enalapril, atenolol and chlorthalidone on blood pressure and kidney function of diabetic patients affected by arterial hypertension and persistent proteinuria. Nephron 1991;58:52–57.

80. Stout RW. Insulin-stimulated lipogenesis in arterial tissue in relation to diabetes and atheroma. Lancet 1968;2:702–703.

81. Stout RW, Bierman EL, Ross R. Effect of insulin on the proliferation of cultured primate arterial smooth muscle cels. Circ Res 1975;36:319–327.

82. Stout RW, Vallance-Owen J. Insulin and atheroma. Lancet 1969;1:1078–1079.

83. Swislocki ALM, Hoffman BB, Reaven GM. Insulin resistance, glucose intolerance and hyperinsulinemia in patients with hypertension. Am J Hypertens 1989;2:419–423.

84. Task Force Report. Prevention of coronary heart disease in clinical practice. Recommendations of the Second Joint Task Force of European and other Societies on Coronary Prevention. Eur Heart J 1998;19:1434–1503.

85. Tuomilehto J, Rastenyte D, Birkenhager WH, et al. Effects of calcium-channel blockade in older patients with diabetes and systolic hypertension. N Engl J Med 1999;340:677–684.

86. UKPDS Study. UK Prospective Diabetes Study Group. Efficacy of atenolol and captopril in reducing risk of macrovascular and microvascular complications in type 2 diabetes: UKPDS 39. BMJ 1998;317:713–20.

87. Viberti G, Mogensen CE, Groop LC, et al. For the European Microalbuminuria Captopril Study Group. Effect of captopril on progression to clinical proteinuria in patients with insulin-dependent diabetes-mellitus and microalbuminuria. JAMA 1994;271:275–279.

88. Zavaroni I, Bonora E, Pagliara M, et al. Risk factors for coronary artery disease in healthy persons with hyperinsulinemia and normal glucose tolerance. N Engl J Med 1989;320:703–706.

89. Zuanetti G, Latini R, Maggioni AP, et al. Effect of ACE inhibitor lisinopril on mortality in diabetic patients with acute myocardial infarction. Circulation 1997;96:4239–4245.

A look into the future

"Angiotensin receptor blockers should be used primarily in patients in whom ACE inhibitors are indicated but who are unable to tolerate them"[9]

Coming to the end of this book presents us with the opportunity of a glimpse into the future. In general terms, coronary heart disease will remain the major cause of heart failure, and will in fact become more rather than less important as other causes of death such as infections, including AIDS, diminish. Greater longevity will mean more, not less cardiovascular disease and heart failure (Fig 12-1). Therefore the progression from risk factors through to heart failure (Fig 12-2) will become the bedrock of prevention of heart failure. This chapter will argue that the growing positive data on ACE inhibitors will increasingly inhibit both the primary and secondary arms that lead to heart failure.

Against this positive scenario some pertinent questions must be asked. First, how would the new angiotensin receptor blockers (AT-1 blockers) compare with the ACE inhibitors? In the era of evidence-based medicine, will the promising claims made for their future be realized? Is there room for combination therapy? Regarding inhibition of the

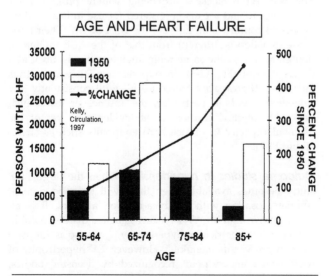

Figure 12-1 Effect of increasing longevity on incidence of heart failure in Australia. From Kelly[10] with permission of the author and the American Heart Association.

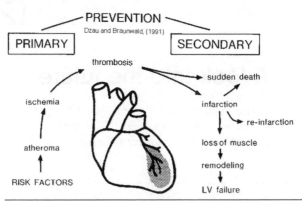

Figure 12-2. A scheme whereby risk factors for coronary artery disease can lead to left ventricular failure, evolved from that proposed by Dzau and Braunwald,[3] with permission of the authors and the American Heart Journal. Note contrasting sites of action of primary and secondary prevention. LV, left ventricular.

renin-angiotensin system, will it always be: the more the better? Second, what are the prospects for improved treatment of heart failure, and will ACE inhibitors continue to be the cornerstone of treatment? Third, what will be the likely new indications for ACE inhibitors in the reasonably near future? Fourth, how does ACE inhibition relate to new aspects of experimental cardiology, such as preconditioning and apoptosis? How will ACE inhibitors fit into the current emphasis on preventative cardiology? What are the large trials currently in progress? Can we guess how they are going to alter our practice in the future?

ANGIOTENSIN RECEPTOR BLOCKERS (AT-1 BLOCKERS)

The new AT-1 blockers are being widely promoted for hypertension, and are also registered for use in heart failure in several countries, though not the USA or UK. Their basic mode of action is different from that of the ACE inhibitors, though acting on the same renin-angiotensin axis albeit at a different level (Fig 12-3). In hypertension, they have thus far shown the capacity to reduce BP with consistently few side-effects, and, in particular, the absence or lower incidence of cough. But there is no evidence as yet of the essential capacity to reduce hard endpoints such as stroke (Table 12-1).

Outcome studies in hypertension. When the large LIFE study becomes available, then there will be good data to compare losartan with the beta-blocker, atenolol. It is already known that an AT-1 blocker is better than atenolol in reducing left ventricular hypertrophy,[23] as also is the case for ramipril versus atenolol.[18] However, LV hypertrophy of itself is not an endpoint recognized by licensing bodies, although known to be an independent risk factor for other cardiovascular diseases.[11] Strictly speaking, information on outcome in hypertension is also lacking in the case of the

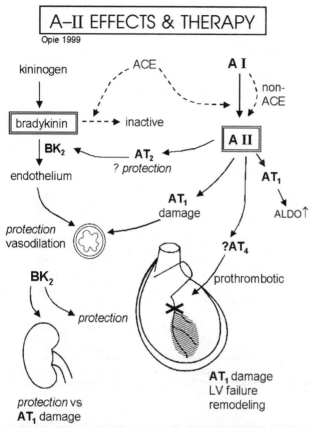

Figure 12-3. *Mechanisms whereby angiotensin II (A II) exerts adverse effects on cardiovascular system. Most of the damaging effects are via the AT-1 receptor, with possible protection via the unopposed AT-2 receptor (see page 7 for controversies). The putative AT-4 receptor may mediate pro-thrombotic effects. Bradykinin (BK) mediates protection by activation of the BK-2 receptor. Fig copyright L.H. Opie, 1999*

ACE inhibitors, except for the CAPPP study[2] in which the short acting agent captopril was used. Yet ACE inhibitors have been used in combination with calcium blocker therapy in two major outcome studies, namely the HOT Study[8] and STOP-2.[21] In the ongoing ASCOT study, the prime therapy for hypertension is amlodipine or atenolol. Perindopril or a diuretic, respectively, may thereafter be added if a second drug is needed.

Thus in the absence of good outcome trial data, the argument rests on the better evidence-based medicine for the ACE inhibitors, versus a very good side effect profile, resembling that of placebo, for the AT-1 blockers. Yet even the ACE inhibitors are strikingly well tolerated, and in still unpublished studies, the withdrawal rate from therapy with ACE inhibition is almost as low as with AT-1 blockers. Combining the ACE inhibitor and an AT-1 blocker, although theoretically sound, is likely to be much more expensive than combining either agent with a diuretic. Decisive comparative anti-hypertensive trials between these two types of agents are not likely to take place, so that indirect arguments will be used to compare them.

TABLE 12-1. COMPARISON OF SOME PROPERTIES OF AT-1
BLOCKERS VERSUS ACE INHIBITORS RELEVANT TO
USE IN HYPERTENSION

Property	AT-1 blocker	ACE inhibitor
Major site of block	AT-1 receptor	Converting enzyme
Major claims, basic science	More complete AT-1 block, AT-2 activity increased	Block of AT-1, AT-2, AT-4, and of bradykinin breakdown
Hypertension: Licensed in USA, UK	Yes	Yes
First line therapy, USA (JNC VI)	No	No
Compelling indications, USA	No	Yes (heart failure, diabetes, post-MI)
First line therapy, WHO	Yes	Yes
Major clinical claims, hypertension	Equal BP reduction to ACE inhibitors, little/no cough**	Well tolerated, years of experience Good quality of life
Effect on LVH, vs beta-blocker	Better (valsartan)	Better (lisinopril, ramipril)
Effect on fibrinogen levels*	No	Yes
Major problem, hypertension: no outcome studies	LIFE underway (vs atenolol)	Used in HOT and STOP-2, often with calcium blocker

LVH = left ventricular hypertrophy; HF = heart failure. *Fogari et al.[6] **Post-marketing information from Australia indicates that cough can develop with losartan.

Special patient groups in hypertension. Despite the lack of formal outcome studies, certain subgroups of hypertensives may be associated with coexisting diseases that are indications for ACE inhibitors in their own right. As AT-1 blockers do not have American licenses for heart failure, post-infarct systolic dysfunction, or diabetic nephropathy, it is understandable that the JNC VI committee regards hypertension associated with these conditions as a *"compelling indication" for ACE inhibition.*[9] "However, in the absence of data documenting equal long-term cardiac and renal protection in patients with these conditions, angiotensin receptor blockers should be used primarily in patients in whom ACE inhibitors are indicated but who are unable to tolerate them."[9] Obese, insulin resistant hypertensives may be another group in whom ACE inhibitors are preferred, because of reduction of insulin resistance and plasma fibrinogen with perindopril but not losartan;[6] confirmatory studies with long term outcome are however required.

Heart failure. Here there is a vast experience with ACE inhibitors (Table 12-2), culminating in the meta-analysis of Flather and Yusuf in which 12,763 patients were followed for 42 months, with a clear mortality reduction of 20%.[5] In contrast, there is thus far only one good trial with an AT-1 blocker with mortality as a secondary end-point, namely the ELITE study in the elderly, with a mean age of 74 years, the majority being hypertensive with an initial BP level of 137/79 mmHg.[4] In contrast with the ACE inhibitor trials, the mean age was usually lower (60 years in SAVE

TABLE 12-2. COMPARISON OF AT-1 BLOCKERS VERSUS ACE
INHIBITORS IN HEART FAILURE, IN REINFARCTION
AND IN STROKE

Property	AT-1 blocker	ACE inhibitor
Heart failure: Licensed in USA, UK	No	Yes
Major clinical claims, heart failure	ELITE study in the elderly, secondary endpoint of mortality better than captopril; study being repeated ELITE II	Many studies with large data base, at least 12,000 patients, definite mortality reduction of 20%, may prevent reinfarction
Post-MI: Major claims	No data, large trials underway	Several large studies, definite protection including LV dysfunction
Diabetic nephropathy: Major claims	No data	Renoprotective in type 1 diabetes independently of hypertension
Major claims, diabetic hypertension, type 2 diabetes	No data	As good as β-blockade in decreasing major vascular end points. Lower diabetes-related mortality.
Prevention of reinfarction	No data	Strongly suggested by several major trials. Under test as primary end-point. Positive in small diabetic trial vs calcium blocker (ABCD)
Prevention of repeat stroke	No trial	PROGRESS, enrolment complete
Prevention of cardiovascular complications in high risk patients without LV failure	No trial	HOPE and EUROPA underway
Major warning in package insert	Pregnancy	Pregnancy
Additional warnings	Hypotension; renal function	Angioedema; hypotension; renal function

and 61 years in the SOLVD treatment trial) and the initial
BP values also lower (113/70 mmHg in SAVE and 125/77
mmHg in SOLVD). Thus, there are substantial differences
in the populations studied in ELITE and in the other trials,
so that the results of ELITE, if confirmed in ELITE II, may
not apply to the populations studied in the ACE inhibitor
trials. Regarding ELITE, according to the 1999 American
Consensus document, "the difference in survival was no
longer significant after adjustment for the multiplicity of
endpoints and interim analyses".[16] In other words, taking
present results at face value, the AT-1 blockers may be better for elderly hypertensives with systolic heart failure, but
the result would have to be confirmed in ELITE II. In contrast, the ACE inhibitors have a vastly greater record of
safety and efficacy in all types of heart failure (Table 12-3).
It will still have to be clarified why the RESOLVD heart
failure trial with the AT-1 blocker, candesartan, was prema-
turely stopped.[19]

TABLE 12-3. COMPARISON OF ELITE WITH OTHER STUDIES OF
HEART FAILURE

	ELITE	SOLVD, SAVE
Clinical situation	Heart failure	Heart failure
Patient numbers	Hundreds	Thousands
Test drug	AT-1 blocker, losartan	ACE inhibitors
Comparator	Captopril	Placebo
Mean age, years	74	61
Hypertensive %	57%	History in 40%
Initial BP, mmHg	137-79	125-77; 113-70
Primary endpoint	Renal function, →	Mortality↓
Secondary endpoint	Mortality↓	CV morbidity↓

CV = cardiovascular

Guesses for the future: ACE inhibitors vs AT-1 blockers.
In hypertension, ACE inhibitors will remain much used
especially those many patients with complications and in
those in whom tight control, as in the HOT study, is judged
to require a multiple drug regime in which ACE inhibition
will play an important role. ACE inhibitors will remain first
line treatment in heart failure. AT-1 blockers will become
one of the standard initial therapies for hypertension, already recognized as possible first line therapy by the 1999
WHO-ISH guidelines.[24] Future recognition by bodies such
as JNC VII will follow. The LIFE study will ensure that AT-
1 blockers compete successfully with beta-blockers in hypertensive left ventricular hypertrophy. The LIFE study
might also lead to LV hypertrophy becoming a licensed indication for AT-1 blockers. These agents will also eat into
the calcium antagonist market, which will remain well
ahead in hypertension in the elderly. However, the total hypertension market will greatly expand, giving each category
of agent greater use in absolute terms. *In heart failure,* AT-1
blockers will, however, always and inevitably be behind
the ACE inhibitors when it comes to the magnitude of the
studies, the experience of clinicians and long term safety.
The combination of these two groups will, however, be
used more and more especially when the results of the Val-
Heft study are out. Finally, the function of the *AT-2 receptor*
will be much better understood.[7A] Agonists of this receptor
will become available, possibly for use in combination with
the other two types of drugs.

NEW PROSPECTS FOR HEART FAILURE

Granted that ACE inhibitors have changed the face of treatment of heart failure, and that in relative terms mortality
after long term treatment has fallen 20%, yet in absolute
terms the residual mortality is still high at 23% over 42
months.[5] This control figure, relating to past trials, may presently be too high. The control all cause mortality in the
most recent trial to be published CIBIS-II, is 17.3%, which is
reduced to 11.8% by bisoprolol (Table 12-4). Thus, a further
reduction of about 33% can be obtained by the addition of

TABLE 12-4. SOME MORTALITY REDUCTIONS WITH TREATMENT
WITH INITIAL ACE INHIBITION AND DIURETICS, AND
WITH ADD-ONS

Therapy	Year	Control Mortality	Mortality Reduction
Enalapril, CONSENSUS	1987	44% over 27 weeks	40% fall
Enalapril, SOLVD	1991	35% over 41 months	16% fall
Captopril, SAVE	1992	25% over 42 months	19% fall
Yusuf meta-analysis	1985–1994	22%, short term, months	23% fall
Yusuf meta-analysis	1992–1995	29%, 30 months	26% fall
Carvedilol	1996	8%, 6 months	? 65% fall
β-blocker meta-analysis	1998	12%, 7 months	32% fall
Spironolactone, RALES	1998	Not known, 36 months	27% fall
Bisoprolol, CIBIS-II	1999	17%, 15 months	34% fall

a beta-blocker, of which the best tested are metoprolol, bisoprolol and carvedilol.[16] Already the 1999 American Consensus document recommends that the standard triple therapy for heart failure with fluid retention should now become the combination of diuretics, an ACE inhibitor, and a beta-blocker.[16]

In RALES, another recent trial that tested the addition of spironolactone to a diuretic and ACE inhibitor, with digoxin being optional, mortality fell by 27%, that is in the same range as the effect of beta-blockade (page 141). There were more patients in severe class IV failure in RALES than in the beta-blocker trials.[16] The addition of low dose spironolactone, being much simpler than the prolonged upward titration of a beta-blocker, is likely to become standard practice in the near future, especially in class III-IV patients. Short-term trials may soon be initiated on the combination of a beta-blocker and spironolactone, always on the background of an ACE inhibitor and a diuretic. Further or alternate combination with an AT-1 blocker may also become commonplace, depending on future trial data. Of the additional agents, endothelin antagonists may be able to swing more patients towards benefit, but there are no outcome trial results at present. For those who can afford it, short term left ventricular assist devices will be a bridge to transplantation or tide the patient through a crisis period.

NEW EXPERIMENTAL CONCEPTS

ACE inhibition may be important in conferring more than vascular protection. Experimentally, ACE inhibitors can confer protection on the myocardium by facilitating *preconditioning*. Thus, with ACE inhibition there is a bradykinin-dependent mechanism that allows a small ischemic insult to generate the same protection that would otherwise require a larger insult, without the added risk of the latter.[14] *Apoptosis*, or programmed cell death, is another experimental process that is also of increasing interest. Apoptosis may play a role in ischemic-reperfusion injury, and in increasing the severity of heart failure as more and more cells disappear into the dead. The renin-angiotensin system, acting via the AT-1 receptor, may promote apoptosis, and ACE-inhibition may theoretically inhibit apoptosis. The latter hypothesis is of importance in that some of the established benefit of ACE inhibitors in heart failure may be mediated in part by decreased myocardial apoptosis.

POSSIBLE NEW INDICATIONS FOR ACE INHIBITORS

The two most likely areas are both in the prevention of vascular disease. First, the PROGRESS study is likely to show a reduction in repeat strokes, because it is already known that the addition of the ACE inhibitor under test, perindopril, decreased the blood pressure, and that stroke incidence is directly related to the blood pressure level. Second, there are a large number of patients under study in HOPE, EUROPA, and other trials that are aimed at preventing cardiovascular events in those at risk (Table 12-5). The reason why the present author makes this prediction rests on both basic science evidence and on meta-analysis. Angiotensin II, acting on the AT-4 receptor, inhibits fibrinolysis, while in humans ACE inhibition can reduce fibrinogen levels. In addition, the unexpected finding, confirmed by meta-analysis, is that myocardial infarction fell by 20% reduction in patients treated by ACE inhibition for heart failure. Possibly diabetic retinopathy may be another new indication. Although another three trials are evaluating the role of ACE inhibitors in the prevention of atherosclerosis (Table 12-6), I predict negative outcomes. There have been negative results with both of the first trial with quinapril,[17] and of part 2 with ramipril.[12] Furthermore, neointimal vascular injury can develop even in AT-1 receptor knockout mice.[7] Perhaps beneficial ACE inhibitor effects on vascular structure (pp 63–64) will be translated into reduced myocardial infarction and stroke, which both correlate with carotid intima-media thickness in humans.[15] Reduced mortality is also likely.[12]

TABLE 12-5. SOME MAJOR TRIALS CURRENTLY TESTING THE HYPOTHESIS THAT ACE INHIBITORS CAN CONFER PROTECTION IN THOSE AT HIGH RISK OF CARDIOVASCULAR DISEASE

Trial and agent	Aim	Numbers	Duration
EUROPA, perindopril	Outcome in stable coronary heart disease	10,500	3.5 years
HOPE, ramipril	Outcome in high risk with 36% diabetics	9,000	Up to 4 years
PEACE, trandolapril	Outcome in coronary disease patients with LV ejection fraction 40% or more	8,100	5–7 years
PROGRESS, perindopril	Prevention of stroke and other major cardiovascular events in those with prior stroke or transient cerebral ischemia	6,000	4 years minimum

TABLE 12-6. CLINICAL TRIALS OF THE EFFECTS OF ACE INHIBITOR THERAPY ON ATHEROSCLEROSIS

Trial Name	Study Drugs	Comments
Simvastatin Coronary Atherosclerosis Trial (SCAT)	Enalapril, simvastatin	This study is evaluating the prolonged use of enalapril and simvastatin on coronary atherosclerosis in > 460 patients with known coronary heart disease
Study to Evaluate Carotid Ultrasound Changes in Patients Treated with Ramipril and Vitamin E (SECURE)	Ramipril, tocopherol (vitamin E)	The SECURE study is a substudy of HOPE; it is specifically examining the effects of ramipril and tocopherol on carotid atherosclerosis in 732 patients at high risk for cardiovascular events (i.e. patients with a previous MI, angina pectoris, multivessel PTCA or CABG, multivessel CHD, peripheral vascular disease or diabetes mellitus with an additional risk factor)
Prevention of Atherosclerosis with Ramipril Therapy-2 (PART 2)	Ramipril	The primary outcome measure is progression of atherosclerosis in carotid arteries. The effects of ramipril 5 or 10 mg/day, or placebo, are being studied in 617 patients with cardiovascular disease.
Plaque-Hypertension Lipid Lowering Italian Study (PHYLLIS)	Fosinopril, hydrochlorothiazide, pravastatin	To determine whether fosinopril (compared to hydrochlorothiazide), pravastatin (compared to diet), or fosinopril plus pravastatin can slow the rate of coronary artery atherosclerosis progression in patients with hypertension and hypercholesterolemia

See Stather[20]

GENE POLYMORPHISM

Exercise training is of increasing importance, not only in postinfarct rehabilitation, but in prevention of obesity and hence of type 2 diabetes, and as part of the lifestyle changes that must accompany the treatment of hypertension. In heart failure, exercise training is increasingly used to give a better quality of life and improved survival (Fig 12-4). In patients almost all already treated by an ACE inhibitor and a diuretic, long term moderate exercise training reduced cardiac deaths substantially.[1] Of great interest are the links between ACE gene insertion, which is associated with a lower ACE activity in body tissues and better response to physical training.[13] Hypothetically, the *II* genotype alters energy metabolism in a favourable way during rigorous physical training. Thus the response to exercise training may be predictable.[13]

It also seems likely that gene techniques will help predict who develops left ventricular hypertrophy or hypertension.[22] It will be a relatively small step from these and other studies[13] to using gene polymorphism to decide which AT receptor is involved, and perhaps to define who will respond best to which type of blockade, by ACE inhibitor or by AT-receptor.

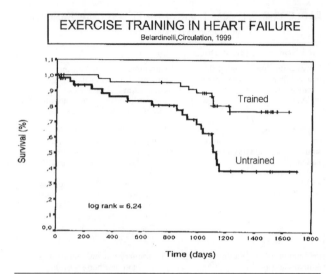

Figure 12-4. Exercise training lessens cardiac death in heart failure patients. Modified from Belardinelli[1] with permission of the author and the American Heart Association.

PREDICTIONS CAN BE WRONG

Of course, predictions and perceptions can be wrong. But it seems likely that we will be using ACE inhibitors more and more, despite the advent of the angiotensin receptor blockers. ACE inhibitors will be regarded as the standard agents to interrupt the progression from risk factors to congestive heart failure (Fig 12-5). At level of basic science, vast efforts are being put into the tissue renin-angiotensin system, the molecular biology of angiotensin II and its various AT receptors, and into the mechanisms of control of cell damage and death by apoptosis and necrosis. Clinically, we will have even more major trials involving many more thousands of patients. Several specific areas stand out.

SPECULATIVE PREDICTIONS

1. *In heart failure,* the primacy of ACE inhibitors will remain as result of the thousands and thousands of patients already studied. Nonetheless, trials with angiotensin receptor blockers may well be positive, and my guess is that a combination of these two types of drugs will become one of the choices in severe heart failure.

2. *In hypertension,* the overall demand for antihypertensive agents that are well tolerated, including ACE inhibitors and AT-1 blockers, is going to leap was the results of the HOT study sink in, and governments realize how cost-effective therapy of hypertension is, especially in the elderly. In hypertension, these drugs will increasingly be part of combination therapy. I favor either the ACE inhibitor-diuretic combination, or the ACE inhibitor-calcium blocker combination which

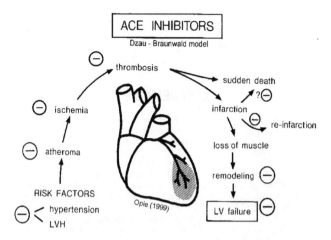

Figure 12-5. roposed sites of action of ACE inhibitors in primary and secondary prevention. ACE inhibitors have an indirect effect in primary prevention by lessening hypertension and by decreasing left ventricular hypertrophy. In addition, it is proposed that they may inhibit experimental atherogenesis. By an antiarrhythmic effect, they may act to prevent sudden death, a possibility that is being tested in postinfarct trials. By lessening wall stress, they may beneficially improve postinfarct remodeling and decrease the incidence of left ventricular failure. The concept of sequential changes leading to a chain of events from risk factors to left ventricular failure is based on Dzau and Braunwald (Fig. 12-2). LVH, left ventricular hypertrophy. Fig © LH Opie, 1999

is under test in the STOP-2 study (results will be out before this book goes to press).

3. *Cardiovascular prevention in high risk patients (post-infarct or diabetic or the elderly)* is becoming a therapeutic target in its own right. The belief of the present author is that ACE inhibitors will play an increasingly important role not only in the treatment of hypertension and heart failure in general, but also in the prevention of cardiovascular complications in high risk patients. For example, we will also be using these agents more and more in diabetic patients to prevent major cardiac, renal and ocular complications. Such vascular protection may not be a specific effect of ACE, but rather of vigorous blood pressure reduction. Nonetheless, the protective effect of ACE inhibitors in diabetic nephropathy is more specific, and a good reason for including an ACE inhibitor as at least one component of the several drugs needed to control blood pressure adequately in the diabetic.

4. *The antithrombotic effect* of ACE inhibitors will probably become clinically applied, as the results of the current prospective studies become available. These trials will, at a guess, put ACE inhibitors into the same preventative league as the beta-blockers and the statins. We already know that heart failure patients without symptoms but with depressed left ventricular function should initially be treated by an ACE inhibitor. In the future, my guess is that trials such as HOPE, PEACE and EUROPA will probably show the importance of

these agents in cardiovascular prevention, in the absence of depressed left ventricular function, and especially in high risk patients.

REFERENCES

1.   Belardinelli R, Georgiou D, Ciance G, et al. Randomized, controlled trial of long-term moderate exercise training in chronic heart failure. Effects on functional capacity, quality of life, and clinical outcome. Circulation 1999;99:1173–1182.

2.   CAPP Study Group. Hansson L, Lindholm LH, Niskanen L, et al. Effect of angiotensin-converting-enzyme inhibition compared with conventional therapy on cardiovascular morbidity and mortality in hypertension: the Captopril Prevention Project (CAPPP) randomised trial. Lancet 1999;353:611–616.

3.   Dzau V, Gibbons GH, Pratt RE. Molecular mechanisms of vascular renin-angiotensin system in myointimal hyperplasia. Hypertension 1991;18 (Suppl II):II-100–II-105.

4.   ELITE Study. Pitt B, Segal R, Martinez F A, et al. On behalf of the ELITE Study Investigators. Randomised trial of losartan versus captopril in patients over 65 with heart failure (Evaluation of Losartan in the Elderly Study, ELITE). Lancet 1997;349:747–752.

5.   Flather MD, Yusuf S, Kober L, et al. Systematic overview of individual patient data fromt he large randomized trials of long term ACE inhibition or therapy in patients with heart failure or left ventricular dysfunction following myocardial infarction. Submitted for publication 1999.

6.   Fogari R, Zoppi A, Lazzari P, et al. ACE inhibition but not angiotensin II antagonism reduces plasma fibrinogen and insulin resistance in overweight hypertensive patients. J Cardiovasc Pharmacol 1998;32:616–620.

7.   Harada K, Komuro I, Sugaya T, et al. Vascular injury causes neointimal formation in angiotensin II type 1a receptor knockout mice. Circ Res 1999;84:179–185.

7A. Horiuchi M, Akishita M, Dzau VJ. Recent progress in angiotensin II type 2 receptor research in the cardiovascular system. Hypertension 1999;33: 613–621.

8.   HOT Study. Hansson L, Zanchetti A, Carruthers SG, et al. Effects of intensive blood-pressure lowering and low-dose aspirin in patients with hypertension: principal results of the Hypertension Optimal Treatment (HOT) randomised trial. Lancet 1998;351:1755–1762.

9.   JNC VI. Joint National Committee on Prevention, Detection, Evaluation and Treatment of High Blood Pressure. The Sixth Report of the Joint National Committee on Prevention, Detection, Evaluation and Treatment of High Blood Pressure. Arch Intern Med 1997;157:2413–2446.

10. Kelly D. Our future society. A global challenge. Circulation 1997; 95:2459–2464.

11. Levy D, Garrison RJ, Savage DD, et al. Prognostic implications of echocardiographically determined left ventricular mass in the Framingham heart study. N Engl J Med 1990;322:1561–1566.

12. MacMahon S, Sharpe N, Gamble G, et al. Long-term effects of the ACE inhibitor, ramipril, on atherosclerosis in patients with coronary heart disease or other occlusive arterial disease. Final results from the Part-2 trial (Abstract). J Am Coll Cardiol 1999;33 (Suppl A):Abstr no. 899-4.

13. Montgomery H, Clarkson P, Barnard M, et al. Angiotensin-converting-enzyme gene insertion/deletion polymorphism and response to physical training. Lancet 1999;353:541–545.

14. Morris SD, Yellon DM. Angiotensin-converting enzyme inhibitors potentiate preconditioning through bradykinin B_2 receptor activation in human heart. J Am Coll Cardiol 1997;29:1599–1606.

15. O'Leary D, Polak J, Kronmal R, et al. For the Cardiovascular Health Study Collaborative Research Group. Carotid-artery intima and media thickness as a risk factor for myocardial infarction and stroke in older adults. N Engl J Med 1999;340:14–22.

16. Packer M, Cohn J. Consensus recommendations for the management of chronic heart failure. Am J Cardiol 1999;83 (2A):1A–38A.

17. QUIET Trial. Cashin-Hemphill L, Holmvang G, Chan RC, et al. Angiotensin-converting enzyme inhibition as antiatherosclerotic therapy: no answer yet. Am J Cardiol 1999;83:43–47.

18. RACE Study. Agabati-Rosei E, Ambrosioni E, Palu CD, et al. On behalf of the RACE Study Group. ACE inhibitor ramipril is more effective than the β-blocker atenolol in reducing left ventricular mass in hypertension. Results of the RACE (Ramipril Cardioprotective Evaluation) study. Journal of Hypertension 1995;13:1325–1334.

19. Richardson M, Cockburn N, Cleland JGF. Update of recent clinical trials in heart failure and myocardial infarction. Europ J Heart Failure 1999; 1:109–115.

20. Stather R. ACE inhibitors in the next millennium: a role in CHD? Inpharma 1998;1161:3–4.

21. STOP Study. Ekbom R, Dahlöf B, Hansson L, et al. Antihypertensive efficacy and side effects of three beta-blockers and a diuretic in elderly hypertensives: a report from the STOP-Hypertension study. J Hypertens 1992;10:1525–1530.

22. Takami S, Katsuya T, Rakugi H, et al. Angiotensin II Type I receptor gene polymorphism is associated with increase of left ventricular mass but not with hypertension. Am J Hypertens 1998;11:316–321.

23. Thurmann PA, Kenedi P, Schmidt A, et al. Influence of the angiotensin II antagonist valsartan on left ventricular hypertrophy in patients with essential hypertension. Circulation 1998;98:2037–2042.

24. WHO-ISH Committee. World Health Organization-International Society of Hypertension. Guidelines for the Management of Hypertension. J Hypertens 1999;17:151–183.

A